Health Promotion in Canada

Health Promotion in Canada

Critical Perspectives on Practice

THIRD EDITION

EDITED BY

Irving Rootman, Sophie Dupéré, Ann Pederson, and Michel O'Neill

Canadian Scholars' Press Inc.
Toronto

Health Promotion in Canada: Critical Perspectives on Practice, Third Edition
edited by Irving Rootman, Sophie Dupéré, Ann Pederson, Michel O'Neill

First published in 1994 by
Canadian Scholars' Press Inc.
180 Bloor Street West, Suite 801
Toronto, Ontario
M5S 2V6

www.cspi.org

Canadian Scholars' Press Inc. gratefully acknowledges financial support for our publishing activities from the Government of Canada through the Canada Book Fund (CBF).

Library and Archives Canada Cataloguing in Publication

Health promotion in Canada : critical perspectives on practice / [edited by] Irving Rootman ... [et al.]. — 3rd ed.

Includes index.
ISBN 978-1-55130-409-0

1. Health promotion—Canada—Textbooks. I. Rootman, I

RA427.8.H45 2012   613'.0971   C2011-907298-X

Text design by Susan MacGregor/Digital Zone
Cover design by Colleen Wormald
Cover image: "15694899 (Spiry Roots)," by Cunfek. From www.istockphoto.com.

Printed and bound in Canada by Webcom

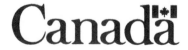

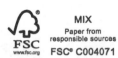

MIX
Paper from
responsible sources
FSC® C004071

Table of Contents

DEDICATION

The editors of this edition would like to honour the past and celebrate the future by dedicating this book to people near and dear to us. Irv would like to express his joy about the birth of his second and third grandsons, Sacha Rootman on January 22, 2008, and Zev Rootman on October 21 (Irv's own birthday), 2009, and his first granddaughter, Navah Rootman, on July 29, 2011. He would also like to dedicate this book to Barb Rootman, his wife and life partner. Sophie would like to express the great pleasure and honour it has been to work on this third edition with Irv, Michel, and Ann, great pioneers in the field of health promotion in Canada. Ann would like to thank her co-editors for their long-standing friendship and the generosity of spirit that has characterized their partnership. She would like to dedicate this work to her life partner, Barry, and to thank him for his steadfast support and love. Michel would like to dedicate this book to his son Sébastien and his partner, Paule Mackrous, who gave him the great joy of a first grandson, Mathias, born on April 22, 2011; may their intellectual and familial projects continue to be blessed with the creativity that has characterized them up to now. Finally, we would all like to dedicate this book to the memory of two people who in different but important ways contributed to promoting the health of the people of Canada. The first is Robin Badgley, a professor and colleague of two of the editors at the University of Toronto (Pederson and Rootman) as well as an author of a key chapter in the first edition of *Health Promotion in Canada*. Robin was both a gentleman and a scholar who established the Department of Behavioural Sciences in the Medical School at the University of Toronto and who guided and inspired several generations of graduate students to take the social sciences seriously in addressing health issues and thereby helped to provide an academic foundation for health promotion in Canada. The second is Jack Layton, who devoted his life to fight directly and indirectly to promote the health of his fellow citizens. May their contributions and lives continue to inspire future generations of health promotion scholars and practitioners.

Acknowledgements

As was the case for the first and second editions of this book, we relied on the collaboration of a large number of contributors in preparing this book. Their enthusiasm and willingness to work with our deadlines, as well as the quality of their work, were both exceptional and inspirational. We clearly found the right people to help us with this book. We are certainly grateful and would like to thank them sincerely for their commitment to this project and to health promotion.

We had the good fortune of working with James MacNevin, who managed this project on behalf of CSPI with professionalism, responsiveness, and flexibility, which we appreciated greatly. We would also like to thank the other staff of CSPI who worked on this book for their help in facilitating its timely publication.

In addition, we would like to gratefully acknowledge the support that we received from various institutions: the Faculté des sciences infirmières de l'Université Laval, which supported the involvement of Michel O'Neill and Sophie Dupéré, and the British Columbia Centre of Excellence for Women's Health, which supported Ann Pederson's involvement. Both organizations also provided some financial assistance toward the creation of the index.

We would also like to thank the external reviewers who provided us with feedback on the draft manuscript and the reviewers who commented on the second edition; all these suggestions have helped us to reflect more critically upon our work and clearly have improved the quality of the final product.

Finally, we would like to thank our families and friends who allowed us to borrow time from them to complete this book, particularly Barb Rootman, Robin Couture, Barry Spruston, and Francine Courchesne.

Preface to the Third Edition

This is the third edition of *Health Promotion in Canada*. These books were written over a span of more than 15 years, and the contents of each reflect a distinct orientation, indicated by the different subtitles of the editions, showing how our approach has evolved over time and how we remain committed to looking at health promotion from a variety of perspectives. In this preface, we review the intent of the two previous editions and then describe our vision of this new edition.

In brief, the first edition was framed as an historical and sociological examination of health promotion as a field in Canada. The second built on this theme, but recognized contributions to theory and practice that had emerged within the field since the first edition. The current book further extends the focus on health promotion practice, offering a review of theory, methods, and promising practices in health promotion in Canada.

Health Promotion in Canada: Provincial, National, and International Perspectives

The first edition, published in 1994 (Pederson, O'Neill, and Rootman, 1994), was mainly a socio-historical analysis of the development of health promotion in Canada over the 20 years following the release of the Lalonde Report (Lalonde, 1974).[1] We looked at health promotion in Canada with a critical eye over those 20 years, particularly the period following the release of the *Ottawa Charter for Health Promotion* in 1986 by the World Health Organization, the Canadian Public Health Association, and Health and Welfare Canada (WHO, 1986). Contrary to most books in the field at that time, we decided to prepare one that reflected "on" health promotion (Pederson, O'Neill, and Rootman, 1994, p. 1) rather than preparing another manual "in" health promotion that provided suggestions on how to design programs or conduct research in the field. With the help of experienced academics and professionals in Canada and elsewhere, we thus analyzed the development of the field from conceptual, national, provincial, and international perspectives.

Based on the discussions in the book, we concluded, among other things, that there was a consensus about what health promotion is and how to go about implementing it; that Canada was an international leader in the field; and that while health promotion was beginning to enter the mainstream of health discourse and activity, it remained marginal in health care and was more of a professional movement than a social movement.

Health Promotion in Canada: Critical Perspectives

Although the first edition of the book was intended for people working in health promotion or related fields in Canada and other countries, it turned out that the largest group of readers was undergraduate students in health sciences in Canada. As a consequence, the second edition, which included Sophie Dupéré as a fourth editor, was specifically directed at this audience, using a style and format appropriate for undergraduate courses while maintaining an orientation that was also designed to interest other readers in Canada and elsewhere. We maintained the approach of analyzing the health promotion field in Canada by adopting a critical perspective. We tried to identify what was critical in the field at the beginning of the twenty-first century in the sense of what was important or crucial in Canada and abroad 13 years after the first edition, with the "inclination to criticize" characteristic of "critical social science" (O'Neill, Pederson, Dupéré, and Rootman, 2007, p. 12). In addition, based on feedback for the first edition suggesting that we should be more explicit about how and why reflecting on the field is crucial for practice, we added a new section on practical perspectives encouraging readers to apply reflexive thinking to their own practice. We also made a deliberate effort to include a team combining newer and more experienced contributors from a variety of backgrounds, including practitioners, policy-makers, and academics, because we wanted the book to showcase a new generation of health promotion. In the final count, the second edition involved a total of 93 authors from 22 countries.

Thus, the 2007 edition of *Health Promotion in Canada* was an entirely new book relative to the 1994 edition. We also worked on a slightly different version that was published in French at almost the same time (O'Neill, Dupéré, Pederson & Rootman, 2006). In 2007 we concluded that among other things, health promotion, although resilient, was still marginal in the Canadian health care system and that day-to-day health promotion practice in Canada remained lifestyle-oriented and focused on individuals' behavioural changes. In addition, Canada continued to have a good international reputation and to play an important role internationally in the field.

Health Promotion in Canada: Perspectives from Practice

The current edition is thus the third iteration of the book. We felt that it was premature to do a comprehensive update on the status of health promotion in Canada as we had done in the first two editions because too little time had passed to understand the full implications of what had taken place since 2007. Instead, we chose to focus this edition on health promotion practice, linking it to health promotion theory, research, evaluation, and ethics. This approach built upon an important development introduced in the second edition, namely, the introduction of a discussion of critical reflective practice. Consequently, about half of the chapters in this edition are updated versions of chapters of the second one and the rest are new, covering topics that we felt were central for health promotion practice.

Thus, even if this edition of *Health Promotion in Canada* is less historical than the previous two, it maintains a critical, interdisciplinary perspective and continues to insert Canadian health promotion within the global context. Its main purpose is to reflect upon health promotion as currently practised in Canada, which is still perceived internationally as a hotbed of innovation and exemplary practices. We want to provide practitioners with an improved understanding of what forces shape their practice, as well as with concrete examples of what we call "promising practices" (i.e., practices that might or might not have been evaluated enough to reach the status of "best practice," but that are nevertheless illuminating and inspiring). We expect the readers, wherever they live around the globe, to draw lessons that can be derived from current health promotion practice in Canada to better understand and transform their own work, whether it is in the intervention, research, teaching, or policy-making domains. We thus maintain our orientation for the book "on" health promotion and not one "in" health promotion (i.e., it is not a how-to book explaining how to develop and or evaluate effective interventions, but rather one that helps to reflect on health promotion as it is practised in Canada).

This edition attempts to convey a number of key messages about the current practice of health promotion in Canada. As was the case in the previous editions, it is guided by some values and principles, many of which are embodied in the *Ottawa Charter for Health Promotion*. Deciding to explore promising practices across Canada 25 years later was indeed a way to celebrate the accomplishments in the field since the release of the *Ottawa Charter*, which obviously does not preclude looking at it today with a critical eye. Although this third edition will appear only in English, in order to show the diversity as well as the similarities of what happens in such a large country, we have again made significant efforts to include anglophone and francophone authors from different provinces, often working in pairs, as well as newer and more experienced contributors from a variety of backgrounds.

The book has 18 chapters and is divided into four parts, each with a short introduction to establish the context. Part I, "Key Contextual, Conceptual, and Theoretical Elements for Understanding Health Promotion Practice," is organized in six chapters. Part II, "Addressing Issues, Populations, and Settings through Health Promotion," contains five chapters. It first provides a discussion in which three key entry points into health promotion practice—issues, settings, and populations—are identified. It also discusses the limitations of each for health promotion practice. Based on this division, teams of contributors have been recruited and asked to discuss key issues, populations, and settings, addressing the general context of their practice in Canada and identifying at least one concrete example of a "promising practice" on their topic. We obviously could not cover every single relevant area of practice, but the sample we made allows us to raise most of what we consider the key issues and lessons to be addressed. We also added a chapter on Aboriginal health promotion to illustrate the unique context of health promotion within this population group.

Part III, "Additional Topics to Consider in Reflecting on Health Promotion Practice," includes six chapters and looks at important elements useful in developing the type of critical reflexive practice we advocate, in addition to providing examples of promising practices.

The final part of the book contains Chapter 18, the concluding chapter by the editors, and an Afterword by Ilona Kickbusch, one of the international driving forces in the field of health promotion. Chapter 18 presents an analysis of our own, continuing to build on the metaphor of the tree and the rhizome proposed by Dr. Kickbusch in the second edition of the book (Kickbusch, 2007). In this chapter we reflect on the perspectives that emerge from the current practice of health promotion in Canada, linking them to the future of the field here and globally. Ilona Kickbusch also comments on recent developments and the future of health promotion in her "Afterword."

There are a few things to keep in mind when reading the book. First, the manuscript was sent to the publisher in July 2011; as the field is constantly evolving, some things might have changed by the time the book is released in 2012. Second, as noted above, the main audience for this book is students, especially undergraduate students in health sciences in Canada. Each chapter thus includes pedagogical elements such as critical thinking questions and additional annotated resources. We are nevertheless convinced that in addition to students, people already working in the field will be interested in reading this book to update themselves on current developments by reflecting critically on their practice.

Finally, as editors we are once more heartened by the continuing support of the numerous colleagues who have written contributions to one or the other editions of this book. We see health promotion as a collective enterprise of working together to improve health. That so many people are willing to work with us, some of them for the third time, to maintain an active dialogue about health promotion in Canada is evidence that, despite the erosion of official support for health promotion in many jurisdictions, there remains an enthusiastic and thoughtful community of scholars and practitioners engaged in the field. For us, it has also been a renewed pleasure to continue the collaboration we've enjoyed as co-editors—for three of us, it has been a few decades. The particular mix of skills, shared work ethic, and curiosity about the field has allowed us to be part of a "dream team."

Irving Rootman, Sophie Dupéré, Ann Pederson, and Michel O'Neill

Vancouver and Quebec City, July 2011

Note

1. The Lalonde Report is a key publication in the field of health promotion. Some dates, events, and key documents such as this one will be constantly referred to in the book. They are presented in detail in Chapter 1.

References

Kickbusch, I. (2007). *Health promotion: Not a tree but a rhizome* (2nd ed.), 363–366. Toronto: Canadian Scholars' Press Inc.

Lalonde, M. (1974). *A new perspective on the health of Canadians.* Ottawa: Health and Welfare Canada.

O'Neill, M., Dupéré, S., Pederson, A. & Rootman, I. (dirs.). (2006). *Promotion de la santé au Canada et au Québec: Perspectives critiques.* Quebec: Les Presses de l'Université Laval.

O'Neill, M., Pederson, A., Dupéré, S. & Rootman, I. (Eds.). (2007). *Health promotion in Canada: Critical perspectives* (2nd ed.). Toronto: Canadian Scholars' Press Inc.

Pederson, A., O'Neill, M. & Rootman, I. (Eds.). (1994). *Health promotion in Canada: Provincial, national, and international perspectives.* Toronto: W.B. Saunders Canada.

WHO. (1986). *Ottawa charter for health promotion.* Ottawa: World Health Organization, Health and Welfare Canada, Canadian Public Health Association.

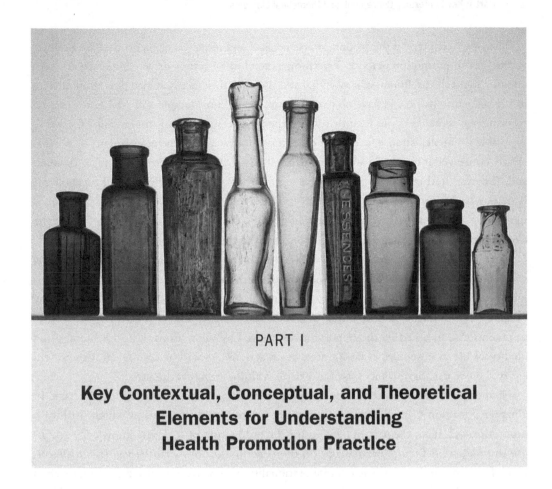

PART I

Key Contextual, Conceptual, and Theoretical Elements for Understanding Health Promotion Practice

This first section of the book contains six chapters that provide basic building blocks for the reader to reflect critically on health promotion as it is currently practised in Canada, 25 years after the famous *Ottawa Charter for Health Promotion* was released.

Chapters 1 and 6 provide *contextual* elements to understanding how the field is positioned in Canada and globally. In Chapter 1, the editors build on several chapters of the previous editions and offer an historical analysis of how health promotion has emerged out of the field of health education, both in Canada and internationally. They also look at how it has evolved since the second edition of the book in 2007 and assesses whether or not Canada's positive reputation on the global health promotion scene, which has been unquestioned for several decades, is still current. In Chapter 6, Ronald Labonté updates one of the important chapters of the second edition and provides key elements to understanding how globalization is affecting health and health promotion. Indeed, there is no place in the world right now, including Canada, and no humane endeavour, including health promotion practice, that is left untouched by the deep changes created by the various dimensions of globalization. The impact of the global fiscal crisis of 2008 is addressed and concrete suggestions are made for actions that can be taken by practitioners to influence these processes upon which they often do not think they can act.

The other chapters of the section offer *conceptual* and *theoretical* elements that are import-ant for health promotion practice. Practitioners tend to be action-driven and often are very dubious about the usefulness of conceptual and theoretical elements, which they think belong to the academic world and have no practical use. In the introduction to Part I of the second edition, two sentences were used that were true in 2007 and are still true today: "Ce qui se conçoit clairement s'énonce facilement et les mots pour le dire arrivent aisément" ("What is clearly conceived is easily said and words to say it come easily"), by French preacher Bossuet; and "There is nothing more practical than a good theory," by American social psychologist Kurt Lewin. Indeed, practitioners' capacity to intervene successfully in health promotion is significantly shaped by their understanding of the world in which they operate and of the elements they should work on. For this, concepts and theories are extremely useful tools.

Thus, in Chapter 2, two of the editors (Rootman and O'Neill) present some of the *central concepts* that frame the field of health promotion: health; health promotion and its distinctions with health education; the special place of the social determinants of health within the array of factors that influence health and illness; the notion of empowerment as a key element of interventions; and, finally, the important role played by the notions of health literacy and quality of life as outcomes of health promotion actions. As will be seen, even if there will always be debates, significant consensus exists on all the concepts discussed.

Chapters 3 to 5 address the issue of *theory* in relation to health promotion practice. In Chapter 3, Simon Carroll addresses at a more general level the ways in which, in health promotion as a field, theory can be used for the production of scientific knowledge and its use in practice. It focuses particularly on the contribution of social theory. In Chapter 4, Reid, Pederson, and Dupéré suggest intersectionality, a contemporary theoretical approach in women's health, as relevant for health promotion. Intersectional theory is proposed to address how diversity in general can be taken into account in health promotion research and practice. Finally, in Chapter 5, Richard and Gauvin show how ecological models can concretely help to plan interventions, noting nevertheless some of the issues and dilemmas that are still chal-lenging this approach, which is at this point one of the best candidates to being the central theoretical model for health promotion as a field.

At the end of this section, the reader should be well equipped to better understand what the field of health promotion is, where it comes from, what some of its key conceptual and theoretical elements are, and how they can be related to practice.

CHAPTER 1

The Evolution of
Health Promotion in Canada

Michel O'Neill, Irving Rootman, Sophie Dupéré, and Ann Pederson

This chapter critically reviews the evolution of health promotion in Canada in the global context. Health promotion emerged in the mid-1980s as an evolution of individually oriented health education practices (providing information on "appropriate" health-related behaviour like tobacco abstinence, adequate diet, proper physical activity, etc.) to which it added environmental and policy concerns. We identify four eras in this evolution: (1) the health education era (prior to 1974); (2) the health promotion development and golden era (1974–1994); (3) the population health era (1994–2007); and (4) the population health promotion era (since 2007). These eras are marked by key events and publications that reflect the emergence of new concepts and approaches to health promotion, as well as shifts in the political climate and support for the field. They are listed in Box 1.1 and will be referred to in the various sections below.

BOX 1.1:

Some Key Milestones of International and Canadian Health Promotion

- 1951: Foundation and first global conference of the International Union for Health Education (IUHE)
- 1974: Release of *A New Perspective on the Health of Canadians,* the famous Lalonde Report
- 1978: The Alma-Ata conference on Primary Health Care, co-organized by the World Health Organization and UNICEF
- 1979: The World Health Assembly of the World Health Organization's adoption of its "Health for All by the Year 2000" resolution
- 1986: First World Health Organization (WHO) international conference on health promotion in Ottawa; release of the *Ottawa Charter for Health Promotion* and of *Achieving Health for All* (also known as the Epp Report)
- 1994: The watershed year between health promotion and population health; publication of two influential books, *Health Promotion in Canada* (Pederson et al., 1994) *and Why Are Some People Healthy and Others Not?* (Evans et al., 1994)
- 2004: Creation of the Public Health Agency of Canada
- 2007: Nineteenth global conference of the International Union for Health Promotion and Health Education (IUHPE), held in Vancouver

---

PRIOR TO 1974: THE HEALTH EDUCATION ERA

Robin Badgley (1994) traced the various types of activities and programs undertaken by the local, provincial, or federal public authorities of Canada from the early 1600s to the middle of the nineteeth century to promote the health of the "colony's" population. He argued that only in the 1880s did the "dissemination of sanitary information" become a concern for the provincial government and the newly established federal government, and that missionary zeal among sanitary reformers, rather than scientifically grounded and well-evaluated interventions, dominated the field for several decades up to the end of World War II. The production of pamphlets and posters, the writing of books and newspaper columns, followed later by the production of film strips and the broadcast of radio messages, occupied most of the time, energy, and resources at the national and regional levels, with scarce public health personnel relaying this information in one-to-one or small group situations at the local level.

Similar developments were concurrently underway in most industrialized countries (e.g., see Green and Kreuter, 1999 for a discussion of developments in the United States), but it was only in the late 1940s and early 1950s that a more systematic and scientific approach to educating the public on health matters began to emerge. In 1951, a group of European and North American public health people, under the leadership of two Frenchmen, Léo Parisot and Lucien Viborel, created what was to become the most important international non-governmental organization in the field—the International Union for Health Education (Modolo & Mamon, 2001)—in response to the need to link those working on health education and to promote the exchange of experience and information on these new ways of working.

From then until the mid-1970s, the dissemination of health education information in the industrialized world was increasingly directed toward the health professional–patient encounter (primarily the doctor–patient relationship) to make sure that the patient understood and used the information provided by health care providers. The general public also became the target of the campaigns of health education specialists, initially in order to encourage the proper use of the health services (especially preventive ones) that governments were establishing in the post–World War II welfare state era. Over time, it became clear that a pattern of so-called "diseases of civilization" was rapidly displacing the earlier pattern of infectious diseases in industrialized countries. When it was observed that the risk factors for these new sources of mortality (e.g., cardiovascular diseases, cancers, accidents) were largely behavioural, these at-risk behaviours themselves (e.g., smoking, sedentary lifestyles, bad eating habits, etc.) became the prime targets of health education.

The 1950s and 1960s witnessed the increasing involvement of social scientists and communication specialists in the development of models to try to understand and predict health-related behaviour and/or in the design of health education campaigns. These scientific developments occurred largely in the United States, which did not undergo the postwar reconstruction of the European nations and thus had greater resources available for such purposes. It was during this period, for instance, that the Health Belief Model was developed (Becker, 1974); the first of a long series of theoretical models of individual health behaviour, it identified key beliefs (like the perceived severity of a problem, the perceived likelihood to be affected by it, etc.) that should be taken into account when educating the public about health matters.

These developments gradually infiltrated the day-to-day practice of health educators in Canada (Badgley, 1994), and were reflected in programs, manuals (e.g., Gilbert, 1963), and the training of personnel. These practices were built upon a deeply rooted, virtually unquestioned belief that educating the public was intrinsically good and the hope that health would improve with the help of science and a more systematic way of conducting health education. All this occurred, however, in a context in which public health and health education services, which were almost the only type of health-related governmental intervention prior to the 1950s, were quickly dwarfed and eventually marginalized as the governments of Western industrialized societies became heavily involved in establishing publicly financed acute medical care systems with the establishment of hospitals, where an increasingly important part of all health care would be provided by a growing diversity of health-related professionals (Gilbert, 1967).

1974–1994: THE HEALTH PROMOTION DEVELOPMENT AND GOLDEN ERA

During the 1970s, it became increasingly obvious that health education was not having the desired effects, and that individuals, though better informed, did not necessarily adopt the healthful behaviours expected of them. A series of events then took place that resulted in significant revision to the way health education was conceived and led to its transformation into health promotion.

International Developments

Internationally, the mid-1970s marked the end of 30 years of sustained growth within the Western postwar economies. This economic situation allowed the "welfare state" to flourish in the 1950s and 1960s. In Canada, as in most Western countries, governments were sufficiently wealthy, and the public was sufficiently supportive, to become involved in insuring the welfare of their populations through the direct or indirect provision of services to fulfill basic needs, notably in the sectors of health and education.

However, a major reorganization of the world economy, triggered by the so-called "oil shocks" of 1973 and 1976, completely changed this picture. This was followed by 20 gloomy years of economic stagnation or minimal growth within the Western economies, which deprived governments of taxation revenues and forced them to borrow heavily to maintain the level of public services they had committed to providing their citizens.

It was in this context that the Lalonde Report, formally entitled *A New Perspective on the Health of Canadians*, was released in 1974. The report received immediate worldwide attention because it was the first document by the central government of a major developed country that advocated for the importance of investing resources beyond health services to improve the health of the population (Lalonde, 1974). As seen in Box 1.2, the "health field concept," introduced in *A New Perspective*, identified four sets of factors—later to be called "determinants of health"—that contributed to the health of populations: human biology, health services, personal lifestyle, and the environment.

BOX 1.2:

Elements of the Health Field Concept

Human Biology
Environment (physical and social)
Lifestyle
Health Care Organization

Source: Lalonde, M. (1974). *A new perspective on the health of Canadians.* Ottawa: Government of Canada.

In the following years, given the deteriorating macro-economic context, almost every Western industrialized country produced its own version of the Lalonde Report, encouraging investment in areas other than health care systems (which were increasingly difficult to finance through public funds). This context also produced a major international expert conference in 1978, co-sponsored by the World Health Organization (WHO)[1] and UNICEF, at which delegates proposed that the world stop investing in costly acute care systems, recognizing that after more than 30 years, such systems had not yielded the expected results in the developed world and had been almost irrelevant for the developing world. The Alma-Ata conference thus suggested a return to the basics—to "primary health care" (PHC)—and to addressing the set of factors described in the Lalonde Report and its counterparts (see Box 1.3).

BOX 1.3:

Primary Health Care as Defined in the Alma-Ata Declaration

1. reflects and evolves from the economic conditions and socio-cultural and political characteristics of the country and its communities and is based on the application of the relevant results of social, biomedical, and health services research and public health experience;
2. addresses the main health problems in the community, providing promotive, preventive, curative, and rehabilitative services accordingly;
3. includes at least: education concerning prevailing health problems and the methods of preventing and controlling them; promotion of food supply and proper nutrition; an adequate supply of safe water and basic sanitation; maternal and child health care, including family planning; immunization against the major infectious diseases; prevention and control of locally endemic diseases; appropriate treatment of common diseases and injuries; and provision of essential drugs;
4. involves, in addition to the health sector, all related sectors and aspects of national and community development, in particular agriculture, animal husbandry, food, industry, education, housing, public works, communications, and other sectors; and demands the coordinated efforts of all those sectors;

---

5. requires and promotes maximum community and individual self-reliance and participation in the planning, organization, operation, and control of primary health care, making fullest use of local, national, and other available resources; and to this end develops through appropriate education the ability of communities to participate;

6. should be sustained by integrated, functional, and mutually supportive referral systems, leading to the progressive improvement of comprehensive health care for all, and giving priority to those most in need;

7. relies, at local and referral levels, on health workers, including physicians, nurses, midwives, auxiliaries, and community workers as applicable, as well as traditional practitioners as needed, suitably trained socially and technically to work as a health team and to respond to the expressed health needs of the community.

Source: UNICEF. (1978). *The Alma-Ata Declaration on Primary Health Care* (p. 2). Retrieved from: http://www.who.int/hpr/NPH/docs/declaration_almaata.pdf

Mindful of these developments, the ministers of health of most countries of the world, gathered in what is called the World Health Assembly of the WHO, voted in 1979 the "Health for All by the Year 2000" (HFA) resolution, which proposed a set of measures in keeping with the spirit of the Lalonde Report and the Alma-Ata Declaration. These measures were further operationalized in a global strategy in 1981 (see Box 1.4).

BOX 1.4:

WHO Global Strategy for Health for All by the Year 2000

The General Assembly,

- Recalling its resolution 34/58 of 29 November 1979 concerning health as an integral part of development,

- Noting with approval World Health Assembly resolution WHA 34.36 of 22 May 1981 by which the thirty-fourth Assembly unanimously adopted the Global Strategy for Health for All by the Year 2000,

- Considering that the Global Strategy fully reflects the spirit of General Assembly resolution 34/58,

- Considering that peace and security are important conditions for the preservation and improvement of the health of all people and that co-operation among nations on vital health issues can contribute substantially to peace,

- Noting further that the Global Strategy is based upon the principles of the Declaration of Alma-Ata on primary health care, which implies an integrated approach to the solution of health care problems and requires the fullest support and involvement of all economic and social development sectors,

- Recognizing that the implementation of the Global Strategy will constitute a valuable contribution to the improvement of overall socio-economic conditions, and thus to the fulfillment of the International Development Strategy for the Third United Nations Development Decade,

1. Endorses the Global Strategy for Health for All by the Year 2000 as a major contribution of Member States to the attainment of the world-wide social goal of health for all by the year 2000 and to the fulfillment of the International Development Strategy for the Third United Nations Development Decade;

2. Urges all Member States to ensure the implementation of the Global Strategy as part of their multisectoral efforts to implement the provisions contained in the International Development Strategy;

3. Also urges all Member States to co-operate with one another and with the World Health Organization to ensure that the necessary international action is taken to implement the Global Strategy as part of the fulfillment of the International Development Strategy;

4. Requests all appropriate organizations and bodies of the United Nations system— including the United Nations Children's Fund, the Food and Agriculture Organization of the United Nations, the International Labour Organisation, the United Nations Development Programme, the United Nations Environment Programme, the United Nations Educational, Scientific, and Cultural Organization, the United Nations Fund for Population Activities and the World Bank—to collaborate fully with the World Health Organization in carrying out the Global Strategy;

5. Requests the Director-General of the World Health Organization to ensure that measures to implement the Global Strategy are taken into account in the review and appraisal of the implementation of the International Development Strategy.

Source: WHO. (1981). November 19, 1981 Sixty-fourth plenary meeting, Resolution 36/43. Retrieved from: http://whqlibdoc.who.int/publications/9241800038.pdf

The Canadian–European Connection

Lavada Pinder (1994) argued that very little happened in Canada following the release of the Lalonde Report until 1978, when the federal government established a Health Promotion Directorate (HPD), thought to be the first national body of its kind anywhere in the world. The directorate focused initially on the lifestyle component (i.e., changing health-related individual behaviour) of the health field concept, although a more comprehensive strategy, including both lifestyles as well as more structural policy measures, was developed in 1982, but was only partially implemented because it was never fully funded.

At about the same time, the European office of the World Health Organization (WHO) in Copenhagen, under the leadership of Ilona Kickbusch, articulated for Europe a fundamental redirection of health education toward health promotion in a small discussion document (WHO-EURO, 1984), written in collaboration with international leaders in the field. This collaboration ultimately led to the first International Conference on Health Promotion, held in Ottawa in 1986.

Another key outcome of this collaboration was the demonstration of the importance of environmental factors in health, which, although identified by the Lalonde Report, had received only limited attention in Canada and elsewhere. The health education community had already begun to articulate its own internal critique during the second half of the 1970s (e.g., Brown & Margo, 1978; Freudenberg, 1978; Labonté & Penfold, 1981), conscious that providing health information alone and focusing on individual behaviour could lead to "blaming the victim" for his or her health problems (Ryan, 1976). Critics argued that changing the environment should become as much a concern for health education as changing individual behaviour if it was to ensure, as Nancy Milio famously suggested, "making the healthiest choice the easiest choice" (Milio, 1986). Social, political, economic, cultural, and physical environments had to become supportive of, rather than barriers to, individual changes if people were going to change how they lived, worked, and played.

The term "health promotion" was a critical signal of this evolution from a traditional, individually focused health education to the ecological, multi-level models that emerged in 1986 with the release of the *Ottawa Charter for Health Promotion*. As will be seen in Chapter 5, these models pay particular attention to global environmental factors without dismissing those operating at the individual, familial, community, or societal levels. This is clear in Kickbusch's own work (1986) (see Figure 1.1), in the *Ottawa Charter* itself (WHO, 1986) (see Figure 1.2), and in the Canadian document *Achieving Health for All* (Epp, 1986), which was launched in Ottawa at the first international health promotion conference.

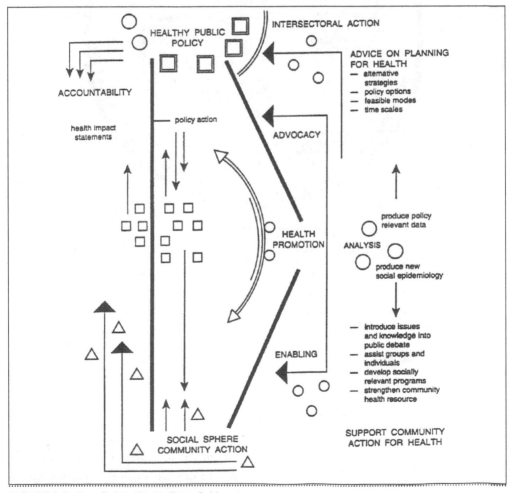

FIGURE 1.1: New Public Health Forcefield

Source: Kickbusch, I. (1986). Health promotion: A global perspective. *Canadian Journal of Public Health, 77,* p. 324.

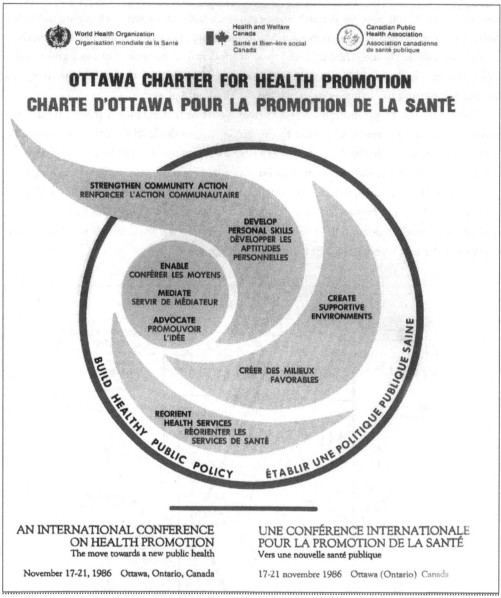

FIGURE 1.2: The *Ottawa Charter*

Source: WHO. (1986). *Ottawa Charter for Health Promotion* cover. Ottawa: World Health Organization, Health and Welfare Canada, Canadian Public Health Association

1986–1994: The Golden Age of Health Promotion

After 1986, health promotion received significant international attention. Following the development of the WHO European program, its main international champion, Ilona Kickbusch, moved to WHO headquarters in Geneva to develop a global health promotion strategy. The second and the third international health promotion conferences, aimed at better understanding two of the strategies proposed in the *Ottawa Charter*—healthy public policy and creating supportive environments—were held in Adelaide, Australia, in 1988 and in Sundsvall, Sweden, in 1991 respectively.

The years immediately following the release of the *Ottawa Charter* and the Epp Report were very important ones for health promotion within Canada. Some additional resources were given to the Health Promotion Directorate of Health and Welfare Canada; programs and initiatives to follow up on the Epp Report were started; and a knowledge development strategy was established. Many of these developments were described in detail in the first edition of this book (Pinder, 1994; Rootman & O'Neill, 1994), as well as two important federal initiatives, the Strengthening Community Health project (Hoffman, 1994) and the Healthy Communities initiative (Manson-Singer, 1994), both of which reflected the flurry of activity of the period. These two strategies aimed at providing local-level entities (communities, municipalities, etc.) with small amounts of monies, allowing them to stimulate health-enhancing community mobilization processes.

1994–2007: THE POPULATION HEALTH ERA

The year 1994 marked the beginning of an era of weakened support for health promotion both in Canada and abroad (O'Neill, Pederson & Rootman, 2000; Pederson, Rootman & O'Neill, 2005). As described below, these had to do with changes in the global and Canadian economic environment and institutions, as well as the emergence of "population health" as a new and very powerful perspective in Canada.

International Developments

Internationally, from the mid-1990s onward, the shift away from the welfare state that began in the late 1980s was clearer. The litany of the rhetoric of balanced government budgets, of deficit reduction, of a diminished role for the state and an increased one for the market, of the necessity of global economic competition in a neo-liberal era—all this was more present and operative than previously. The dominance of this economic view of the world over the more social one that the welfare states had promoted for several decades had consequences. For example, the United Nations' system organizations (such as WHO) lost influence while transnational corporations and economic global institutions, such as the World Bank, the International Monetary Fund, and the World Trade Organization, became increasingly powerful.

In the second edition of this book, Ron Labonté (2007) argued that these global tendencies, in conjunction with the collapse of the former communist world in the early 1990s, which left the US virtually alone to define the "new world order," had important consequences for the evolution of health promotion. Among other things, he suggested that the field needed to align itself with global social movements for health and justice, build empowering partnerships linking poorer nations with wealthier ones, and participate in debates on how globalization affects global health equity (Labonté, 2007, p. 216). Most importantly, he suggested that health promoters need to acknowledge and address the indefensible economic practices that undermine the health of people throughout the world, an argument that he maintains in Chapter 6 of this book.

In the concluding section of the second edition of this book, Ilona Kickbusch (2007) also argued that several of the key institutions that had been instrumental in the birth of health promotion almost abandoned it after 1994. For example, after the Sundsvall conference in 1991, instead of continuing its pattern of hosting international conferences almost every other year to address the three remaining strategies of the *Ottawa Charter* (strengthening community action, developing personal skills, and reorienting health services), the WHO was forced to hold them at irregular intervals and on topics that addressed the interests of the host countries rather than its overall strategy. The Djakarta (1997), Mexico (2000), and Bangkok (2005) conferences each reflected this new order of things. Consequently, the global health promotion community publicly voiced its concern about the WHO's lack of commitment at the Mexico conference (Mittelmark et al., 2001) and about the inclusion of the private sector as a key partner in the *Bangkok Charter* (see the debate in the series *From Ottawa to Vancouver* of the electronic journal *Reviews of Health Promotion and Education Online (RHP&EO)* at http://www.vhpo.net/). The fear was that if governments, which had been the main mechanism through which key health-enhancing policies were adopted for decades from the global to the local levels, were putting health promotion matters in the hands of private corporations whose main interest is to maximize the profits for their shareholders, the common good and the public's health would be at risk.

The Rise of Population Health in Canada

At virtually the same time as the first edition of this book was released, another book was published that contributed to a significant change in the status and practice of health promotion in Canada. Edited by Canadian and American health economists, the book, entitled *Why Some People Are Healthy and Others Are Not* (Evans, Barer & Marmor, 1994), as well as a previous paper (Evans & Stoddard, 1990), helped to put the concept of "population health" on the health policy agenda in Canada and then elsewhere. These publications and masterful presentations to federal/provincial/territorial (F/P/T) meetings in Canada led the federal government to abandon its international and Canadian leadership in health promotion in the mid-1990s as the population health approach gained greater currency. As described by Pinder (2007), among the indicators of the downgrading of health promotion were the replacement of the Health Promotion Directorate by a Population Health Directorate in 1995 and the federal Cabinet's adoption, in 1997, of the population health approach to guide health policy. In addition, several provinces adopted a population health approach in their policy development and F/P/T Advisory Committee on Population Health was established in 1992. The key elements of the population health approach are presented in Figure 1.3. They gained a lot of currency among politicians because they were presented in a kind of economic language by high-profile, politically well-connected scholars of major Canadian universities, whereas health promotion was couched in a social language less popular at that time and promoted by lower profile scholars and practitioners.

Nevertheless, health promotion did not disappear entirely at the federal or provincial levels. For example, as shown in Figure 1.3, Health Canada made a serious effort to integrate

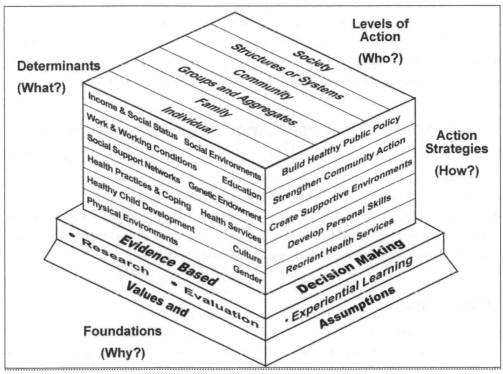

FIGURE 1.3: Population Health Promotion Framework

Source: Hamilton, N. & Bhatti, T. (1996). Retrieved July 12, 2011 from http://www.courseweb.uottawa.ca/pop8910/Outline/Models/Hamilton-Bhatti.htm.

population health and health promotion into a common framework (Hamilton & Bhatti, 1996) and the department did maintain and produce programs built on the foundation established in the first two decades of health promotion. Health promotion concepts and approaches were also integrated into federal, provincial, and territorial (F/P/T) strategies, and at least two provinces established ministries or departments of health promotion. In addition, Health Canada, and subsequently the Public Health Agency of Canada, provided funding and support for the Canadian Consortium for Health Promotion Research to facilitate work on projects and to organize the nineteenth world conference of the IUHPE in Vancouver in 2007. As indicated in the second edition of this book (Rootman, Jackson & Hills, 2007), the network of Canadian university-based research centres in health promotion, six of which were funded by the precursor of the Canadian Institutes of Health Research (CIHR), was also very successful in obtaining funding for health promotion research projects from CIHR and other research-funding programs and agencies. Finally, the Public Health Agency of Canada, established in 2004, created an internal Centre for Health Promotion shortly afterwards.

Thus, even though health promotion was eclipsed by "population health" from 1994 to 2007, it was still active as a field in Canada when the second edition of the book was published and released at the IUHPE Conference in July 2007. Leadership of the field had shifted, however, from the government to the academic sector. In fact, there were reasons for optimism about the future of health promotion at that time, not least of which was the opportunity that the IUHPE global conference presented to showcase Canadian accomplishments in the field and to consolidate Canada's reputation as an international leader in the field.

2007 AND BEYOND: THE POPULATION HEALTH PROMOTION ERA

Four years is not a very long time in terms of the development of a field. It is certainly too short to know the long-term significance of any changes that have taken place since the conference in Vancouver. However, it is possible to identify international and national developments that have already led to or are likely to have significant effects on health promotion. They are included in the last section of the conclusion to this book, where their consequences for the immediate future of the field here and abroad are also discussed.

CONCLUSION

Thus, health promotion is not dead in Canada even though its infrastructure (ministries, agencies, academic units, etc., formally labelled "health promotion") appears to have been weakened considerably over the past few years. To use a metaphor that was suggested in the second edition of the book by Ilona Kickbusch (2007) and taken up by the authors of its final chapter (Dupéré et al., 2007), health promotion in Canada, as in many countries, increasingly appears to be acting like a rhizome rather than a tree. That is, it is becoming more like a "system that has many roots, that is connected and heterogenic; it does not respect territory but expands continuously ... " (Kickbusch, 2007, p. 363). Interesting examples of this might be the increasing adoption of the term "population health promotion,"[2] both health promotion and population health seemingly having found their respective and integrated niche, as well as the spread of health promotion concepts such as "health literacy" to other fields.[3]

So the story continues as we see the field changing both nationally and internationally and evolving in ways that we would never have predicted 20 years ago when we began planning the first edition of *Health Promotion in Canada*. One thing is clear, though: Health promotion in Canada seems to be resilient because of its value base, the strength of the scientific base it has helped develop, and because of the strong network of people and organizations that are still involved.

Notes

1. The World Health Organization is a specialized technical agency of the United Nations system where national governments of most countries of the world get together to decide on general global health-related orientations, which they are then free to apply or not.
2. For example, the British Columbia 2010 Public Health Summer School used the term "population health promotion" rather than "health promotion" to describe its program. (See http://www.phabc. org/modules/Summer_School_reg/files/Program_2011_BC_Public_Health_Summer_School.pdf).

3. For example, the Canadian Medical Association, in partnership with other organizations, has developed a health literacy curriculum module that incorporates a health promotion perspective. (See http://mdcme.ca/mymdcme.asp)

References

Badgley, R. (1994). Health promotion and social change in the health of Canadians. In A. Pederson, M. O'Neill & I. Rootman (Eds.), *Health promotion in Canada* (pp. 20–39). Toronto: W.B. Saunders.

Becker, M.H. (1974). *The health belief model and personal health behavior.* Thorofare: Charles B. Slack.

Brown, R.E. & Margo, G.E. (1978). Health education: Can the reformers be reformed? *International Journal of Health Services, 8*(1), 3–26.

Commission on the Social Determinants of Health (CSDH). (2008). *Closing the gap in a generation: Health equity through action on the social determinants of health.* Geneva: World Health Organization.

Dupéré, S., Ridde, V., Carroll, S., O'Neill, M., Rootman, I. & Pederson, A. (2007). Conclusion: The rhizome and the tree. In M. O'Neill et al. (Eds.), *Health promotion in Canada* (2nd ed.) (pp. 371–389). Toronto: Canadian Scholars' Press Inc.

Epp, J. (1986). *Achieving health for all: A framework for health promotion.* Ottawa: Health and Welfare Canada.

Evans, R.G., Barer, M.L. & Marmor, T.R. (1994). *Why are some people healthy and others not? The determinants of health of populations (social institutions and social change).* New York: Aldine de Guyter.

Evans, R.G. & Stoddard, G.L. (1990). Producing health, consuming health care. *Social Science and Medicine, 31*(12), 1347–1363.

Freudenberg, N. (1978). Shaping the future of health education: From behavior change to social change. *Health Education Monographs, 6*(4), 372–377.

Gilbert, J. (1963). *L'éducation sanitaire.* Montreal: Presses de l'Université de Montréal.

Gilbert, J. (1967). The grandeur and decadence of health education. *Canadian Journal of Public Health, 58,* 355–358.

Green, L.W. & Kreuter, M. (1999). *Health promotion planning: An educational and ecological approach* (3rd ed.). Mountain View: Mayfield.

Hamilton, N. & Bhatti, T. (1996). *Population health promotion: An integrated model of health and health promotion.* Ottawa: Health Promotion Development Division, Health Canada.

Hoffman, K. (1994). The strengthening community health program: Lessons for community development. In A. Pederson, M. O'Neill & I. Rootman (Eds.), *Health promotion in Canada* (pp. 123–139). Toronto: W.B. Saunders.

Kickbusch, I. (1986). Health promotion: A global perspective. *Canadian Journal of Public Health, 77,* 321–326.

Kickbusch, I. (2007). Health promotion: Not a tree but a rhizome. In M. O'Neill, A. Pederson, I. Rootman & S. Dupéré (Eds.), *Health promotion in Canada: Critical perspectives* (pp. 363–366). Toronto: Canadian Scholars' Press Inc.

Labonté, R. (2007). Promoting health in a globalizing world: The biggest challenge of all? In M. O'Neill et al. (Eds.), *Health promotion in Canada* (2nd ed.) (pp. 207–222). Toronto: Canadian Scholars' Press Inc.

Labonté, R. & Penfold, S. (1981). Canadian perspectives in health promotion: A critique. *Health Education, 19*(3–4), 4–10.

Lalonde, M. (1974). *A new perspective on the health of Canadians.* Ottawa: Government of Canada.

Manson-Singer, S. (1994). The Canadian healthy communities project: Creating a social movement. In A. Pederson, M. O'Neill & I. Rootman (Eds.), *Health promotion in Canada* (pp. 107–122). Toronto: W.B. Saunders.

Milio, N. (1986). *Promoting health through public policy* (2nd ed.). Ottawa: Canadian Public Health Association.

Mittelmark, M.B., Akerman, M., Gillis, D., Kosa, K., O'Neill, M., Piette, D., et al. (2001). Mexico conference on health promotion: Open letter to WHO director general, Dr. Gro Harlem Brundtland. *Health Promotion International, 16*(1), 3–4.

Modolo, M.A. & Mamon, J. (2001). *A long way to health promotion through IUHPE conferences (1951–2001).* Perugia: University of Perugia, Inter-university Experimental Center for Health Education.

O'Neill, M., Pederson, A. & Rootman, I. (2000). Health promotion in Canada: Declining or transforming? *Health Promotion International, 15*(2), 135–141.

O'Neill, M., Pederson, A., Rootman, I. & Dupéré, S. (Eds.). (2007). *Health promotion in Canada: Critical perspectives.* Toronto: Canadian Scholars' Press Inc.

Pederson, A., O'Neill, M. & Rootman, I. (Eds.). (1994). Health Promotion in Canada: Provincial, national and international perspectives. Toronto: W.B. Saunders Canada.

Pederson, A., Rootman, I. & O'Neill, M. (2005). Health promotion in Canada: Back to the past or towards a promising future? In A. Scriven & S. Garman (Eds.), *Promoting health: Global perspectives* (pp. 255–265). London: Palgrave Macmillan.

Pinder, L. (1994). The federal role in health promotion: Art of the possible. In A. Pederson et al. (Eds.), *Health promotion in Canada* (pp. 374–387). Toronto: W.B. Saunders.

Pinder, L. (2007). The federal role in health promotion: Under the radar. In M. O'Neill et al. (Eds.), *Health promotion in Canada* (2nd ed.) (pp. 92–106). Toronto: Canadian Scholars' Press Inc.

Rootman, I., Jackson, S. & Hills, M. (2007). Developing knowledge for health promotion. In M. O'Neill et al. (Eds.), *Health promotion in Canada* (2nd ed.) (pp. 123–138). Toronto: Canadian Scholars' Press Inc.

Rootman, I. & O'Neill, M. (1994). Developing knowledge for health promotion. In A. Pederson, M. O'Neill & I. Rootman (Eds.), *Health promotion in Canada: Provincial, national, and international perspectives* (pp. 139–153). Toronto: W.B. Saunders.

Ryan, W. (1976). *Blaming the victim* (rev. ed.). New York: Vintage Books Edition.

UNICEF. (1978). *The declaration of Alma-Ata.* International Conference on Primary Health Care. Alma-Ata: United Nations Children's Fund and World Health Organization.

WHO. (1981). *November 19, 1981 64th plenary meeting, Resolution 36/43.* Retrieved from: http://www.un-documents.net/a36r43.htm

WHO. (1986). *Ottawa Charter for Health Promotion.* Ottawa: World Health Organization, Health and Welfare Canada, Canadian Public Health Association.

WHO. (2009). Closing the gap in a generation: Health equity through action on the social determinants of health. Final report of the Commission on social determinants of Health. Geneva. Retrieved from http://www.who.int/social_determinants/thecommission/finalreport/en/index.html .

WHO-EURO. (1984). *Health promotion: A discussion document on the concept and principles. ICP/HSR 602 (m01).* Unpublished manuscript, Copenhagen. Retrieved from: http://heapro.oxfordjournals.org/content/1/1/73.citation

Critical Thinking Questions

1. What have been the four main periods in the evolution of health promotion in Canada?
2. Can we consider the *Ottawa Charter for Health Promotion* a Canadian document? Why or why not?
3. Why did the Lalonde Report receive so much international attention?

4. Do you think 2007 was the beginning of a new era in Canadian health promotion? Why or why not?

5. Do you think that Canada is an international leader in health promotion? Why or why not?

Resources

Further Readings

Critical Public Health. (2008). Special issue on Health Promotion, 18(4), 431-540.

In this special issue, the recent situation of health promotion is addressed with a critical eye at the global level, as well as in several countries (Canada, Australia, England) or continents (Africa).

O'Neill, M., Pederson, A., Rootman, I. & Dupéré, S. (2007) (Eds.). *Health promotion in Canada: Critical perspectives* (pp. 363–366). Toronto: Canadian Scholars' Press Inc.

The second edition of the book, which analyzes the 1994–2007 period of Canadian health promotion and presents views of health promotion by provincial, territorial, and international authors.

Pederson, A., O'Neill, M. & Rootman, I. (Eds.). (1994). *Health promotion in Canada: Provincial, national, and international perspectives.* Toronto: W.B. Saunders.

The first edition of the book, which analyzes the 1974–1994 period of Canadian health promotion.

Relevant Websites

International Union for Health Promotion and Education (IUHPE)

www.iuhpe.org/

The International Union for Health Promotion and Education is the only global organization entirely devoted to advancing public health through health promotion and health education. This site is an important source for news and events in health promotion in three languages (English, Spanish, French).

Reviews of Health Promotion and Education Online

www.rhpeo.net/

The website of IUHPE'S electronic journal, the *Reviews of Health Promotion and Education Online* (RHPEO).

World Health Organization

www.who.int/healthpromotion/conferences/en

WHO's website on global health promotion conferences, including charters, declarations, etc., as well as the complete text of the *Alma-Ata Declaration on Primary Health Care* and the report of the Commission on the Social Determinants of Health (2009).

CHAPTER 2

Key Concepts in Health Promotion

Irving Rootman and Michel O'Neill

Introduction

A concept is "an abstract idea."[1] Concepts are critical for both research and practice and help to define what a field is about, stimulate theory-building, and are the primary elements of the theories that are built. In addition, they also reflect the values that guide a field. All of this is certainly true for health promotion. Thus, this chapter discusses some of the key concepts that help to define the field. In particular, it covers the following concepts: health, health promotion, social determinants of health, empowerment, health literacy, and quality of life. In doing so, it draws on some chapters from the previous two editions and adds new material from other sources. It reflects the evolution in thinking about health promotion and the dynamic nature of this field of study and practice.

The Concept of Health

Health is a fundamental concept for many fields, including medicine, nursing, public health, and health promotion. There are many competing concepts of health (Rootman & Raeburn, 1994; Raeburn & Rootman, 2007). Examples of different views of health from different perspectives are shown in Box 2.1. Probably the most influential for health promotion is the definition of health in the World Health Organization's Constitution as "a state of complete physical, mental, and social well-being, and not merely the absence of disease and infirmity" (WHO, 1946), although some critics have questioned the use of the term "state" rather than "process," and others have argued that it puts no boundaries on what is encompassed and therefore no limits on expenditure (Rootman & Rayburn, 1994).

Another internationally influential concept of health for health promotion was "the health field concept" (Lalonde, 1974), which suggested that health was determined by more than just health services. It listed four broad contributory categories of factors or "elements," later to be called determinants, making up the "health field," namely: human biology, environment, lifestyle, and health care organization.

For health promoters, it was the introduction of lifestyle and environment into the health discourse that was memorable, especially the notion of "lifestyle," a concept that dominated Canadian and international health promotion thinking and action for at least a decade after the Lalonde Report and still lingers on. However, as mentioned in Chapter 1, during the 1980s, there was a move away from individualistic behavioural views of health promotion to more

---

BOX 2.1: _____

Some Definitions of Health

Academic definition: "involves the interplay of biological, psychological and social aspects of the person's life" (Sarafino, 1990, p. 16).

Bangkok Charter definition: [Health promotion] "offers a positive and inclusive concept of health as a determinant of the quality of life and encompassing mental and spiritual well-being" (World Health Organization, 2005, p. 1).

Holistic definition: "an ongoing sense of finely tuned wellness, which involves not only excellent care of the physical body but also care of ourselves in such a way that we nurture our capacity to be mentally alert and creative as well as emotionally stable and satisfied ... " (quoted in Alster, 1989, p. 78).

Medical definition: "The normal physical state, i.e., the state of being whole and free from physical and mental disease or pain, so that the parts of the body carry on their proper function" (Critchley, 1978, p. 784).

Native American definition: "living in total harmony with nature and having the ability to survive under exceedingly difficult circumstances" (Spector, 1985, p. 181).

Ottawa Charter definition: "a resource for everyday life, not the objective of living. Health is a positive concept emphasizing social and personal resources, as well as physical capacities" (World Health Organization, 1986, p. 1).

WHO definition: "health is a state of complete physical, mental, and social well-being and not merely the absence of disease and infirmity" (World Health Organization, 1946, p. 1).

---

social and policy views. In Canada, the mid-1980s were important for Hancock's influential introduction of concepts like the "Mandala of Health" (Hancock & Perkins, 1985). In 1986, the *Ottawa Charter for Health Promotion* was released, with its framing of health as a "resource for living" and its emphasis on a broad social determinants model of health (WHO, 1986). This social model of health was echoed in the 1986 Canadian government document *Achieving Health for All: A Framework for Health Promotion* (Epp, 1986), albeit with a more personal and friendly tone (using concepts like "self-help" and "mutual aid"), and a strong emphasis on equity. In 1989, Raeburn and Rootman combined the health concepts of the Lalonde health field concept and the *Ottawa Charter* (Raeburn & Rootman, 1989), and in 1993, Labonté (1993) took up the issue of subjective and objective views of health.

While there are many ways of looking at health, its common conceptual feature is that the term is related to a broad domain of life that can be differentiated from other broad domains, such as economics, politics, justice, and education. The distinctive feature of this domain, however, is that it relates to integration of the human organism's condition, well-being, and functioning. Thus, it was suggested in 1994 that the following statement describes a concept of health that could be of use by Canadian health promoters:

Health as perceived in a Canadian health promotion context has to do with the bodily, mental and social quality of life of people as determined in particular by psychological, societal, cultural and policy dimensions. Health is seen by Canadian health promoters as being enhanced by a sensible lifestyle and the equitable use of public and private resources to permit people to use their initiative individually and collectively to maintain and improve their own well-being, however they may define it. (Rootman & Raeburn, 1994, p. 69)

Thirteen years later, these same authors took another look at the concept of health and the dilemmas that it generated, and it was concluded that a new concept was necessary for the twenty-first century to reinvigorate health promotion and make it more relevant to the present and the future. The following was suggested as a possible definition, underpinning and giving direction to health promotion practitioners:

In the health promotion domain, health is equivalent to healthiness and is related to concepts of resilience and capacity. It refers primarily to mental and physical dimensions of healthiness, has strong experiential and social aspects, and is determined by many internal and external factors, including those of a personal, collective, environmental, political, and global nature. (Raeburn & Rootman, 2007, p. 28)

It was hoped that this statement would lead to articulation of a strong, positive, exciting, and relevant concept of health that would take the field of health promotion forward in the twenty-first century.

As a step leading in this direction, a paper was published about the same time in *Health Promotion International* (Eriksson & Lindström, 2008), which argued that Antonovsky's salutogenic theory of health could become a key one for the field. The authors suggested that the focus on factors supporting well-being, in contrast to ones that cause disease, could make an important contribution to health promotion theory and practice. The high profile that salutogenesis received at the twentieth Global Conference on Health Promotion, held in Geneva in the summer of 2010,[2] reinforces the fact that it is currently one of the key conceptual developments of what health is about.

BOX 2.2:
_____

Salutogenesis

The term "salutogenesis" was put forward by Aaron Antonovsky in the early 1980s to describe an approach to human health emphasizing the factors supporting health and well-being, rather than those that cause disease. He developed this concept from his research on how people survive, adapt, and overcome even the most difficult life-stress experiences, such as living in a concentration camp. He hypothesized that a stress factor will be either pathogenic, neutral, or salutary, depending on what he called *generalized resistance resources* (GRRs). According to

> him, these GRRs helped people make sense of and manage events. He postulated that a person's sense of coherence determines whether stress will harm him or her.

Source: Lindström, B. & Eriksson M. (2010). The hitchhiker's guide to salutogenesis: Salutogenic pathways to health promotion. Helsinki: Folkhälsan Research Centre. Retrieved from: http://www.salutogenesis.fi/eng/Publications.18.html

The Concept of Health Promotion

As is the case for "health," there are also many different concepts of "health promotion" and, not surprisingly, much confusion among them (O'Neill & Stirling, 2007). In order to sort out this confusion, it is important to distinguish between two ways in which the words "health promotion" are used: (1) as a *discourse* on the place of health in societies, and (2) as a *specialized field of intervention* within the broader field of public health. Thus, it has been suggested that the expression *the promotion of health* be used for the discourse that can be undertaken by anybody and that the expression *health promotion* be restricted to the specialized field of practice (O'Neill & Stirling, 2007).

This distinction is well illustrated by contrasting two of the best-known definitions of the field, the one from the *Ottawa Charter for Health Promotion*: "The process of enabling people to increase control over, and improve, their health" (WHO, 1986, p. 1), with the one by Green and Kreuter: "[...] any planned combination of educational, political, regulatory and organizational supports for actions and conditions of living conducive to the health of individuals, groups or communities" (2005, p. 462).

The Promotion of Health

The *Ottawa Charter* definition, as well as most governmental health policy documents in Canada or around the world since the mid-1970s, are typical of the reflections on what health is or should be; on the place health should have in societies; and on who should undertake health-promoting, health-restoring, or health-maintaining endeavours, hence the idea of naming this a discourse on *the promotion of health*, which is nothing but the old public health discourse that has been around for centuries (Fassin, 2000). This reflects upon what health is in societies or populations; what produces or hinders it; and what can be done to improve it, reduce the risk of losing it, or restore it when compromised. It is in this perspective that health promotion (as symbolized by the *Ottawa Charter*) has been identified as the "third public health revolution" of humankind (Breslow, 1999) after the first, which had tackled infectious diseases, and the second, which addressed chronic illnesses. The health promotion era, according to Breslow, embarks on the journey toward health rather than engaging in a battle against diverse types of diseases. This shift in thinking is illustrated in Figure 2.1, where we can see that with the evolution of humankind, of the epidemiological patterns of disease, and of the technological means available, the various functions of public health have successively developed in a series of layers like sediments, the latter not displacing but building on top of the former, which still needs support by the previous ones to continue to function properly.

The discourse on the promotion of health in *modern* societies, which is symbolized by the *Ottawa Charter*, is usually referred to as the "new" (Ashton & Seymour, 1988; Martin & McQueen, 1989) or the "ecological" public health (Chu & Simpson, 1994; Kickbusch,

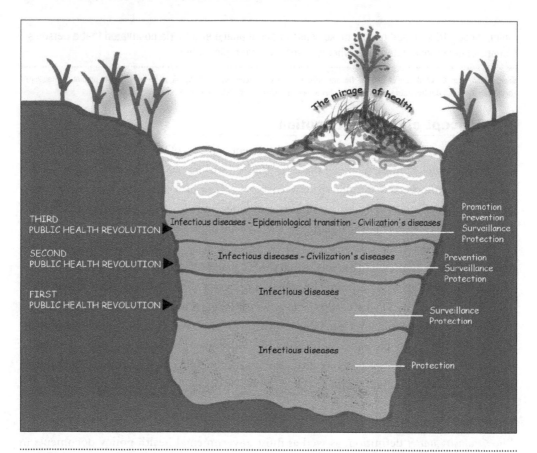

FIGURE 2.1: Sedimentation Approach to Public Health throughout Human History

Source: Adapted from Potvin, L. (2005). Présentation dans le séminaire doctoral SAC-66008, Université Laval, October 17, 2005, and Breslow, L. (1999). Breslow, L. (1999). From disease prevention to health promotion. *JAMA, 281*(11), 1030-1033.

1989) in order to differentiate it from the more classical discourse of "hygiene" or "old" public health. We thus argue that population health, as it emerged in Canada in 1994 and as discussed at length in Chapter 1, was but a variation of this new public health discourse on *the promotion of health* and that "in general, the proponents of population health can be seen as allies [of health promotion] in the move towards the new public health, particularly since overall, neither framework has significantly challenged the dominance of biomedicine in the health field" (O'Neill, Pederson & Rootman, 2000, p. 141).

Health Promotion

Conversely, Green and Kreuter's definition is more in line with the idea that *health promotion* is a specialized subarea, or essential function, of the public health sector of health systems, which, according to the Pan-American Health Organization, aims at "the promotion of changes in lifestyle and environmental conditions to facilitate the development of a culture of health" (2002, p. 67). We thus argue that what really defines health promotion is its focus on the *planned change* of lifestyles and life conditions having an impact on health, using a variety of specific strategies, including health education, social marketing, and mass communication on the individual side, as well as political action, community organization, and organizational development on the collective side.

Given this view, the planned change skills and other specific competencies (see Chapter 13) of properly trained health promoters can be used at whatever stage in the natural history of any illness or health problem (thus in primary or secondary prevention, in acute care, in rehabilitation, or in tertiary prevention) and at any level, from the individual to the societal, including the family and the community. Moreover, even if the value base (empowerment and participation of populations, social justice, etc.) of the *Ottawa Charter* can be used to work with these *health promotion* skills, they can also be used by other groups, working with other value bases. Finally, in order to be as effective as possible, planned change *health promotion* interventions must apply strategies that are knowledge-based or even evidence-based when that type of information is available. The relationship between *the promotion of health* and *health promotion* is illustrated in Figure 2.2.

We thus propose that the words "new public health" or "ecological public health" should be used when we talk about the discourse on the promotion of health, and the expression

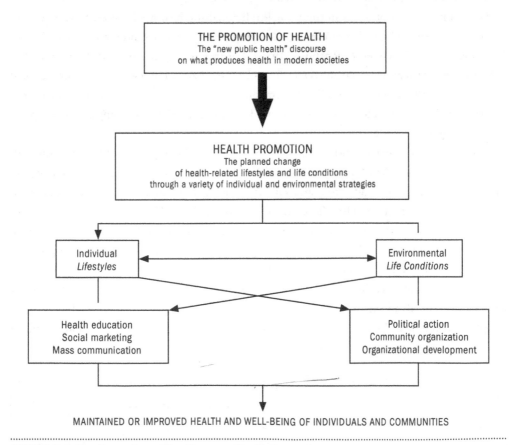

FIGURE 2.2: The Promotion of Health versus Health Promotion

Source: Adapted and modified from O'Neill, M. & Stirling, A. (2007). The promotion of health or health promotion? In M. O'Neill, S. Dupéré, A. Pederson & I. Rootman (Eds.), *Health promotion in Canada: Critical perspectives* (p. 42). Toronto: Canadian Scholars' Press Inc.

"health promotion" reserved to designate the specific planned change skills needed to achieve the results desired by the "new public health" discourse. Whether or not the field will adopt this advice remains to be seen.

Health Promotion versus Health Education

Furthermore, in trying to clarify the boundaries of health promotion as a field, it is helpful to compare it with another closely related field, namely, health education (O'Neill & Stirling, 2007). As noted in Chapter 1, health promotion emerged as an evolution of health education, which had formalized itself at the beginning of the 1950s and worked from then on to influence individual health-related behaviours. However, at the end of the 1970s, many health educators realized that trying to influence individual behaviours without altering the environments in which they occurred produced limited results. In the mid-1980s, the field as a whole thus relabelled itself "health promotion" to signify that from then on, just working to change individual lifestyles was no longer a viable option. A much broader way of looking at things, soon to be called "ecological" (see Chapter 5 of this book), was suggested as required to understand and influence health-related behaviours.

For many, the transition from traditional individualistic health education toward a more ecologically oriented health promotion, requiring practitioners to intervene at a variety of levels, was difficult (Green & Raeburn, 1988). For instance, it was only at the very end of 1993 that the main professional and scientific global organization in the field, the International Union for Health Education (IUHE), decided to follow the trend and rename itself the International Union for Health Promotion and Education (IUHPE), keeping the two expressions within its new title.

Even today, in several countries like the US or France, the words "health education" still have more currency than "health promotion," sometimes used to designate the old version of individualistic health education, and sometimes used to designate the new enlarged field called "health promotion" elsewhere. We can thus say that: "Health education comprises consciously constructed opportunities for learning involving some form of communication designed to improve health literacy, including improving knowledge, and developing life skills which are conducive to individual and community health" (Nutbeam, 1998, p. 354).

Box 2.3, co-authored by the former editor of *Health Education Research*, one of the most important journals in the field, shows that the debate is far from over. Nevertheless, most people working in health promotion take the view that health education is one strategy within the larger field of health promotion.

BOX 2.3:

Health Education: Resurrection and Reinvention

The following simple equation encapsulates a "revitalized" definition of health education:
Health promotion = Health education × healthy public policy.

An essential weakness of pre-Ottawa health education was its apparent lack of awareness of the importance of the social and environmental determinants of disease in its blinkered emphasis on the individual. However, health promotion's justifiable attempts to remedy this myopic view have tended to ignore the importance of education in overcoming political barriers in pursuit of *Healthy Public Policy*. Education without policy is emasculating; on the other hand, policy without education is virtually unattainable. Technically, health education involves a planned attempt to provide the conditions necessary for efficient learning, including those learning outcomes centrally involved in empowering communities. Accordingly, we assert the importance of providing community members, through health education, with specific skills (e.g., assertiveness), recognize that it is highly desirable for them to enlist the support of coalitions, and, finally, believe in media advocacy in order to generate indignation and community action.

Other Key Concepts in Health Promotion

There are a number of other key concepts in health promotion and a discussion of some is presented below. The specific concepts discussed are: social determinants of health, empowerment, health literacy, and quality of life. They were selected because they are considered by many in the field to be core to the practice of health promotion and are frequently used by people working in the field.

Social Determinants of Health

Among the various sets of determinants that have an impact on health, the social ones have gained significant currency in health promotion over the past few years, partly as a result of work done in Canada. The history of this idea has been traced to the political economist Friedrich Engels and to the physician and politician Rudolf Virchow in the nineteenth century (Raphael, 2009), both of whom drew attention to the links between social conditions and health. More recent contributions have been made by British politicians and researchers, as well as Canadian politicians (Lalonde, 1974; Epp, 1986) and public health officials (Canadian Public Health Association (2000, 2001).

The term "social determinants of health" made its debut only fairly recently in a book by British researchers (Blane, Brunner & Wilkinson, 1996), which expanded on the environmental determinants of health in the health field concept of the Lalonde Report. Work has also been done by the Canadian Institute for Advanced Research (Evans, Barer & Marmor, 1994) and Health Canada (1998) to outline various determinants of health, many of which are social in nature. A pivotal national conference in 2002 on the social determinants of health identified 12 key social determinants of health (see Box 2.4) and led to the definition of "social determinants of health" as "the economic and social conditions that shape the health of individuals, communities, and jurisdictions as a whole" (Raphael, 2009, p. 2).

Attention has been drawn internationally to the social determinants of health by the WHO Commission on the Social Determinants of Health (CSDH, 2008). Although it does not provide a simple declarative definition of "social determinants of health" in its report, a WHO backgrounder on the work of the commission defines it as "the circumstances in which people are born, grow up, live, work and age, and the systems put in place to deal with illness" (WHO, 2010, p. 2).

BOX 2.4:
_____

The Social Determinants of Health Framework

The following 12 social determinants of health were identified by the organizers of the York University conference on the social determinants of health:

- Aboriginal status
- Early life
- Education
- Employment and working conditions
- Food security
- Gender
- Health care services
- Housing
- Income and its distribution
- Social exclusion
- Social safety net
- Unemployment and employment security

Source: Raphael, D. (2009). *Social determinants of health* (2nd ed.) (p. 7). Toronto: Canadian Scholars' Press Inc.

Mikkonen and Raphael (2010) subsequently added "Race" and "Disability" to the list of social determinants

Empowerment

Empowerment is another important concept and value for health promotion. In fact, it has been suggested that "the primary criterion for determining whether or not a particular initiative should be considered to be health promoting, ought to be the extent to which it involves the process of enabling, or empowering individuals or communities" (Rootman et al., 2001, p. 14). Similarly, the authors of this statement suggested that "health promotion is fundamentally about ensuring that the individuals and communities are able to assume the power to which they are entitled" (pp. 13–14). Although some people working in the field do not routinely apply the criterion of empowerment to their work, perhaps because they have constraints that limit their capacity to act in empowering ways, it is widely acknowledged by many, if not most, as a cardinal principle and value of health promotion. This is, in part, because of its relevance as a mechanism for reducing inequities in health, which is a fundamental goal of health promotion.

The concept of empowerment was developed in the field of community psychology in the 1980s where it was defined by Rappaport as "a mechanism by which people, organizations and communities gain mastery over their lives" (1987, p. 122). It was also picked up in the field of nursing with a similar definition (Gibson, 1991). Rissel added to the concept in health promotion by distinguishing between psychological and community empowerment. He defined the former as "a feeling of greater control over their own lives which individuals experience following active membership in groups or organizations, and may occur without participation in collective political action" (Rissel, 1994, p. 41). He suggested that "community empowerment" "includes a raised level of psychological empowerment among its members, a

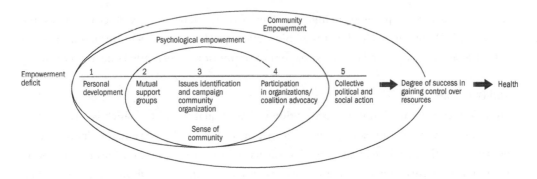

FIGURE 2.3: Model of the Critical Components of Community Empowerment and the Process by Which It May Be Achieved

Source: Rissel, C. (1994). Empowerment: The holy grail of health promotion. *Health Promotion International, 9*(1), 43.

political action component in which members have actively participated, and the achievement of some redistribution of resources or decision-making favourable to the group or community in question" (Rissel, 1994, p. 41). He further added to the understanding of the concept by putting forward a conceptual framework outlining a process through which psychological and community empowerment can lead to health, both at the individual and community levels.

Subsequently, empowerment has been defined as a "social action process for people to gain mastery over their lives in the context of changing their social and political environment to improve equity and quality of life" (Minkler, Wallerstein & Wilson, 2008, p. 295). As did Rappaport, the authors of this definition added "organizational empowerment" as another level of empowerment to consider (Minkler, Wallerstein & Wilson, 2008, p. 295), located between individual and community empowerment.

Health Literacy

Health literacy is increasingly becoming a core concept in health promotion (Rootman, Frankish & Kaszap, 2007). Although it first appeared in the health education literature in 1974 (Simonds, 1974), it wasn't picked up by health promotion until the later 1990s in a paper by Kickbusch (1997), as well as in a glossary of health promotion terms by Nutbeam (1998) and in a paper in which he argued (Nutbeam, 2000) that health literacy is a key outcome of health education activity for which people in health promotion and education should be held accountable. Although Nutbeam did not indicate why it was a key outcome of health education, presumably it may have been because literacy is widely acknowledged as a key outcome of education.

The concept of health literacy made its first appearance in Canada in 2000 at the first Canadian Conference on Literacy and Health and has become an area of increased research and practice since the second Canadian conference in 2004 and the report of the Canadian Expert Panel on Health Literacy (Rootman & Gordon-El-Bihbety, 2008). Although there is still some controversy over the definition of health literacy, the following one put forward by the Canadian Expert Panel on Health Literacy is becoming more widely used in this country and, to some extent, in others: "the ability to access, understand, evaluate and communicate information as a way to promote, maintain and improve health in a variety of settings across the life-course" (Rootman & Gordon-El-Bihbety, 2008, p. 11). Chapter 8 of this book discusses health literacy as one of the key issues that health promotion is currently concerned about.

Quality of Life

A final key concept used in health promotion is that of quality of life, which is often seen as the ultimate outcome of health promotion. Although again, there are many definitions of quality of life, the one developed by the University of Toronto's Centre for Health Promotion research unit on this topic was "*The degree to which a person enjoys the important possibilities of his or her life*" (Quality of Life Research Unit, 2010). This concept of quality of life is represented in nine life sectors grouped as Being, Belonging, and Becoming, as shown in Figure 2.4.

In this model, "Being" consists of physical, psychological, and spiritual components; "Belonging" of physical, social, and community components; and "Becoming" of practical, leisure, and growth components.

The concept of quality of life fits well in health promotion because it is both positive and inclusive (Raeburn & Rootman, 2007). Possibly for these reasons, it was included explicitly in the *Bangkok Charter for Health Promotion* (World Health Organization, 2005).

Conclusion

This chapter has discussed a number of key concepts in health promotion. Others could have been included. However, we believe that the chapter has presented a sufficient number of the concepts central to the field to provide the reader with a good sense of what its major concepts and conceptual issues currently are. Additional ones are also introduced throughout this book.

Notes

1. Retrieved from: http://oxforddictionaries.com/definition/concept
2. Retrieved from: http://www.iuhpeconference.net/

References

Alster, K.B. (1989). *The holistic health movement*. Tuscaloosa: University of Alabama Press.

Ashton, J. & Seymour, H. (1988). *The new public health*. Philadelphia: Open University Press.

Blane, D., Brunner, E. & Wilkinson, R. (Eds.). (1996). *Health and social organization*. London: Routledge.

Breslow, L. (1999). From disease prevention to health promotion. *JAMA, 281*(11), 1030–1033.

Canadian Public Health Association. (2000). *Reducing poverty and its negative effects on health: Resolution passed at the 2000 CPHA Annual Meeting*. Retrieved from: http://www.cpha.ca/uploads/resolutions/2000_e.pdf

Canadian Public Health Association. (2001). *CPHA policy statements*. Retrieved from: http://www.cpha.ca/uploads/policy/conditions_e.pdf

Chu, C. & Simpson, R. (1994). *Ecological public health: From vision to practice*. Toronto: Centre for Health Promotion, University of Toronto.

Being	*Who One Is*
Physical Being	· physical health
	· personal hygiene
	· nutrition
	· exercise
	· grooming and clothing
	· general physical appearance
Psychological Being	· psychological health and adjustment
	· cognitions
	· feelings
	· self-esteem, self-concept, and self-control
Spiritual Being	· personal values
	· personal standards of conduct
	· spiritual beliefs

Belonging	*Connections with One's Environments*
Physical Belonging	· home
	· workplace/school
	· neighbourhood
	· community
Social Belonging	· intimate others
	· family
	· friends
	· co-workers
	· neighbourhood and community
Community Belonging	· adequate income
	· health and social services
	· employment
	· educational programs
	· recreational programs
	· community events and activities

Becoming	*Achieving Personal Goals, Hopes, and Aspirations*
Practical Becoming	· domestic activities
	· paid work
	· school or volunteer activities
	· meeting health or social needs
Leisure Becoming	· activities that promote relaxation and stress reduction
Growth Becoming	· activities that promote the maintenance or improvement of knowledge and skills
	· adapting to change

FIGURE 2.4: Centre for Health Promotion Quality of Life Model

Source: Quality of Life Research Unit, University of Toronto website. Retrieved from: http://www.utoronto.ca/qol/concepts.htm

Commission on the Social Determinants of Health (CSDH). (2008). *Closing the gap in a generation: Health equity through action on the social determinants of health.* Geneva: World Health Organization.

Critchley, M. (Ed.). (1978). *Butterworth's medical dictionary.* London: Butterworth's.

Epp, J. (1986). *Achieving health for all: A framework for health promotion.* Ottawa: Health and Welfare Canada.

Eriksson, M. & Lindström, B. (2008). A salutogenic interpretation of the Ottawa Charter. *Health Promotion International, 23*(2), 190–199.

Evans, R.G., Barer, M.L. & Marmor, T.R. (1994). *Why are some people healthy and others not? The determinants of health of populations.* New York: Aldine de Guyter.

Fassin, D. (2000). Comment faire de la santé publique avec des mots. Une rhétorique à l'œuvre. *Ruptures, revue transdisciplinaire en santé, 7*(1), 58–78.

Gibson, C.H. (1991). A concept analysis of empowerment. *Journal of Advanced Nursing, 16,* 354–361.

Green, L.W. & Kreuter, M.W. (2005). *Health program planning: An educational and ecological approach* (4th ed.). Boston & Toronto: McGraw-Hill Higher Education.

Green, L.W. & Raeburn, J.M. (1988). Health promotion: What is it? What will it become? *Health Promotion, 3*(2), 151–159.

Hancock, T. & Perkins, F. (1985). The Mandela of health: A conceptual model and teaching tool. *Health Education, 24*(1), 8–10.

Health Canada. (1998). *Taking action on population health: A position paper for health promotion and programs branch staff.* Ottawa: Health Canada.

Kickbusch, I. (1989). *Good planets are hard to find.* Copenhagen: FADL Publishers.

Kickbusch, I. (1997). Think health: What makes the difference? *Health Promotion International, 12,* 265–272.

Labonté, R. (1993). *Community health and empowerment.* Toronto: Centre for Health Promotion.

Lalonde, M. (1974). *A new perspective on the health of Canadians.* Ottawa: Government of Canada.

Lindström, B. & Eriksson, M. (2010). *The hitchhiker's guide to salutogenesis: Salutogenic pathways to health promotion.* Helsinki: Folkhälsan Research Centre. Retrieved from: http://www.salutogenesis.fi/eng/Publications.18.html

Martin, C.J. & McQueen, D.V. (Eds.). (1989). *Readings for a new public health.* Edinburgh: Edinburgh University Press.

Mikkonen, J. & Raphael, D. (2010). *Social determinants of health: The Canadian facts.* Toronto: York University School of Health Policy and Management. Retrieved from: http://www.thecanadianfacts.org/

Minkler, M., Wallerstein, N. & Wilson, N. (2008). Improving health through community organization and community-building. In K.M. Glanz, B.K. Rimer & K. Viswanath (Eds.), *Health behavior and health education: Theory, research, and practice* (4th ed.) (pp. 287–312). San Francisco: Jossey-Bass.

Nutbeam, D. (1998). Health promotion glossary. *Health Promotion International, 13,* 349–364.

Nutbeam, D. (2000). Health literacy as a public health goal: A challenge for contemporary health education and communication strategies into the 21st century. *Health Promotion International, 15,* 259–267.

O'Neill, M., Pederson, A. & Rootman, I. (2000). Health promotion in Canada: Declining or transforming? *Health Promotion International, 15*(2), 135–141.

O'Neill, M. & Stirling, A. (2007). The promotion of health or health promotion? In M. O'Neill, S. Dupéré, A. Pederson & I. Rootman (Eds.), *Health promotion in Canada: Critical perspectives* (pp. 32–45). Toronto: Canadian Scholars' Press Inc.

Pan-American Health Organization (PAHO). (2002). *Public health in the Americas.* Technical publication no. 589. Washington: Pan-American Health Organization.

Pederson, A., Rootman, I. & O'Neill, M. (2005). Health promotion in Canada: Back to the past or towards a promising future? In A. Scriven & S. Garman (Eds.), *Promoting health: Global perspectives* (pp. 255–265). London: Palgrave.

Potvin, L. (2005). Presentation at doctoral seminar SAC-66008, Université Laval, October 17, 2005.

Quality of Life Research Unit. (2010). *Concepts.* Retrieved from: http://www.utoronto.ca/qol/concepts.htm

Raeburn, J. & Rootman, I. (1989). Towards an expanded health field concept: Conceptual and research issues in a new era of health promotion. *Health Promotion International, 3*(4), 383–392.

Raeburn, J. & Rootman, I. (2007). A new appraisal of the concept of health. In M. O'Neill, S. Dupéré, A. Pederson & I. Rootman (Eds.), *Health promotion in Canada: Critical perspectives* (pp. 1–16). Toronto: Canadian Scholars' Press Inc.

Raphael, D. (Ed.). (2009). *Social determinants of health* (2nd ed.). Toronto: Canadian Scholars' Press Inc.

Raphael, D. (Ed.). (2010). *Health promotion and quality of life in Canada.* Toronto: Canadian Scholars' Press Inc.

Rappaport, J. (1987). Terms of empowerment/exemplars of prevention: Toward a theory for community psychology. *American Journal of Community Psychology, 15*(2), 121–148.

Rissel, C. (1994). Empowerment: The holy grail of health promotion. *Health Promotion International, 9*(1), 39–47.

Rootman, I., Frankish, J. & Kaszap, M. (2007). Health literacy: A new frontier. In M. O'Neill, S. Dupéré, A. Pederson & I. Rootman (Eds.), *Health promotion in Canada: Critical perspectives* (pp. 61–74). Toronto: Canadian Scholars' Press Inc.

Rootman, I., Goodstadt, M., Potvin, L. & Springett, J. (2001). A framework for health promotion evaluation. In I. Rootman et al. (Eds.), *Evaluation in health promotion: Principles and perspectives* (pp. 7–38). Copenhagen: European Regional Office of the World Health Organization.

Rootman, I. & Gordon-El-Bihbety, D. (2008). *A vision for a health literate Canada: Report of the expert panel on health literacy.* Ottawa: Canadian Public Health Association.

Rootman, I. & Raeburn, J. (1994). The concept of health. In A. Pederson, M. O'Neill & I. Rootman (Eds.), *Health promotion in Canada: Provincial, national, and international perspectives* (pp. 139–152). Toronto: W.B. Saunders Canada.

Sarafino, E.P. (1990). *Health psychology: Biopsychosocial interactions.* New York: John Wiley & Sons.

Simonds, S.K. (1974). Health education and social policy. *Health Education Monographs, 2*(Suppl. 1), 1–10.

Spector, R.E. (1985). *Cultural diversity in health and illness.* Norwalk: Appleton-Century-Crofts.

World Health Organization. (1946). *Constitution.* Geneva: World Health Organization.

World Health Organization. (1986). *Ottawa Charter for Health Promotion.* Ottawa: Canadian Public Health Association.

World Health Organization. (2005). *Bangkok Charter for Health Promotion.* Geneva: World Health Organization. Retrieved from: www.who.int/healthpromotion/conferences/6gchp/bangkok_charter/en/index.html

World Health Organization. (2010). *Backgrounder 3: Key concepts.* Retrieved from: http://www.who.int/social_determinants/final_report/key_concepts_en.pdf

Critical Thinking Questions

1. What concept of health do you prefer? Why? Do you think it is an appropriate concept for health promotion?

2. If you had to define health promotion to the following people, what would you say to: your uncle Jack in a family gathering; a graduate student in physics; or Ms. Jones at the neighbourhood community centre?

3. Explain the difference between the promotion of health and health promotion. Do you believe it is a useful distinction or not? Why?

4. What is the relationship between health education and health promotion? Do you think they should be separate fields or integrated into one?

5. Which of the other concepts discussed in this chapter do you think are most central in health promotion?

Resources

Further Readings

Antonovsky, A. (1979). *Health stress and coping.* San Francisco: Jossey Bass; and Antonovsky, A. (1987). *Unravelling the concept of health.* San Francisco: Jossey Bass.

These two books raise the question of what creates "health" rather than "disease." Antonovsky suggests and discusses the term "salutogenesis" to encourage more thinking and research about the determinants of health rather than of disease. Lindström and Erickson (2010) have also recently published a book on the concept and Lindström has also established a research centre in Finland built around salutogenic research.

Bunton, R. & MacDonald, G. (Eds.). (2004). *Health promotion: Disciplines and diversity* (2nd ed.). London & New York: Routledge.

One of the key books to reflect on whether or not health promotion can be considered a discipline.

Contandriopoulos, A.P. (2005). A "topography" of the concept of health. In R. Lyons (Ed.), *Social Sciences and Humanities Health Research* (pp. 13–15). Ottawa: Canadian Institute of Health Research.

This is an interesting article about the concept of health that considers contributions from the social sciences and humanities to thinking about the concept. Also in the same volume is a one-page article (p. 120) by Contandriopoulos and other Canadian colleagues on a proposed project to integrate approaches and perspectives about the concept of health from the social and life sciences.

Green, L.W. & Kreuter, M.W. (2005). *Health program planning: An educational and ecological approach* (4th ed.). Boston & Toronto: McGraw-Hill Higher Education.

If you had to buy just one book in health promotion in your life, it should be this one for its positioning of the field, as well as for its famous PRECEDE-PROCEED planning framework.

Raphael, D. (Ed.). (2010). *Health promotion and quality of life in Canada.* Toronto: Canadian Scholars' Press Inc.

This book contains a series of papers produced by the University of Toronto Centre for Health Promotion's Quality of Life Unit, as well as other papers written for the volume. It explores the integral link between quality of life and public policy choices.

Relevant Websites

Click4HP

www.lsoft.com/scripts/wl.exe?SL1=CLICK4HP&H=YORKU.CA

Click4HP is a listserv that was established by the Ontario Health Promotion Clearinghouse in 1996 and is operated by York University. It has an archive of discussions that have taken place since it was established on a wide range of health promotion topics, including the concept of health.

What Is "Real" Health Promotion?

www.web.ca/~stirling/c4hpreal.htm

An edited compilation of more than 30 postings made during September 1996 on Click4HP about "What is real health promotion?"

CHAPTER 3

Social Theory and Health Promotion

Simon Carroll

Introduction

Embarking on a chapter with such an ambitious title is perilous. To pretend to adequately cover the breadth of developments in the field of health promotion relevant to "social theory" and vice versa, even over the past 10 years, would be to overreach. Nevertheless, ironically, to get to the bottom of what needs to be considered, we have to start on a tangent that has even more risk at its heart.

I start with the end, by prefacing the chapter with what I take to be its central conclusion: What marks health promotion as an ambiguous, contradictory, and at times even nebulous field of thought and practice is its problematic relationship with its own theoretical basis. Health promotion has and uses many "theories," yet it is nearly silent, though less so recently (McQueen & Kickbusch, 2007) on just what should constitute its own theoretical basis. As we shall see, this is partly due to a conception of "theory" handed down from a narrowly positivistic empiricism that sees "theories" exclusively as analytical devices constructed to help *explain* specific empirical phenomena. There is nothing inherently wrong with this narrowly empiricist interpretation of "theory," and certainly health promotion, in practice, has need of understanding and using all sorts of specific empirical theories (e.g., epidemiological theories about the causes of disease in populations; psychological theories of behaviour change; theories of community coalition-building). Indeed, other publications have taken this approach to theory very seriously (DiClemente, Crosby & Kegler, 2002). However, we must begin with a deeper issue: What is theory and how should health promotion relate to it?

A corollary to the conclusion prefaced above is that health promotion is—unlike medicine, disease prevention, or even population health (see Hancock, 1994, Chapter 2 for conceptual distinctions)—almost exclusively about *social action* broadly interpreted. Of course, all the other activities are or involve *social* activities; however, for health promotion, it is not just the application of its knowledge that involves understanding the social world, it is the theoretical core of its knowledge that is *essentially social in nature*. The argument here is that health promotion is about *social* change, and that even when it is concerned with individuals, it is about individuals as *social* beings. Health is produced socially; individual health behaviours can only be understood, never mind changed, within a social context (Kickbusch, 1989). In this guise, this chapter takes a position close to the perspective on theory offered by McQueen and Kickbusch in their more recent book, *Health & Modernity: The Role of Theory in Health Promotion* (McQueen & Kickbusch, 2007).

The implication of this perspective for health promotion is that we have to think very differently about "theory" than is typical within the received tradition of empirical science. In fact, the type of theorization necessary for health promotion is more akin to the traditions of philosophical and social theory than to theory as it is often interpreted within the sciences. Such a departure from the orthodox scientific[1] understanding of "theory" is difficult to manage, particularly for a field so institutionally dominated by its relations with the biomedical sciences and epidemiology, and even the positivistic orthodoxy of certain psychological and sociological approaches to social science.[2] Yet, if we cannot move from this narrow interpretation of theory, then the hopes of understanding what health promotion is really about—and, even more so, what it *should* be about—will be unrealized.

Before delving more deeply into the vexing problem of how theory relates to health promotion, something should be said about how "methodology" fits into this picture. There is an unfortunate tendency to think of "methods" and "theories" as separate entities that operate independently in the grand enterprise of science. Nothing could be further from the truth. All scientific methods are built on theoretical presuppositions. We can use thermometers to "read" temperature only because we assent to a series of theoretical suppositions concerning the material arrangements used to construct the thermometer, among many other considerations. Similarly, we use instruments such as a social survey based on a series of theoretical assumptions about people's responses to questions, how language works, their intentions and behaviours, along with broader conceptions of "society, the individual and the relationship between them" (Ackroyd & Hughes, 1992, p. 8). In fact, the important distinction (though often conflated) between *methodology* and *methods* is built upon this insight. A *methodology* is the logical or "theoretical" justification for the use of a specific method or methods to answer particular types of research questions. Thus, when we talk about different ways to theorize about health promotion, we are at the same time talking about what kind of methodological implications these different theoretical conceptions have for the field. This chapter will directly address certain methodological issues that have recently captured the imagination of health promoters. Nevertheless, the reader should keep in mind that there is a constant dialectic between theoretical and methodological concerns, and that in many ways, the real distinction is within a broader understanding of "theory" that considers both *ontological* and *epistemological* questions, with both these concepts being more directly connected to issues of methodology. In other words, "theory" in health promotion is about what health promotion's object or field (ontological) is, and how we know about it (epistemological), and thus what the rationale or (methodological) justification is for using a particular set of methods for acquiring this knowledge. Having now introduced two quintessentially philosophical terms (ontology and epistemology), we can move to what theory is about from a philosophical perspective.

Philosophy and Social Theory

"Theory" is a loaded term in philosophy. In fact, it represents the key distinguishing feature of the being, knowledge, and activity of the philosopher. It constitutes the ground upon

BOX 3.1:

Key Philosophical Terms: Ontology

Ontology is the study of "being," "existence," or "reality." In other words, it is the study of that which "is." However, ontology is the abstract conceptualization of being, meaning that it is not concerned with the facts pertaining to a particular thing, but rather to the nature of existence itself. That is, it wants to know what kind of things exist in general, and whether there are certain fundamental beings. It is interested in questions such as: What things are essential and what things are merely accidental or contingent? What does it mean for something to have an *identity*, and when does a thing cease to be, as opposed to merely changing? It also asks other general questions, such as: Is reality eternal or is it in constant flux? Is reality stratified into different levels and, if so, what are they? To understand why these very abstract questions can be important, even in such concrete subject areas as health promotion, we have to be aware that how we think the world is structured has a profound influence on how we think about the world and how we act in it. For example, if you see the essence of the social world as fundamentally unchanging and eternal (e.g., "The poor will always be with us," "People are basically greedy"), you approach social problems and whether and how to solve them in a very different way than someone who sees even basic aspects of social life as open to change.

BOX 3.2:

Key Philosophical Terms: Epistemology

Epistemology is the study of the nature of "knowledge," including how we attain it and the extent of its scope and limitations. Epistemology addresses three fundamental questions: What is knowledge? How is knowledge acquired? How do we know what we know? The first question is concerned mainly with defining knowledge and establishing criteria for whether a person can be said to have knowledge of something. The second question concerns where knowledge comes from and how it is attained, with the main traditional dividing line being between those who accept that knowledge can come from *a priori* reasoning or "intuition," and those who believe that the only reliable knowledge has to come from experience. Many further divisions have developed over time in philosophy concerning this question, but it is important to know that the vast majority of what we call "empirical science" is based on the assumption that we can gain knowledge only through experiencing the world, particularly by way of perceiving "sense impressions." The final question addresses the problem of skepticism, or how any of our claims to knowledge can be warranted. For the purpose here, it is important to understand that epistemology is influenced by our ontological assumptions and vice versa. If you do not believe in the existence of an ontological level of reality where ideas have an independent existence (as Plato did), then it is very hard to admit that one can derive knowledge from ideas alone; conversely, if the only way to access knowledge is through sense impressions, then any talk of different levels of reality makes no sense, as the only level we can rationally access is the world of empirical experience. Furthermore, as shown in Box 3.3, how we understand both ontology and epistemology has much to do with the type of *methodology* we might use to discover new knowledge.

BOX 3.3:

Key Philosophical Terms: Methodology

Methodology is the logic or reasoned justification for following certain principles or rules of inquiry and for the use of particular methods for collecting and analyzing data. Methodology is not simply a description of the various *methods* available to the inquirer; rather, it is the philosophically coherent combination of theory and method that are required to answer a particular sort of researchable question. To understand how methodology is connected to ontology and epistemology, imagine one starts with a particular research question. First, one has to know what we are assuming about the nature of the phenomenon under inquiry: What type of thing(s) is it? Second, we have to know how we might come to know about this phenomenon: What is the source of knowledge we will need to access in order to better understand it? Finally, given our answers to these questions, we can construct a rationale for using specific procedures for attaining this knowledge that are consistent with our ontological and epistemological assumptions. Is this how every inquiry is actually constructed? Rarely. However, without this type of reflection, we often proceed with methodological strategies that incorporate these ontological and epistemological assumptions without us consciously acknowledging them.

---

which philosophers, since Plato and Aristotle, have defined the essence of what it is to be a philosopher or "lover of wisdom"; it is what distinguishes philosophical knowledge from other forms of knowledge; and it is what marks the difference between philosophical activity and practical or, as Aristotle put it, "utilitarian" activity. It is "loaded" because, as Plato and Aristotle knew very well, the possibility of an activity with no immediate practical utility that could be carried out only by people with the leisure and thus support provided by the rest of society was in desperate need of justification. So, what was this justification? Well, it wasn't just that theoretical or "contemplative" activity was worthwhile; it was that it was superior to all other forms of activity! Thus, from its very beginnings, "theory" was an essentially hubristic and condescending occupation (as Socrates found to his cost). Nevertheless, what has been handed down from the Greeks is the notion that theory is about understanding the first principles or "causes" of phenomena. It was about discovering "why" things worked the way they did, as opposed to just that they worked. Yet, it also set up a lasting, and in many ways damaging, hierarchical contrast between superior "theory" on the one hand, and infer-ior "practice" on the other. It is no coincidence that these great philosophers had political theories that favoured the aristocracy, given their penchant for denigrating practical work as a lower form of existence (Meiksins Wood, 2008). It is a good warning to health promoters enamoured (as I am) with "theory," particularly in a field dominated by practitioners (and ones who have often been historically subordinated to a distinctly aristocratic medical caste) to be mindful and reflectively critical of theory's pretensions.

Nevertheless, what lessons can health promotion derive from the philosophical tradition, the originators of the "theoretical attitude"? First, we have to briefly consider the development of the conception of "theory," and reason itself, within the philosophical tradition; then we can trace how social theory is really a further development of, and origin-ated from, philosophical reflection, and in particular, out of the tradition of "critical reason" as it was fully formed in the Enlightenment and post-Enlightenment. This genealogy is important because another basic argument made in this chapter is that health promotion is constituted as a *social critique* of public health. That is, health promotion's basic orientation is as an emancipatory project in the tradition of critical social theory. This is not an original insight, as some health promotion researchers have long argued something analogous (Eakin, Robertson, Poland et al., 1996). However, too often what gets articulated as "concepts and principles" of health promotion, such as those found in the *Ottawa Charter for Health Promotion* (WHO, 1986), are not understood as foundational *theoretical* positions; this is problematic as these positions make very specific philosophical assumptions linked to important traditions in post-Enlightenment thought.

It should be made clear that what is argued here is *not* that all people identifying themselves as health promoters would recognize the peculiar genealogy of thought I am about to reconstruct as *the* theoretical basis for health promotion. Rather, what is argued is that if one follows through on certain foundational premises of health promotion, as set out in the *Ottawa Charter* (a declared bias to begin with, but one that I think is both compatible with this book and with Canadian health promotion generally), one is led, logically, to a very particular tradition of thought. If health promotion is essentially tied to the tradition of thought we call "critical social theory," what does that mean? The tradition of critical reason, since Kant, is the story of a constantly evolving, dialectical movement of reason, aimed at a critique of existing society, with the goal of the emancipation of human beings from a variety of arbitrary and (collectively) self-imposed restrictions on their ability and capacity to flourish and express themselves equitably, freely, and authentically. How and why is health promotion a part of this, admittedly grandiose, project?

First, it takes some historical perspective to understand how deeply embedded health promotion is in modernity. Following many others, health promotion can best be seen as a kind of "third revolution" of public health (Breslow, 1999; Potvin & McQueen, 2007). Key to understanding this revolution is to follow the shift within public health from a focus on individual behaviour change to a focus on the social context of health and on the levers of societal change that are necessary if one wants to transform the lives of populations for the better. Now, there is little doubt that public health, particularly as a societal movement, but also as a field of knowledge, is deeply embedded in the whole historical development of modern society. In fact, many of the most prominent theorizations of modernity give a pride of place to public health in the narrative of how a self-consciousness of the possibility of societal "improvement" came into being (Porter, 2000). For thinkers like Foucault, the appearance of "society" as an object of reflection is itself coincident with the development of the concepts of "population," "statistics," "political arithmetic," and many others that inaugurate reflections on how to manage the state as not simply bounded territories with certain resources, but as containing populations with specific, measurable characters, such as wealth and health (Foucault, 1980, 2000, 2008). John Graunt's famous "Bills of Mortality," epidemiological science's prototype, is at once a precursor to public health and a peculiar mode of societal self-consciousness, premised on the notion that societies were objects that could be strengthened and improved with the use of reason. At the core of public health's story is an almost perfect embodiment of the dilemmas and contradictions at the heart of the development of modern societies; public health is a grand tradition that is driven by the great Enlightenment themes of improvement, progress, freedom, and reason, while at the same time being caught up with all the less positive modern tropes,[3] such as bureaucratization, rationalization, domination, and a hubristic scientism. The modern health promotion movement arrives with a series of other "second wave" critical social movements, such as environmentalism, feminism, and the peace movement, as part of a general trend of "postmodern" critique that puts advanced, industrial societies under intense scrutiny and, in many cases, finds the modern experiment wanting (cf. Labonté, 1994). Although health promotion itself is probably less a social movement and more a kind of para-bureaucratic tendency (Stevenson & Burke, 1991), it shares with the *Zeitgeist* a deep suspicion of the social engineering approach to an increasingly administered society, and a strong attachment to participatory democratic principles. Yet despite its attachment to these more postmodern themes, health promotion is still tied to some fundamental commitments that one can identify only with the values of the Enlightenment and modernity. It is how it negotiates the ambiguous legacy of modernity that frames health promotion from a social-theoretical perspective.

To more carefully consider how this tradition of critical thought unfolds in relation to our contemporary situation, we need to move more directly to an analysis of some of the guiding thematic disputes within the realm of critical social theory understood broadly.[4]. Some of these guiding themes, it will be seen, constitute central problems for health promotion theory and the appropriate methodological strategies that are necessary to meet these challenges.

Social Theory and Health Promotion

In this section, I begin to address some of the central animating themes in social theory and demonstrate how they are connected to core dilemmas for health promotion research and practice. The three key themes that I explore are: (1) class and status; (2) the dialectic of rationalization; and (3) the duality of structure and agency. These themes all have strong relevance to health promotion and the point is not to resolve these debates or contradictory perspectives for health promotion, but to explore their dialectical development in order to give the reader a deeper sense of the types of theoretical tensions that drive social theory, and thus the types of theoretical questions that should drive, at least an important part of, future debates within the field of health promotion.

Class and Status

Ironically, although contemporary health promotion is awash with references to the link between social inequality and inequitable health outcomes, there is little, if any, direct confrontation with one of the central questions of social theory: What are the main causal mechanisms underlying social inequality? Within the sociological tradition in particular, this constitutes the main differences between followers of Marx and followers of Weber, along with further substantial disputes within these two social theoretical traditions. Why is this important to health promotion? Well, if health promotion aims to change society in order to reduce social inequity and thereby health inequity (surely one of its main goals and, arguably, increasingly the central goal), it requires a clear-headed approach to understanding what causes these inequities in the first place in order to be effective at changing them for the better. This inquiry is a different one from social epidemiological disputes concerning which types of social variables (e.g., income, education, SES, Gini coefficients (measure of inequalities), etc.) have the most impact on health, although these empirical findings are complementary and informative. Rather, what is at stake is to understand the underlying, dynamic mechanisms that create and reproduce relatively stable group differences in income, wealth, housing, education, health, and many other characteristics.

For Marx, it was clear that the basic driving force of social inequalities was the division of societies into antagonistic "classes," defined by their relationship to the means of the material reproduction of those societies (Marx, 1976, 1981). In Western societies in particular, stages of social development were divided into different sets of class relations of production, from classical ancient societies based on the relationship between slave owners and slaves, to feudal societies based on the relationship between landlords and serfs, to modern capitalist societies based on the relationship between the bourgeois owners of capital and the free wage labourers forced to sell their labour for subsistence. Marxist theory has developed in many forms since Marx, and there have been many different approaches to interpreting his concept of class (Olin Wright, 2009), yet key to understanding this perspective is to avoid identifying classes primarily using different brackets of income or different occupational strata. For Marxists, it is the *dynamic* of class struggle in capitalist societies over the division of surplus value between capital and labour that is the most powerful force underlying the generation of social inequalities more broadly. What does this mean? When we look only at different snapshots of income differentials or other social inequalities, we may miss some underlying trends and tendencies that form the main tectonic shifts in social relations and cause ripple effects throughout the social structure. A prime example is how over the past 40 years there has been a steady yet massive shift of wealth and power to the capitalist class, and at the same time a receding set of public institutions and resources (often collectively referred to as the "welfare state") that acted as a bulwark against rampant inequality in the previous post–World War II era. The Marxist explanation for this inexorable trend is based on two mutually reinforcing tendencies: one, the objective pressures on capital accumulation and the rate of profit, causing a need for the system to undergo several crises of "creative destruction" in order to restore profitability; second, a subjective defeat of working-class institutions, particularly labour unions, that had acted as resources to defend working-class gains and a share in the expansion of social productivity.[5] In other words, the capitalist class has been relatively successful in passing on the costs of various economic crises to the workers and to come out the other end of these crises in a strengthened position for renewed profitability. One need not look far from current news headlines to find ample evidence that substantiates some of these insights.

To summarize, Marxists see class, and a particular version of that concept, as the key driving force behind the generation of social inequality. There are certain features of this perspective that are important to keep in mind in relation to health promotion. First, taking a Marxist or Marx-inspired perspective on social inequality means taking a medium- to long-term view because it focuses on what are seen as the fundamental underlying economic forces that affect all other levels of society. How deterministic a view this is depends on how you conceptualize and theorize the relationship between these basic economic drivers and other levels and spheres of the social world. However, for health promoters, the message is that having a real impact on social inequality may require some basic shifts in the relationships between owners of capital and those employed by them. This does not mean that nothing positive can be done short of social revolution, but it does mean having a more sanguine view of the possibilities of social change within a system that so powerfully drives those very inequalities we aim to ameliorate.

While the Weberian approach to class and status differs substantially from the Marxist approach (though not as much as many think: Sayer, 1991), both share a common characteristic that is missing from the more familiar social epidemiological conception of class and status as the hierarchical stratification of social *attributes* and *conditions* (Olin Wright, 2009). Both Marx's and Weber's conceptions of class and Weber's concept of status are deeply connected to *relations of power*. For Marx, the power relations are domination and exploitation, whereas for Weber they are relations of exclusion and distinction. This is a key theoretical point as this *relational* aspect of class and status underlies both the inherent antagonism and the dynamism of class and status-divided societies. Marxist analysis demonstrates the antagonism between the overall distribution of economic surplus between profits and wages, and the relations of domination within the workplace between employers and employees; Weberian analysis points to the forms of closure and exclusion that privileged classes impose on subordinate classes in the marketplace, along with the forms of authority established through social distinction between different status groups in the population. Both approaches tell us about fundamental social forces that drive change and conserve power in modern society, as well as expose deep rifts and contradictions at the heart of those societies. While for Marx the fundamental axis of power was the ownership and control of the means of production, for Weber it was control of property and marketable assets or services.

In order to understand how these classic sources of social theory are still relevant to contemporary health promotion, we can look briefly at health promotion researchers' attempt to apply the work of more recent social theorists working from within the broad tradition of class and status analytical frameworks. One of the more interesting problems that health promotion has confronted in trying to think through the *social* aspect of its revolution in public health is how to deal with so-called "lifestyles." It is indisputable that there is a direct causal relationship between certain individual health-related behaviours (e.g., poor diet, lack of exercise, smoking) and negative health outcomes. However, health promotion, since the *Ottawa Charter*, has recognized that there is a connection between these behaviours and social stratification; in other words, there is consistent evidence that negative health-related behaviours are associated disproportionately with lower socio-economic strata. This has led to two reciprocal conclusions: (1) that more has to be done to understand the *social* causation of these "risk factors"; and, conversely, more has to be done to understand how to effectively intervene to change those behaviours.[6] Many health promoters have become disenchanted with the traditional, individual-psychological focus of many behaviour change strategies, along with the tendency for these approaches to implicitly endorse a narrative of victim-blaming. An alternative approach is to reconsider the notion of "lifestyles" from a sociological or social theory perspective (Kickbusch, 1989; Frohlich, Corin & Potvin, 2001; Abel, 2007). Kickbusch's article was prescient, but mainly outlined a framework to start thinking in different terms about how so-called "lifestyles" had to be conceptualized as socially produced and therefore understanding what those social mechanisms were was part of health promotion's agenda. Over the past 10 years, Frohlich, Abel, and other colleagues have separately and together started to flesh out in more specific theoretical terms just what approaches to social theory might be most helpful in understanding what they have come to call "collective lifestyles." This approach is more concretely addressed in the Frohlich et al. chapter in this volume; however, here we will examine more closely the theoretical arguments behind this move and place them in the historical context of social theory that has been discussed above.

These health promotion researchers used Pierre Bourdieu, a key thinker and famous sociologist, to develop the notion of collective lifestyles. While Bourdieu created his own original theoretical perspective, there is no doubt that he was deeply indebted to both Marx and Weber, and perhaps more to the latter. Bourdieu's conception of how classes reproduced themselves in society was a deeply relational one. For Bourdieu, as for Weber, the social field(s), a system of social positions, was a site of constant power struggles over what Bourdieu called economic, social, cultural, and symbolic capital. Like Weber, he was critical of the Marxist tendency to focus solely on the economic sphere of class struggle and subordinate all other levels of society to this struggle. Bourdieu was primarily occupied with a particular question: Why was it that subordinate classes and status groups in society tended to be resigned to their fate in the social hierarchy? Using his concepts of *habitus*, *field*, and *capital*, Bourdieu offered an explanatory framework that allowed us to conceptualize how individuals internalize social structure through the interaction between the fields of action they operate in, the various forms of capital, and their "habitus," which was the set of mainly unreflective dispositions forming both the medium and outcome of their practical activities. For example, Bourdieu demonstrated that musical tastes, diet, sport preference, and many other social variables were clearly aligned as inherited dispositions according to what part of the class structure an individual came from, rather than as the result of conscious individual choices.

Abel argues that in terms of thinking about "collective lifestyles," a key concept is that of cultural capital (Abel, 2007). For Bourdieu, cultural capital consisted of educational attainment, clothing, food habits, musical taste, exercise habits, and even bodily comportment. Instead of conceiving all these as a set of individual choices made consciously, Bourdieu understood them as primarily dispositions or habits that one was automatically socialized into as part of being in a particular social strata, group, or class fraction. Crucially, and following Weber and Marx, these forms of capital are the object of relational power struggles, such that their "value" is relative to the scarcity that can be maintained by excluding access through forms of social closure to subordinate social strata. One critical conclusion Bourdieu came to was that subordinate groups or classes suffer from "symbolic violence," where some cultural tastes and habits come to be "valued" as better than others, and also happen to be the tastes and habits of the group that is superior in wealth and status. Oppressed groups accept this valuation and thus legitimize their subordinate status as part of the "natural order" of things. Thus they "refuse what they are denied." The implications this has for generating change in the social habits of disadvantaged and so-called "at-risk" populations from a health perspective are very far-reaching. As can be seen in a recent study by Frohlich and colleagues, these different attitudes can have drastically divergent implications for policies such as anti-tobacco legislation (Frohlich, Poland, Mykhalovskiy et al., 2010).

There are two significant concerns with the theoretical framework of Bourdieu, despite its potentially fruitful line of inquiry for health promotion. First, Bourdieu's theoretical framework tends toward a deeply pessimistic scenario when it comes to emancipatory change due to his social epistemology. According to Bourdieu, we are highly constrained by the fact that much of social inequality is deeply ingrained and internalized through unreflective habit, making it extraordinarily difficult to overcome, as we reproduce these inequalities as a matter of course, even if we consciously intend to reduce them. On the other hand, people would say that Bourdieu offers us a salutary realism that asks us to work that much harder to be reflexive practitioners in developing social change and, furthermore, even if his concept of habitus tends toward the more deterministic end of the structure/agency spectrum we discuss below, we need something like his concept of habitus as a mediating concept between praxis and social structure (Sayer, 2005; Mouzelis, 2007). A more serious critique is that developed by Andrew Sayer (2009), who argues that Bourdieu over-sociologizes human interaction to the extent where a positive empirical focus leaves no room for normative or evaluative questions as all interaction is reduced to strategic manoeuvres to accumulate capital, including the move of moral reasoning itself. One can see how this can become problematic in terms of distinguishing between "symbolic violence" and legitimate moral reasoning. For example, Frohlich et al. (2010) point to serious differences in how anti-smoking legislation in relation to public space affects different social groups, and there is no doubt that a certain amount of symbolic violence is inflicted upon subordinate and marginalized groups. However, does this mean that being identified with this symbolic violence automatically taints all the evaluative reasoning behind the implementation of smoking bans? Don't we methodologically deny subordinate classes a certain universal capacity for moral reflection if we paint them as inevitably incapable of doing anything but taking up their habitual disposition of self-identifying as smokers? In their study, Frohlich et al. have examples that seem to find that middle-class smokers invite the imposition of smoking bans, and this is interpreted as being consistent with their ambiguous relationship to other aspects of their cultural capital that tells them that smoking is incompatible with their lifestyles. However, we don't want to conflate this explanation with situations where the distinction is between a self-interested particularism that is concerned only with "my smoking habit," and an other-oriented moral argument that says that my smoking habit shouldn't harm others who choose not to take that risk with their health, and we certainly don't want to identify one or the other stance exclusively with a particular social class. Health promoters, when citing theorists such as Bourdieu or Anthony Giddens, should be aware and explicit about the context of these theorists' work as part of a long-term continuity of sociological reflection on class. Without this awareness, the inherently political implications of their work, as well as an understanding of the underlying social causes of inequality, will be lost.

The Dialectic of Rationalization

The second major theme of the social theory of modernity is the dialectic of rationalization. Since Immanuel Kant's three *Critiques* (of pure reason; of practical reason; and of judgment), within Western philosophy there has been a tradition of critiquing the limits and boundaries of reason. One constant theme has been the potential or actual contradictions between an instrumental, means-ends calculating reason, a practical-moral reasoning based on a substantive values-based orientation to action, and a rationality of aesthetic judgment based on distinctions of taste. Different thinkers have developed this theme in a variety of ways. Followers of Kant have tended to think of modernity as having become differentiated into different "value-spheres," with each type of reason legislating over its own appropriate societal jurisdiction (with pure theoretical reason governing the sciences and other purely cognitive interests, practical reason governing politics and the law, and aesthetic reason governing the arts and other areas of cultural production). Others have been concerned about the domination of one type of reason over the others, with either more or less pessimistic extrapolations of where modern societies' developmental trajectory is heading (Marcuse, 1991; Horkheimer & Adorno, 2002). Martin Heidegger (1993) and his followers developed the ultimate extreme of the pessimistic approach, where a totalizing domination of instrumental reason is traced back as a fundamental original sin of Western philosophy starting with Plato and ending with the critique of Western reason *in toto* as "logocentrism" by Derrida (1976). Foucault developed his own critique of Western reason in a series of penetrating analyses of different modern institutions, such as the hospital, the prison, and the therapeutic relationship dominated by psychoanalysis, but also more generally he analyzed the relationship between power, knowledge, and what he came to term a "biopolitics of health" (2008). An attempt to develop a more balanced approach to the legacy of the Enlightenment and modernity through a positive reconstruction of the history or modern reason has been the life work of Habermas (1984, 1987, 1998), who also happens to be the philosopher who most closely engaged with the sociological tradition and who most explicitly linked the tradition of critical theory to that discipline. How we understand our relationship with the history of Western rationality can have a deep influence on how we do health promotion. Particularly in relation to instrumental reason, our relative optimism or pessimism about its potential for resolving societal problems will lead us in very specific directions in terms of the types of programs we develop or the types of processes we use in doing our work.

In social theory more directly, many writers have taken up Max Weber's original analysis of what he called contradictions between formal reason (*Zweckrationalitat*) and substantive reason

(*Wertrationalitat*). Weber outlined how all the major modern institutions—including capital-ism, rational-legal authority, legal systems, bureaucracy, science, and technology—embodied a contradiction between a formal, instrumental reason aimed at intervening in society to make it more efficient and effective through a generic cost-benefit, calculative rationality, and a substantive reason that judges outcomes based on concrete and particular values (Weber, 1978, 2002). Weber argued that there is a constant dialectic of *rationalization* in modern society that makes formal reason's interventions the basis of ambiguous substantive consequences, some of which are judged as negative, which then calls for further instrumental interventions. A typical example relevant to health promotion and public health is the problem of redressing the results of social inequalities by intervening with a variety of programs of social support, only to have the negative unintended consequence of creating dependency and disempowering local communities.

This dilemma is one that is indirectly addressed in Raeburn and Rootman's book, *People-Centred Health Promotion* (1998), in which the authors make clear the potential ambiguities of shifting from a focus on individual-level, over-psychologizing interventions to macro-level, over-socializing interventions and end up squeezing people living in communities out of the equation. The question here goes to the core of the stated health promotion values of *participation* and *empowerment*. It is also a key distinguishing feature of health promotion from a much more state-centred, utilitarian tradition in public health (Hills & Carroll, 2009). Two negative consequences of traditional public health approaches to health promotion issues can be seen in both the bureaucratic formal rationality of state-run programs that take little account of local context and often undermine community empowerment and participation, and in the excesses of scientism that appear in the formal rationality of evaluation techniques emerging from the academy. Despite the stated intentions of redressing inequities in many of these programs, often unintended consequences are generated that substantively undermine core values, such as empowerment and participation, never mind those programs that also undermine the value of equity itself. For example, parenting programs that focus on redressing "poor parenting skills" without acknowledging the broader social issues that these parents may be dealing with can both undermine the parents' self-confidence and self-esteem and ignore their potential input and knowledge, thereby doing damage to the value of participation and empowerment; conversely, parents with less social barriers who take better advantage of the program's narrow focus on knowledge and skills can have disproportionately positive gains, thereby undermining the value of equity (with the people the most in need receiving the least benefits). As we will pick up in the final section, the Weberian theme of rationalization is also intimately tied to how we consider the dualism of structure and agency for, as Habermas has warned, there is a danger in not recognizing the autonomy of the communicative life-world and subsuming it entirely under the rubric of a systems rationality.

Agency and Structure: Dualism or Duality?

The whole history of social theory has been taken up with a cleavage around the issue of what the nature of sociality and social action is: What is its ontology? In other words, what kind of thing is society? What is it made up of? Does it have special "social" substances, or is it just the collective properties of individual people? Philosophically, this is intertwined with several older debates, such as free will (or "voluntarism") vs. determinism, individualistic vs. holistic explanation, and the micro- vs. macro-level opposition and/or linkage. While both Marx and Durkheim tended to defend a structural or functionalist holism, Weber and other more phenomenologically inspired thinkers tended to look at social order as constituted by social interaction, with the "unit act," as Talcott Parsons was to put it, as the foundational concept. Thus, most of social theory's history has been built on a major internal dualism between those who looked to social structure as the primary lever of explanatory value, and those who focused almost entirely on the interaction setting as the locus for the production of social order. Much ink has been spilt on this dualism, with a fair amount of commentary consisting of straw-man caricatures of the opposing position. Structuralists and functionalists are accused of entirely wiping the individual human agent off the face of the social theory map, while interactionists are accused of a myopic, blinkered attitude to structures and in particular of ignoring the powerful constraints they impose on human action. Rather than focus any further on the merits of each polarized position, we can look at a more recent example of an approach that has tried to convert this dualism into a more balanced "duality of structure and agency," as Giddens (1984) has coined the phrase. We will then end by briefly considering how "complexity theory" can add to this debate.

Before moving on to consider Giddens's attempted resolution, we should note why this particular theme is so crucial for health promotion. In order to avoid falling into the trap Raeburn and Rootman warned against in their previously cited text, we have to negotiate carefully how we reconcile the need to integrate insights concerning structural constraints on human agency and choices with the imperative not to treat social actors as "cultural dupes," thereby undermining their autonomy and dignity, and thus destroying the potential for participation and empowerment, which health promoters rightly emphasize. The twin dangers are, on the one hand, acceding to a victim-blaming voluntarism that tragically overemphasizes people's ability to make simple choices concerning their own health-related lifestyles and, on the other, so powerfully developing a narrative of structural constraint that the possibility of change and resistance recedes into some never feasible, impractical utopian future. It also matters a lot how this "dualism" is conceptualized because depending on what pole of the dualism gets emphasized, strategic priorities for intervention and engagement become initiated. For example, if the argument falls on the side of the importance of structure and macro-level institutional phenomena, then a focus will tend to offer prescriptions that advocate for large-scale public policy changes at the expense of more micro-level community engagement; conversely, if the argument focuses on the importance of agency and local action, then we tend to focus on individual behaviour change and community development at the expense of taking into account the need for broader supportive environments and macro-level healthy public policy. In other words, the structure/agency dualism is closely tied in health promotion to whether or not an integrated approach to the *Ottawa Charter* strategies will be implemented: If the dualism holds, then battles over which strategies are more important takes place; if we can truly transcend the dualism and think of it as a duality, then it is much easier to conceptualize the integrated, multi-level, multi-strategy approach that has been consistently advocated for over the past decade or more.

Anthony Giddens's approach to resolving this constitutive dualism is perhaps the best-known contemporary effort to do so, and his theory of "structuration" is still a popular source for those who do not want to choose sides in the old polarizing debates. Giddens's efforts developed out of a long-term concern he had about the cleavages in social theory between those who emphasized an objectivist, often functionalist reading of social structure as the basic causal force in social life, and those who held that social action was really about subjective meaning and understanding. The so-called "theory of structuration" is not really a substantial social theory at all, but is rather an "ontological framework for the study of human social activities" (Giddens, 1991). It is essentially a conceptual recategorization of classical social thought in an attempt to reconcile the above-mentioned dualism. It is important to grasp this lesson as health promoters, locked as they are into a deeply applied field of research, may be too quick to jump from the rarified theoretical atmosphere of structuration theory into a definite empirical application of Giddens's conceptual framework. The issue is that Giddens's "theory" works much better as a sort of sensitizing conceptual device that allows us to avoid certain ontological assumptions about how sociality works than as some concrete methodological guide to carrying out health promotion research or, for that matter, any specific social research endeavour at all!

The key conceptual manoeuvre that Giddens employs in his attempt to transcend the dualism of structure and agency is in his use of *time* and *space* as categories that relativize social agency and social structure. For Giddens, the relative durability of social systems and social institutions has to do with systematic patterns of social activity (thus agency) as they are distributed across time and space; hence, social structure is both the medium and outcome of social activity. In acting as a medium, structure is both constraining and enabling in relation to social action. He argues that the process of modernization has built increasingly distanciated societies, where the effects of social action and institutions are spread across larger expanses of time and space, reducing the relative import of face-to-face interactions in the structuring of societies. Conversely, new mediums of communication have also enormously increased the amount of social interaction that is possible across great distances by compressing the amount of time it takes to engage in those interactions. A second innovation of structuration theory was to incorporate the concepts of *power* and *domination* into his theoretical framework. In Giddens's terms, modern societies have both increased the level and effectivity of administrative "power" in terms of its ability to transform and act, along with an increase in the potential for relations of domination, particularly through the use of knowledge.

While Giddens's work is still seen as a substantial contribution, many theorists have suggested that he has failed to fully transcend the dualism of structure and agency at the conceptual level (Mouzelis, 1995; Jessop, 2001), while from the very beginning, empirical researchers have felt there is little positive methodological guidance in structuration theory in how to conduct better research (Storper, 1985). This is not to discourage the use of Giddens's work;

however, health promoters should recognize that within the field of sociology itself, and for social theorists themselves, there is just as little consensus on how to move forward in conceptualizing the ontological and epistemological aspects of the social world as there was when Giddens published his theory. In particular, theorists concerned with producing adequate accounts of social structure are not convinced that Giddens's use of language as the exemplary social institution as the basis for conceptualizing structure was helpful. Nor are theorists of social action satisfied with his account of agency. Following Mouzelis's (1995) critique of Giddens, arguably health promoters should retain the tension in social theory represented by the dualism of structure and agency or, in older terms, between social interaction and social institutions. Many key questions that health promotion must address require *both* an analysis of key patterns of social interaction (such as with "collective lifestyles"), as well as systemic analyses of social institutions, including how governmental institutions, markets, and networks function to coordinate social action on broader scales. The duality of structure is a key insight shared by many contemporary thinkers, but this insight alone will not by itself produce substantive knowledge of important health promotion issues.

One other emerging theoretical approach to resolving the dualism between structure and agency is *complexity theory* (see Chapter 7). Originating from work in a variety of fields (general systems theory, cybernetics, chaos theory, non-linear dynamics, information theory), scientists began, in the late 1980s, to coalesce around a series of general propositions concerning how complex systems worked (Waldrop, 1992). While it is impossible here to explicate the full range of theoretical and methodological implications of complexity theory, it is important to grasp the potential insight it can bring to the structure/agency problem. The core dilemma for the social theorist is to offer a persuasive explanation for how it is that relatively enduring social institutions and structural characteristics arise out of the complex interactions of individual human agents (the so-called "micro-macro linkage"). While almost everyone will accede to the proposition that there is no ontological gap between social institutions and social action (in other words, social activity produces social structure), a key dispute is around whether or not social institutions are *nothing but* the aggregate results of individual human agency. Or, more strongly, can social structure be *reduced* to the properties of individual agents? This is a profound epistemological question. How do we know about social structure? Can we predict what it will look like by examining only the interaction of individuals? Methodological individualists in the social sciences tell us that if you accede to the ontological proposition mentioned above, then there can be nothing left over or extra after you take account of all the individual activities. Yet, methodological holists point out that there clearly are properties that certain social structures or institutions have that an individual human agent does not. Thus far, the methodological individualist has been left with a reductionism that seemed satisfactory in terms of its parsimony, yet wanting in terms of its ability to explain the full development of complex social institutions or systems; conversely, the holist could wax lyrically about the irreducible complexity of social systems, yet be open to legitimate criticism concerning the nebulous extra quality that pertained to social orders that one could not find in the individuals who made it up.

Complexity theory offers a way out of this dilemma or paradox. Through the concept of "emergence" (Sawyer, 2005), it offers a rigorously systematic way of demonstrating how individual components of a system interact to create enduring orders, including social institutions, norms, and role structures, except these orders are created through iterations of interaction that cannot be *reduced* to the original properties of the system in its initial state (including all its individual components). This resolution does not undermine the basic ontological argument of the methodological individualists that social orders are produced by social interaction; rather, it shifts the emphasis to the epistemological failure of the methodological individualist's reductionist program. It argues first that genuinely novel properties are indeed generated by the interaction of individual agents, none of whom have these properties, in part or in whole, prior to the set of relevant interactions. Second, it argues that because this is the case, it has a radical methodological implication: that the static, linear, predictive models that social science has relied so heavily on have to be superseded by new models that *simulate* social systems by allowing artificial, computer-based interactions to take place over time, with changing parameters that attempt to realistically reflect variable social environments.

Interestingly, this new theoretical manoeuvre tends to sidestep the traditional debate over the ontology of the social, turning the question of the "micro-macro linkage" and the agency/structure debate into an epistemological and methodological question to be resolved through experiment with these new forms of modelling. Thus, the question of whether complexity theory solves the grand theoretical dilemmas of social science is turned into the question of whether the findings it produces have some practical relevance to better understanding how the social world works. For that answer we have to wait.

Conclusion

To summarize, health promotion must engage much more deeply with social theory in the coming decade as it attempts to turn its original youthful intuitions into a mature and substantial field of inquiry. I have argued here that much of this theoretical reflection will not necessarily translate into immediate empirical results. In fact, the approach to social theory advocated is one that critically embraces its legacy in the philosophical tradition, a tradition that understands the series of conceptual debates outlined above as constitutive oppositions in a dialectical progression that works by deepening our understanding of the social world through rigorous reflection rather than by way of a narrative of positive transcendence of the debates themselves. Thus, instead of seeing social theory as a *cul-de-sac* of endless, stagnant disputation, it is to be seen as a rich resource of conceptual innovation, opening up new vistas of inquiry and reinvigorating old questions and offering novel answers.

Another conclusion is that as health promotion begins to more seriously take up the question of social theory, it needs to connect to its fundamental core as a mode of societal critique, concerned with applying reflexive reason to basic questions of power, equity, values, resources, capabilities, and general human flourishing. In doing so, it can avoid falling into the trap of using social theory in a purely instrumental fashion as just one other argumentative resource in what are largely academic exercises. As health promotion becomes more comfortable using social theory, it will find that it can substantially enhance its intellectual resources for engaging in broader societal debates beyond the narrow health sector, a perspective that will become increasingly necessary if health promoters are to match their research and advocacy to their rhetoric, particularly in relation to social inequality and health inequity.

Notes

1. Though this use of "science" is typically a peculiarity of the English-speaking world, as in German, for example, the word for "science", *Wissenschaft*, tends to mean any systematic scholarly inquiry.
2. In fact, when it comes to empirical research, much of social science is inherently skeptical of the type of theorizing discussed in this chapter, and still trundles along happily, churning out the type of "abstracted empiricism" that Wright Mills (1959) warned of so many years ago.
3. They are "tropes" in the sense that they have become metaphors for modern society as a whole: as in "the bureaucratic society," "the rationalist society," etc.
4. In this argument, I do not equate the generic term "critical social theory" with the narrower identification of the former with the specific set of ideas that developed out of the Frankfurt School of critical theory (Jay, 1973; Benhabib, 1986; Bernstein, 1995; Rush, 2004), although the latter is certainly one of the more productive and important traditions to consider.
5. Interestingly, the fact that these trends have not been universal in either direction or strength adds to the evidence of their effect on social inequality. It is now clear that countries and societies that retained strong working-class institutions and a relatively generous welfare system have endured fewer increases in social inequality than we have seen in societies more heavily influenced by neo-liberalism and attacks on labour and the welfare state (Esping-Anderson, 1990; Pinch, 1997; Pierson, 1999; Goodin, Heady, Muffels & Dirven, 2000; Jenson & Sineau, 2003).
6. See Frohlich et al. in this volume for a detailed account of this rationale.

References

Abel, T. (2007). Cultural capital in health promotion. In D. McQueen & I. Kickbusch (Eds.), *Health & modernity: The role of theory in health promotion* (pp. 43–73). New York: Springer.

Ackroyd, S. & Hughes, J. (1992). *Data collection in context.* Longman: London.

Benhabib, S. (1986). *Critique, norm, and utopia: A study of the foundations of critical theory.* New York: Columbia University Press.

Bernstein, R. (1995). *Habermas & modernity.* Cambridge: MIT Press.

Breslow, L. (1999). From disease prevention to health promotion. *Journal of the American Medical Association, 281*(11), 1030–1033.

Derrida, J. (1976). *Of grammatology.* G. Spivak (Trans.). Baltimore: Johns Hopkins University Press.

DiClemente, R., Crosby, R. & Kegler, M. (2002). *Emerging theories in health promotion practice and research.* San Francisco: John Wiley & Sons.

Eakin, J., Robertson, A., Poland, B., Coburn, D. & Edwards, R. (1996). Towards a critical social science perspective on health promotion research. *Health Promotion International, 11*(2), pp. 157–165.

Esping-Anderson, G. (1990). *The three worlds of welfare capitalism.* Princeton: Princeton University Press.

Foucault, M. (1980). *Power/knowledge: Selected interviews & other writings.* C. Gordon (Ed.). New York: Pantheon Books.

Foucault, M. (2000). *Aesthetics: Essential works of Foucault 1954–1984*, vol. 2. J. Faubion (Ed.). Penguin Books: London.

Foucault, M. (2008). *The birth of biopolitics: Lectures at the College de France, 1978–1979.* New York: Palgrave MacMillan.

Frohlich, K., Corin, E. & Potvin, L. (2001). A theoretical proposal for the relationship between context and disease. *Sociology of Health & Illness, 23,* 776–797.

Frohlich, K., Poland, B., Mykhalovskiy, E., Alexander, S. & Maule, C. (2010). Tobacco control and the inequitable socio-economic distribution of smoking: Smokers' discourses and implications for tobacco control. *Critical Public Health, 20*(1), 35–46.

Giddens, A. (1984). *The constitution of society: Outline of the theory of structuration.* Cambridge: Polity Press.

Giddens, A. (1991). Structuration theory: Past, present, and future. In C. Bryant & D. Jary (Eds.), *Giddens's theory of structuration: A critical appreciation.* (201–221) London: Routledge.

Goodin, R., Heady, B., Muffels, R. & Dirven, H. (2000). The real worlds of welfare capitalism. In C. Pierson & F. Castles (Eds.), *The welfare state reader, Part II: Debates and issues* (pp. 171–188). Oxford: Blackwell Publishers.

Habermas, J. (1984). *The theory of communicative action,* vol. 1: *Reason and the rationalization of society.* T. McCarthy (Trans.) Boston: Beacon Press.

Habermas, J. (1987). *The philosophical discourse of modernity: Twelve lectures.* Cambridge: MIT Press.

Habermas, J. (1998). *Between facts and norms.* W. Rehg (Trans.). Cambridge: MIT Press.

Hancock, T. (1994). Health promotion in Canada: Did we win the battle but lose the war? In A. Pederson, M. O'Neill & I. Rootman (Eds.), *Health promotion in Canada: Provincial, national & international perspectives.* (350–373) Toronto: W.B. Saunders.

Heidegger, M. (1993). *Basic writings: From being and time (1927) to the task of thinking (1964).* D. Farrell Krell (Trans.). San Francisco: HarperCollins Publishers.

Hills, M. & Carroll, S. (2009). Health promotion, health education and the public's health. In R. Detels, MA. Lansang, & M. Gulliford, (Eds.) Oxford *textbook of public health, 5th Edition.* (pp.752-766). Oxford: Oxford University Press.

Horkheimer, M. & Adorno, T. (2002). *Dialectic of enlightenment.* Palo Alto: Stanford University Press.

Jay, M. (1973). *The dialectical imagination: A history of the Frankfurt School and the Institute of Social Research, 1923–1950.* Berkeley: University of California Press.

Jenson, J. & Sineau, M. (2003). *Who cares? Women's work, child care, and welfare state redesign.* Toronto: University of Toronto Press.

Jessop, R. (2001). Institutional re(turns) and the strategic-relational approach. *Environment and Planning A, 33,* 1213–1235.

Kickbusch, I. (1989). Approaches to an ecological base to public health. *Health Promotion International, 4,* 265–268.

Labonté, R. (1994). Death of program, birth of metaphor: The development of health promotion in Canada. In A. Pederson, M. O'Neill & I. Rootman (Eds.), *Health promotion in Canada: Provincial, national & international perspectives.* (72–90). Toronto: W.B. Saunders.

Marcuse, H. (1991). *One-dimensional man.* London: Routledge.

Marx, K. (1976). *Capital,* vol. 1. London: Penguin Classics.

Marx, K. (1981). *Capital,* vol. 3. London: Penguin Classics.

McQueen, D. & Kickbusch, I. (2007). *Health & modernity: The role of theory in health promotion.* New York: Springer.

Meiksins Wood, E. (2008). *Citizens to lords: A social history of Western political thought from antiquity to the Middle Ages.* London: Verso.

Mouzelis, N. (1995). *Sociological theory: What went wrong?* London: Routledge.

Mouzelis, N. (2007). Social causation: Between social constructionism and critical realism. Available at: http://mouzelis.gr/wp-content/uploads/2010/05/Mouzelis_Social_Causation.pdf

Olin Wright, E. (Ed.). (2005). *Approaches to class analysis.* Cambridge: Cambridge University Press.

Olin Wright, E. (2009). Class patternings. *New Left Review, 60.* (101–116).

Pierson, C. (1999). The welfare state: From Beveridge to Borrie. In H. Fawcett & R. Lowe (Eds.), *Welfare policy in Britain: The road from 1945* (pp. 208–224). London: MacMillan Publishers Ltd.

Pinch, S. (1997). *Worlds of welfare: Understanding the changing geographies of social welfare provision*. London: Routledge.

Porter, R. (2000). *The Enlightenment*. New York: Palgrave.

Potvin, L. & McQueen, D. (2007). Modernity, public health, and health promotion: A reflexive discourse. In D. McQueen & I. Kickbusch (Eds.), *Health & modernity: The role of theory in health promotion* (pp. 12–20). Springer: New York.

Raeburn, J. & Rootman, I. (1998). *People-centred health promotion*. New York: John Wiley & Sons.

Rush, F. (2004). (Ed.). *The Cambridge companion to critical theory*. Cambridge: Cambridge University Press.

Sawyer, R. (2005). *Social emergence: Societies as complex systems*. Cambridge: Cambridge University Press.

Sayer, A. (2005). *The moral significance of class*. Cambridge: Cambridge University Press.

Sayer, A. (2009). Chapter 3: "Bourdieu, ethics, and practice," published by the Department of Sociology, Lancaster University, Lancaster, UK. Retrieved from: http://www.lancs.ac.uk/fass/sociology/papers/sayer_chapter3_bourdieu_ethics_&_practice.pdf

Sayer, D. (1991). *Capitalism and modernity: An excursus on Marx and Weber*. London:Routledge.

Stevenson, H. & Burke, M. (1991). Bureaucratic logic in new social movement clothing. *Health Promotion International, 6*, 281–289.

Storper, M. (1985). The spatial and temporal constitution of social action: A critical reading of Giddens. *Environment and Planning D: Society and Space 3*(4), 407–424

Waldrop, M. (1992). *Complexity: The emerging science at the edge of chaos*. New York: Touchstone.

Weber, M. (1978). *Economy and society: An outline of interpretive sociology*. Berkeley: University of California Press.

Weber, M. (2002). *The Protestant ethic and the spirit of capitalism: And other writings*. P. Baehr & G. Wells (Trans.). New York: Penguin Books.

WHO. (1986). *Ottawa Charter for Health Promotion*. Ottawa: World Health Organization, Health and Welfare Canada, Canadian Public Health Association.

Wright Mills, C. (1959). *The sociological imagination*. New York: Oxford University Press.

Critical Thinking Questions

1. How should we think about the concept of "theory" in relation to health promotion?
2. How do you think class and status affect health inequities and the efforts to reduce or eliminate them?
3. What are the real dangers of "rationalization" for health promotion interventions?
4. Should health promotion be a critical social theory? Why or why not?
5. What are the implications of social theory for the concepts of 'empowerment' and 'participation'?

Resources

Further Readings

Berman, M. (1988). *All that is solid melts into air: The experience of modernity*. New York: Penguin.

> One of the truly great and accessible discussions of the process of modernity and how it has affected social change for over 200 years, this is a key text for understanding the cultural dilemmas at the heart of modern capitalist societies. For health promotion, it offers an example of how to think about the ironic and contradictory aspects of modern social life without falling into despair.

Harvey, D. (2002). Agency and community: A critical realist paradigm. *Journal for the Theory of Social Behaviour, 32*(2), 164–194.

This is a key theoretical article, from a critical realist perspective, that addresses the problem of structure vs. agency. Harvey is one of the most important social theorists of the past 40 years.

Nettleton, S. (2006). *The sociology of health and illness.* Cambridge: Polity Press.

This book is a recent summary and synthesis of sociological approaches to health and illness. Much of the book is relevant to health promotion, particularly Chapter 9, in which Nettleton directly addresses contemporary sociological critiques of health promotion.

Raeburn, J. & Rootman, I. (1998). *People-centred health promotion.* New York: John Wiley & Sons.

As indicated by its title, this book emphasizes the importance of "people" in health promotion. It focuses particularly on the "community" as the key locus for health promotion and suggests methods to "empower" people where they live. The book also emphasizes the role of "culture" and "spirituality" in health promotion, but also uses case studies to show how to translate idealism about health promotion into health-enhancing action. It presents a vision for a society based on health promotion values.

Thorogood, N. (2002). What is the relevance of sociology for health promotion? In R. Bunton & G. Scambler (Eds.), *Health promotion: Disciplines, diversity, and developments* (pp. 53–75). London: Routledge.

This is a dedicated chapter on health promotion and sociology in an important collection. Some key theoretical issues are covered, including social stratification, health promotion values and ideology, and lay perspectives on health.

Relevant Websites

Health Sociology Review

http://hsr.e-contentmanagement.com/

An international, scholarly peer-reviewed journal, *Health Sociology Review* explores the contribution of sociology and sociological research methods to understanding health and illness; to health policy, promotion, and practice; and to equity, social justice, social policy, and social work.

International Journal of Health Services

http://www.baywood.com/journals/previewjournals.asp?id=0020-7314

The journal contains articles on health and social policy, political economy and sociology, history and philosophy, and ethics and law in the areas of health and health care. It provides analysis of developments in the health and social sectors of every area of the world, including relevant scholarly articles, position papers, and stimulating debates about the most controversial issues of the day. It is of interest to health professionals and social scientists interested in the many different facets of health, disease, and health care.

Social Theory & Health

http://www.palgrave-journals.com/sth/index.html

The theorization of health issues is crucial both for understanding and as a guide for action. By providing a forum for academics and practitioners to engage with the theoretical development of the health debate, *Social Theory & Health* aims to develop the theoretical underpinnings of health research and service delivery. The journal is of interest to scholars of health-related sociology, nursing, health and clinical psychologists, health and public policy analysts, and theorists in related disciplines.

Sociology of Health and Illness

http://www.blackwellpublishing.com/shil_enhanced/

Sociology of Health and Illness is an international journal that publishes sociological articles on all aspects of health, illness, medicine, and health care. This journal is particularly open to theoretical approaches to health and supports diverse methodological perspectives.

CHAPTER 4

Addressing Diversity and Inequities in Health Promotion:
The Implications of Intersectional Theory

Colleen Reid, Ann Pederson, and Sophie Dupéré

> Theory is a tool to think with.[1]
> —Dorothy Smith

Introduction

Many have argued that health promotion's theoretical base is still largely dominated by biomedical, psychological, and behavioural models and call for the development of more social theories (Potvin, Gendron, Bilodeau & Chabot, 2005; see chapters 3 [S. Carroll] and 7 [Poland & Frohlich]) and expanded academic alliances to enrich its theoretical base (Ziglio, Hagard & Griffiths, 2000). Vigilance is required, however, to ensure that the exchange of concepts and theories between disciplines is done rigorously. While interdisciplinary exchanges can be potentially enriching, such "transfers" from one field to another occur frequently without an in-depth understanding of their theoretical and epistemological basis, as has been the case with the introduction of the concept of social capital into public health (Forbes & Wainwright, 2001; see Moore, Haines, Hawe & Shiell, 2006 for a full discussion of the theoretical and policy implications of mistranslating the concept of social capital). Of any concept or theory, it should be asked: Whose is it? How is it constructed and reconstructed? Whose interests does it serve? (Noffke, 1998). As humans we always operate from a theoretical position, whether implicit or explicit. What is fundamentally important is that we continue to ask and answer these questions while becoming increasingly explicit about naming our theoretical positions and, in turn, how concepts become operationalized in our research, practice, and policy.

In this chapter we argue that health promotion could learn from more dialogue and exchange with feminist scholarship by presenting intersectionality as an important theoretical contribution from women's studies and other fields (McCall, 2005; Weber & Parra-Medina, 2003) that could help health promotion grapple with diversity and the persistence of health inequities. Through drawing mainly on developments in the field of women's health over the past 40 years, we propose intersectionality as a contemporary approach that could increase the theoretical rigour and enhance health promotion practice and policy both within and beyond women's health. We caution, however, against a superficial adoption of intersectional theory into health promotion research and practice, arguing instead that health promotion advocates should adopt a critical stance toward the contributions that intersectional theory offers to the field and deliberately seek opportunities to test and refine the theory from the perspective of health promotion research, practice, and policy.

Limitations of Current Approaches to Health Promotion to Addressing Persistent Health Inequities: The Case of Gender

A number of important concerns persist in Canadian society about the effects of gender (Canadian Feminist Alliance for International Action, 2003). Examples include: the high percentage of Canadian women who live in poverty and report poor health status; the persistence of violence against Canadian women; the diminished status of immigrant and refugee women; the vulnerability of Aboriginal women who are the "poorest of the poor"; or the educational underachievement of boys, to name a few. With its continual focus on lifestyle change—despite rhetoric addressing the elements of the *Ottawa Charter*—health promotion may have contributed to the persistence of health inequities by perpetuating the advantages that certain groups in Canadian society have in accessing information, organizing themselves for change, and creating the conditions to support healthier living.

Fifteen years ago, British sociologists Daykin and Naidoo (1995) suggested that health promotion rested on and perpetuated certain aspects of gender inequities (Pederson, Ponic, Greaves et al., 2010). In particular, they argued that health promotion held women responsible for their own health and the health of others, and employed the techniques of health education and social marketing to encourage women to adopt healthy lifestyles without regard for the individual and structural constraints of power, income, race, and education, among others, that limited women's ability to take action on health issues. Since then, scholars have recognized that health promotion has contributed to gender inequities in other ways. These include perpetuating a confusion regarding the differences between sex and gender (see Box 4.1) and the tendency to see both as dichotomies (Clow, Pederson, Haworth-Brockman & Bernier, 2009); failing to recognize gender as a social determinant of health (Benoit, Shumka, Phillips et al., 2009); homogenizing and isolating social categories such as gender, class, and ethnicity rather than focusing on power relations and associated values such as social justice (Reid, Ponic, Hara et al., 2011); and contributing to an overall ambiguity regarding theoretical approaches and underpinnings with respect to health inequities (Hankivsky, Reid, Varcoe et al., 2010).

Recently, the World Health Organization (WHO) has taken a step toward addressing health inequities. The final report of the Commission on the Social Determinants of Health, *Closing the Gap in a Generation: Health Equity through Action on the Social Determinants of Health*, (CSDH, 2008), argues that many persistent and avoidable health inequities remain between and within countries. The report outlines a global agenda for health equity with three overarching recommendations, none of which refers to increasing individual health-promoting behaviours. Instead, the report recommends: (1) improving daily living conditions; (2) tackling the inequitable distribution of power, money, and resources; and (3) measuring and understanding the problem and assessing the impact of action. Within these recommendations, an essential action highlighted by the report pertains to addressing gender inequities that are seen as unfair, ineffective, and inefficient. "By supporting gender equity, governments, donors, international organizations and civil society can improve the lives of millions of girls and women and their families" (CSDH, 2008, p. 16).

However, the WHO Commission's report is generally thin on specific recommendations for addressing inequities related to gender and offers only a partial view of the contribution of gender to health. The WHO report offers a framework that identifies gender as an intermediate factor that is shaped by other more fundamental ones such as socio-economic status and policy, as well as cultural and societal norms and values. Other scholars have argued, however, that gender must be understood as a fundamental determinant of health that structures access to key resources. Benoit and Shumka (2009) are proponents of such a view and suggest that sex and gender shape access to education, employment, child care, safe neighbourhoods, and health services—themselves determinants of health. Importantly, Benoit and Shumka's framework identifies other key aspects of social location such as social class, race, ethnicity, age, immigrant status, and geographic location as fundamental determinants of health as well. Acting together, these determinants shape access to resources and ultimately health behaviours, morbidity, and mortality. Understanding the relationships among the determinants of health is important for action to reduce health inequities arising from gender. It is critical that actions be taken to tackle gender-related inequities and their consequences both directly and indirectly in order to reduce the health inequities that are a consequence of them. That is, action should be taken to reduce gender-related inequities themselves, not simply expecting action on other factors to trickle down to improve gender-related inequities. Health promotion research and practice in Canada therefore needs to take bold action (Raphael, 2008). Theoretical innovations to improve knowledge and praxis, such as the uptake of recommendations arising from Benoit and Shumka (2009), are needed to enable us to embrace the complex interplay of health determinants and to understand how they intersect and mutually reinforce each other.

Lessons from the Women's Health Movement

The women's health movement and health promotion share important core values, priorities, and approaches to practice. Those in the women's health field have long embraced a positive conceptualization of health (Thurston & O'Connor, 1996), and perceived health as a continuum that extends throughout the life cycle and that is critically and intimately related to the conditions under which women live. Moreover, women's health activists and scholars have long recognized the link between the social location of a person or group and their health and advocated for both individual and community empowerment to improve health (see, for example, Morrow et al., 2007; Armstrong & Deadman, 2009).[2]

Questions asked early in the women's health movement and that continue to inform women's health research and gender and health research can be instructive for health promotion theory and praxis. For over four decades this broad field has grappled with substantive challenges, including: raising consciousness around "the personal is political"; drawing attention to the increasing medicalization of women's health and loss of control over health decision-making; debating the distinct influences and interactions between biology and social structure; examining the uniqueness of women's issues versus the many diversities and differences among women; and understanding the relevance of gender to men's experiences, while expanding analytic categories to understand diverse men's and women's experiences.

Disentangling sex and gender, describing the interactions of sex and gender and their

---

BOX 4.1:

Distinguishing Sex and Gender

Sex "is a multidimensional biological construct that encompasses anatomy, physiology, genes, and hormones that together create a human 'package' that affects how we are labelled" (Johnson et al., 2007, pp. 4-5). *Gender* "is a social construct that is culturally based and historically specific [and] refers to the socially prescribed and experienced dimensions of 'femaleness' or 'maleness' in a society, and is manifested at many levels" (Johnson et al., p. 5).

---

effects, and situating this analysis in the context of other oppressions has become increasingly important to understanding women's health (Greaves, 2009). Johnson, Greaves, and Repta (2007) argue that including the concepts of sex and gender in research leads to a variety of benefits, such as increased rigour and validity of research, cost savings, greater social justice, and the potential to save lives. It makes important political statements as well. For example, the arguments embedded in a sex- and gender-based analysis reflect the values of inclusiveness and equity, and are based on historical claims for redress for women (Greaves, 2009).

Indeed, while we posit that advances in the field of women's health can be instructive to health promotion and critique health promotion's slow uptake of theories and concepts, the field of gender and women's health has been marred by some limitations. While theoretical advances are sophisticated and complex, there remains a tendency to essentialize[3] the category of "woman," to see gender as primarily affecting women, and to ignore or pay scant attention to men and masculinities. As well, there are those who would argue that some women's health advocates give too much primacy to gender over other key social determinants of health (Hankivsky et al., 2010), or fail to recognize and acknowledge this as a limitation in their work.

The Potential Contributions of Intersectional Theory: Expanding Understandings and Approaches

Many argue that gender is distinct from but interactive with other social features like social class or race/ethnicity. All these social factors combine to determine power relations in society that lead not only to inequities between women and men, but also to inequities among different groups of women and different groups of men (Ostlin, George & Sen, 2003).

Intersectional theory is based on the idea that "different dimensions of social life cannot be separated into discrete or pure strands" (Brah & Phoenix, 2004, p. 76). When attempting to understand social inequities, an intersectional analysis focuses on social relationships of power instead of focusing on access to resources. An intersectional analysis examines social experiences and how they intersect at multiple forms of oppression, and what happens at these intersections (McCall, 2005).

BOX 4.2:

Intersectionality

Intersectionality is a new paradigm that brings to the forefront the complexity of social locations and experiences for understanding differences in health needs and outcomes. It refers to "the interaction between gender, race and other categories of difference in individual lives, social practices, institutional arrangements, and cultural ideologies and the outcomes of these interactions in terms of power" (Davis, 2008, p. 68). Key assumptions of intersectionality include:
1. The pursuit of social justice is the main objective.
2. The conceptualization of identity resists essentializing one group or assuming shared similar perspectives.
3. The recognition that social categories of difference, such as gender, race, age, and so on, are complex, fluid, and flexible.
4. Power and a consideration of systems of domination are central to the analysis.

Source: Hankivsky, O., Cormier, R., with De Merich, D. (2009). *Intersectionality: Moving women's health research and policy forward.* Vancouver: Women's Health Research Network.

Intersectional theory was developed most prominently by Black feminist social scientists, emphasizing the simultaneous production of race, class, and gender inequity, such that in any given situation, the unique contribution of one factor might be difficult to measure (Collins, 1989; Fonow & Cook, 1991). This approach—an alternative to earlier models that assumed that advantage and disadvantage simply accumulate to produce "double jeopardy"—suggests that the content and implications of gender and race as socially constructed categories vary as a function of each other (Mullings & Schulz, 2006). For example, whiteness and blackness are gendered, and masculinity and femininity are "raced" within particular cultural contexts. Hence it is often difficult to pinpoint how the interaction, articulation, and simultaneity of race, class, and gender affect women and men in their daily lives, and the ways in which these forms of inequity interact in specific situations to condition health (Mullings & Schulz, 2006).

Intersectional theory suggests that we need to move beyond seeing ourselves and others as single points in some specified set of dichotomies—male or female, White or Black, straight or gay, scholar or activist, powerful or powerless. Rather, "we need to imagine ourselves as existing at the intersection of multiple identities, all of which influence one another and together shape our continually changing experience and interactions" (Brydon-Miller, 2004, p. 9). Intersectional scholarship arose primarily to better understand and address the multiple dimensions of social inequity, including class, race/ethnicity, gender, sexual orientation, age, and disability. Intersectionality is an analytical tool and framework that can be used both at micro and macro levels. At a micro level, it aims to understand the effects of the structural inequities on individual lives by focusing on the interplay between social categories and multiple sources of power and privilege. At a macro level, it seeks to understand how multiple power systems (i.e., institutions) are implicated in the production, organization, and sustainability of inequities. It provides a social structural analysis of inequity (Bilge, 2009).

What distinguishes intersectionality from a social determinants of health approach is that an intersectional analysis does not seek to simply add categories to one another (e.g., gender, race, class, sexuality), but instead strives to understand what is created and experienced at the intersection of two or more categories (Hankivsky et al., 2010). In so doing, it recognizes the multidimensional and relational nature of social locations and places lived experiences, social forces, and overlapping systems of discrimination and subordination at the centre of analysis (Hannan, 2001). In this way an intersectionality analysis captures several levels of difference (Hankivsky et al., 2010).

While the flexibility of intersectionality may be beneficial in some respects, its elasticity may lend itself to the theory's superficial appropriation. Some argue that it has been used in a reductionist and simplistic way. For example, it has not been always accompanied by an analysis that is actually intersectional (Knapp, 2005). There has also been a tendency to use intersectionality in "micro-level" analyses, which focus on the narration of social identities to the exclusion of macro socio-structural analyses of inequities (Collins, 2009, cited by Bilge, 2009). Other authors raise cautions about its use and have highlighted potential limits to its ability to explain power (see Bilge, 2009). Indeed, intersectional theory is still in its early stages of development and further theoretical and methodological development is needed. Nevertheless, we feel that greater consideration of the theory of intersectionality could enhance the ability of health promotion to recognize and address diversity in research, policy, and practice.

Intersectionality: A Theory to Guide Health Promotion Research and Practice

Intersectional frameworks have much to offer health promotion research and practice. For example, intersectionality can help us see through and beyond defined population groups, targeted settings, and specific health issues. It can move us beyond taken-for-granted assumptions and expectations that have characterized much of health promotion to date. For example, Matsuda (1991) writes of "asking the other question": "When I see something that looks racist, I ask 'Where is the patriarchy in this?' When I see something that looks sexist, I ask, 'Where is the heterosexism in this?'" (p. 1189). In a recent study conducted by Reid et al. (2011) that involved South Asian and Aboriginal women, they "asked the other question" and adopted research strategies and an analytic sharpness to avoid seeing these women's experiences as the product of their gender or ethnicity alone. Indeed, "if we fail to ask the other question, what assumptions are being made, and what is lost?" (Reid et al., 2011, p. 104).

A few authors (Hankivsky et al. 2010; Cole, 2008; Weber, 2007; Hankivsky & Cormier, with De Merich, 2009) provide some useful questions for conducting an intersectional analysis that can deepen the typical questions asked of health promotion practice and research:

- Who is the "target population" for the study or intervention? Why was this group chosen, and how do they identify themselves? Who is being compared to whom? Why?
- What issues are of central importance to the researchers, practitioners, and people themselves? How were they identified? Are issues of domination and exploitation being examined? How will the issue of power be at the centre of all analyses?
- How will human commonalities and differences be recognized without resorting to broad generalizations, stereotypical categories, or obliviousness to historical and contemporary patterns of inequity?
- How do researchers and practitioners ensure that they are not seeing what they want to see?
- Are the perspectives of all key stakeholder groups such as policy-makers, grassroots activists, and community groups, including multiply oppressed communities, represented?
- Is the research or intervention framed within the current cultural, societal, and/or situational context?

Posing these questions health promotion research and practice will improve the work conducted—the range of the issues raised will be broader and dealt with in more depth, the nature of the work conducted will expand, and new and previously unexamined dimensions of both will shift the kinds of issues raised in the work, as well as change the nature of health promotion itself.

While posing these questions is an important step forward for health promotion research and practice, we must be mindful that by virtue of intersectionality's complexity, it is a challenging framework to work with: there is no "one size fits all" approach (for specific examples, see Hankivsky et al., 2010).

Implications for Health Promotion Practice

Even as intersectionality continues to advance as a theory and methodology, we want to consider the challenge of "operationalizing" an intersectional analysis to further and enhance the practice of health promotion. In order to consider this challenge, we asked ourselves: What would interventions look like, or how would they be different, if we applied an intersectional analysis? What might this mean for health promotion practice? We developed the following insights and invite health promotion researchers and practitioners to join this conversation:

- *Change outlook on individual characteristics:* An intersectional analysis would shift our focus from "immutable" individual characteristics (e.g., sex, ethnicity) to "mutable social realities" (e.g., those that can be targeted by intervention). Gender and race are not simply biological categories but also social ones (Krieger, 2003). Rather than adopting rigid categories of "populations," we would focus on the interplay between and among social categories.
- *Reframe the concept of health:* An expanded conception of health would include refocusing on a broad framework of social relations and would locate health in families and communities and not only in individual bodies. This is consistent with contemporary reflections on the health promotion field (see Chapter 2) as well as intersectional analyses.

- *Shift the focus of intervention:* An intersectional analysis invites us to target not only the individual but also to take into consideration and even address explicitly social structures, social processes, and the underlying relationships of power. This will involve developing more upstream interventions and policies (i.e., taking action on the "causes of the causes"—the macro determinants of health, such as poverty) (see Chapter 7) and adopting ecological (see Chapter 5) and multi-sectoral approaches. Additionally, an intersectional analysis would deepen understandings of health by adopting a framework of power and oppression and conceptualizing alternative health interventions.

- *Recognize multiple and diverse perspectives through holistic and community-based approaches:* A holistic perspective invites us to examine social experiences, how they intersect at multiple strands of oppression, and what happens at these intersections (McCall, 2005). It encourages us to bring together multiple and diverse stakeholders and to view research and practice as mutual and reciprocal. Holistic and community-based approaches foster broad-based participation of stakeholders, intersectoral practice, the creation of coalitions and strategic alliances, and increased forms of activism. Additionally, such approaches will help operationalize intersectionality in terms of unpacking the "nuts and bolts" of running an initiative or research project.

- *Encourage reflexive practice:* Intersectional theory invites us to pay attention to social processes, social dynamics, and the role of power in producing and sustaining social inequities. It also encourages the researcher-practitioner to connect her or his personal and political identities, and to become aware of her or his own power and privilege. Adopting a reflexive practice (see Chapter 11) can help prevent health researchers and practitioners from unknowingly perpetuating, sustaining, and reinforcing harmful stereotypes (Reid & Herbert, 2005).

These recommendations are consistent, we believe, with most of the advice given elsewhere in this book about how to strengthen the foundations of health promotion to enhance its effectiveness.

Conclusions

To address the mounting critiques of the atheoretical nature of health promotion research and practice, as well as calls for health promotion, public health, and health science researchers to increase the theoretical rigour of their work in order to better inform and direct practice and policy, we advocate intersectional theory because it challenges us to think about conceptualizations of the content, context, and boundaries of social groups (Mullings & Schulz, 2006). Yet we see two important challenges—to push health promotion researchers, practitioners, educators, and advocates to understand the complexity and diversity of health through an intersectional analysis, and to develop strategies for moving a more theoretically informed health promotion into the mainstream. There is an opportunity and appetite for health promotion to pay attention to the more nuanced and complex understandings of health inequities, as well as women's and men's health, that have been recently advanced by many feminist and intersectional scholars. Intersectional analysis reminds health promotion researchers, theoreticians, and practitioners that we must have a theory of power if we are to understand health inequities and redress them. The field of health promotion in turn reminds intersectional scholars that ongoing attention is needed to adapting intersectional frameworks for policy development and day-to-day practice. Health promotion's tradition of action and engagement can be useful to those who may get caught up in critiquing and theorizing at the expense of practice. By learning from one another, the fields of health promotion and intersectionality can both contribute to reducing health disparities and improving health.

Notes

1. Dorothy E. Smith is professor in sociology and the author of *The Everyday World as Problematic: A Feminist Sociology* and *The Conceptual Practices of Power*. She has written about prevailing discourses of sociology, political economy, philosophy, popular culture, and feminist theory and practice. She is reputed to have made this point in her presentations.
2. Recently feminist and intersectionality scholars have acknowledged the importance of understanding gender—the experience of being feminine or masculine—for both women and men. However, the women's health movement arose from examinations of women's experiences of health and health care. Some examples used in this chapter, however, come from the women's health movement and therefore focus only on women's health.
3. To essentialize is to apply a homogenizing view of a fixed category that specifies the "essential" properties or characteristics of all women (Ristock & Pennell, 1996).

References

Armstrong, P. & Deadman, J. (Eds.). (2009). *Women's health: Intersections of policy, research, and practice.* Toronto: Women's Press.

Benoit, C. & Shumka, L. (2009). *Gendering the health determinants framework: Why girls' and women's health matters.* Vancouver: Women's Health Research Network.

Benoit, C., Shumka, L., Phillips, R., Hallgrímsdóttir, H., Kobayashi, K., Hankivsky, O., Reid, C. & Brief, E. (2009). Explaining the health gap between girls and women in Canada. *Sociological Research Online, 14*(5). Retrieved from: http://www.socresonline.org.uk/14/5/9.html

Bilge, S. (2009). Théorisations feminists de l,intersectionnalité. *Diogène, 1*(225), 70–88.

Brah, A. & Phoenix, A. (2004). Ain't I a woman? Revisiting intersectionality. *Journal of International Women's Studies, 5*(3), 75–86.

Brydon-Miller, M. (2004). The terrifying truth: Interrogating systems of power and privilege and choosing to act. In M. Brydon-Miller, P. Maguire & A. McIntyre, *Traveling companions: Feminism, teaching, and action research* (pp. 3–19). Westport: Praeger.

Canadian Feminist Alliance for International Action. (2003). *Canada's failure to act: Women's inequality deepens.* Ottawa: Canadian Feminist Alliance for International Action. Retrieved from: www.fafia-afai.org/en/node/164

Clow, B., Pederson, A., Haworth-Brockman, M. & Bernier, J. (2009). *Rising to the challenge: Sex- and gender-based analysis for health planning, policy, and research in Canada.* Halifax: Atlantic Centre of Excellence for Women's Health.

Cole, E. (2008). Coalitions as a model for intersectionality: From practice to theory. *Sex Roles, 59*(5–6), 443–453.

Collins, P.H. (1989). The social construction of Black feminist thought. *Signs: Journal of Women in Culture and Society, 14*(4), 745–773.

CSDH. (2008*). Closing the gap in a generation: Health equity through action on the social determinants of health*. Geneva: World Health Organization. Retrieved from: http://whqlibdoc.who.int/hq/2008/WHO_IER_CSDH_08.1_eng.pdf

Davis, K. (2008). "Intersectionality as buzzword: A sociology of science perspective on what makes a feminist theory successful." *Feminist Theory*. 9:67–85.

Daykin, N. & Naidoo, J. (1995). Feminist critiques of health promotion. In R. Bunton, S., Nettleton & R. Burrows (Eds.), *The sociology of health promotion: Critical analyses of consumption, lifestyle, and risk* (pp. 59–69). London & New York: Routledge.

Fonow, M.M. & Cook, J.A. (1991). Back to the future: A look at the second wave of feminist epistemology and methodology. In M.M. Fonow & J.A. Cook (Eds.), *Beyond methodology: Feminist scholarship as lived research* (pp. 1–15). Bloomington: Indiana University Press.

Forbes, A. & Wainwright, S.P. (2001). On the methodological, theoretical, and philosophical context of health inequalities research: A critique. *Social Science and Medicine, 53*(6), 801–816.

Greaves, L. (2009). Women, gender, and health research. In P. Armstrong & J. Deadman (Eds.), *Women's health: Intersections of policy, research, and practice* (pp. 3–20). Toronto: Women's Press.

Hankivsky, O., Cormier, R., with De Merich, D. (2009). *Intersectionality: Moving women's health research and policy forward*. Vancouver: Women's Health Research Network.

Hankivsky, O., Reid, C., Varcoe, C., Clark, N., Benoit, C. & Brotman, S. (2010). Exploring the promises of intersectionality for advancing women's health research. *International Journal for Equity in Health, 9*(5). Retrieved from: http://www.equityhealthj.com/content/9/1/5

Hannan, C. (2001). Gender mainstreaming—a strategy for promoting gender equality: With particular focus on HIV/AIDS and racism. Paper presented at the NGO Consultation in preparation for the forty-fifth session of the Commission on the Status of Women, NYU Medical Center, New York.

Johnson, J., Greaves, L. & Repta, R. (2007). *Better science with sex and gender*. Vancouver: Women's Health Research Network.

Knapp, G. (2005). Race, class, gender: Reclaiming baggage in fast travelling theories. *European Journal of Women's Studies, 12*(3), 249–265.

Krieger, N. (2003). Genders, sexes, and health: What are the connections—and why does it matter? *International Journal of Epidemiology, 32*(4), 652–657.

Matsuda, M.J. (1991). Beside my sister, facing the enemy: Legal theory out of coalition. *Stanford Law Review, 43*(6), 1183–1192.

McCall, L. (2005). The complexity of intersectionality. *Signs: Journal of Women in Culture and Society, 30*(3), 1771–1800.

Moore, S., Haines, V., Hawe, P. & Shiell, A. (2006). Lost in translation: A genealogy of the "social capital" concept in public health. *Journal of Epidemiology and Community Health, 60*, 729–734.

Morrow, M., Hankivsky, O. & Varcoe, C. (Eds.). (2007). *Women's health in Canada: Critical perspectives on theory and policy*. Toronto: University of Toronto Press.

Mullings, L. & Schulz, A.J. (2006). Intersectionality and health: An introduction. In A.J. Schulz & L. Mullings (Eds.), *Gender, race, class, and health: Intersectional approaches* (pp. 3–17). San Francisco: Jossey-Bass.

Noffke, S. (1998). What's a nice theory like yours doing in a practice like this? And other impertinent questions about practitioner research. Keynote address presented at the second International Practitioner Research Conference, Sydney, Australia.

Ostlin, P., George, A. & Sen, G. (2003). Gender, health, and equity: The intersections. In R. Hofrichter (Ed.), *Health and social justice: Politics, ideology, and inequity in the distribution of disease* (pp. 132–156). San Francisco: Jossey-Bass.

Pederson, A., Ponic, P., Greaves, L., Mills, S., Christilaw, J., Frisby, W., Humphries, K., Jackson, B.E., Poole, N. & Young, L. (2010). Igniting an agenda for health promotion for women: Critical perspectives, evidence-based practice, and innovative knowledge translation. *Canadian Journal of Public Health, 101*(3), 259–261.

Potvin, L., Gendron, S., Bilodeau, A. & Chabot, P. (2005). Integrating social theory into public health practice. *American Journal of Public Health, 95*(4), 591–595.

Raphael, D. (2008). Grasping at straws: A recent history of health promotion in Canada. *Critical Public Health, 18*(4), 483–495.

Reid, C. & Herbert, C. (2005). "Welfare moms and welfare bums": Revisiting poverty as a social determinant of health. *Health Sociology Review, 14*(2), 161–173.

Reid, C., Ponic, P., Hara, L., Kaweesi, C. & Ledrew, R. (2011). Performing intersectionality: The mutuality of intersectional analysis and feminist participatory action research. In O. Hankivsky (Ed.), *Health and intersectionality inquiry in Canada.* 92–111.Vancouver: UBC Press.

Ristock, J.L. & Pennell, J. (1996). *Community research as empowerment: Feminist links, postmodern interruptions.* Toronto: Oxford University Press.

Thurston, W.E. & O'Connor, M. (1996). *Health promotion for women: A Canadian perspective.* Paper prepared for the Canada–USA Women's Health Forum, August 9–11, 1996, Ottawa, Ontario.

Weber, L. (2007). Through a fly's eyes: Addressing diversity in our creative, research, and scholarly endeavours. Paper presented at the inaugural celebration of GREAT Day (Geneseo Recognizing Excellence, Achievement, and Talent), State University of New York at Genesceo.

Weber, L. & Parra-Medina, D. (2003). Intersectionality and women's health: Charting a path to eliminating health disparities. In M.T. Segal & V. Demos (Eds.), *Gender perspectives on health and medicine: Key themes* (pp. 181–230). London: Elsevier.

Ziglio, E., Hagard, S. & Griffiths, J. (2000). Health promotion development in Europe: Achievements and challenges. *Health Promotion International, 15*(2), 143–154.

Critical Thinking Questions

1. How is gender a distal, or macro, determinant of health?
2. What can the women's health movement and health promotion learn from each other?
3. What is intersectional theory?
4. How can the application of intersectional theory inform health promotion practice? What kinds of questions would be raised in using intersectional theory?
5. How can intersectional theory help address health inequities in general?

Resources

Further Readings

Greaves, L. (2009). Women, gender, and health research. In P. Armstrong & J. Deadman (Eds.), *Women's health: Intersections of policy, research, and practice.* (pp. 3–20). Toronto: Women's Press.

This chapter provides an overview of women's health, women's health research, and the women's health movement. The author outlines the history of women's health, describes key concepts in women's health research such as sex, gender, gender-based analysis, and gender mainstreaming, and outlines methodological and measurement issues in research. The author concludes with a description of what the future holds for women's health and posits new directions for the field.

Hankivsky, O. (forthcoming). *Health inequities in Canada—Intersectional frameworks and practices.* Vancouver: UBC Press.

This is the first Canadian edited volume to focus on intersectionality frameworks and health inequities. It brings together, for the first time, interdisciplinary scholars from nursing, medicine, sociology, anthropology, social work, political science, women's studies, and health sciences to profile leading-edge research, facilitate dialogue, and inform research, policy, and practice. This book makes a significant contribution to exploring intersectionality-type approaches emerging in the Canadian context for identifying and responding to health inequities.

Morrow, M., Hankivsky, O. & Varcoe, C. (2007). *Women's health in Canada: Critical perspectives on theory and policy.* Toronto: University of Toronto Press.

In the introduction to this edited volume, the authors outline the trends that have marked research into women's health in Canada. They attribute the emphasis on woman-centred approaches to health research to the second wave of feminist thought, and point to contributions and drawbacks of sex and gender analysis. These last approaches are discussed in comparison with gender-neutral approaches, which have been traditionally used in health research to the exclusion of gender-specific needs. However, these approaches are contrasted with emerging intersectional approaches, which help to highlight the experience of gender simultaneously with the experiences of class, race, sexual orientation, and other forms of social difference. The other chapters in this volume provide a contemporary analysis of theory and methods, the social determinants of health, and key issues in women's health.

Schulz, A.J. & Mullings, L. (2006). *Gender, race, class, and health: Intersectional approaches.* San Francisco: Jossey-Bass.

This volume aims to provide opportunities for dialogue or mutual exchange across the disciplines and paradigms that inform empirical efforts to understand and address inequalities in health. It brings together an interdisciplinary group of scholars from the social sciences and public health to examine the ways that gender, race, and class are mutually constituted and interconnected. The goal is to inform theory, research, and practice focused on the elimination of health disparities. The volume is divided into five parts: (1) intersectionality and health; (2) race, class, gender, and knowledge production; (3) the social context of health and illness; (4) structuring health care: access quality and inequality; and (5) disrupting inequality.

Relevant Websites

Centre for the Study of Gender, Social Inequities, and Mental Health

http://www.socialinequities.ca/

The Centre for the Study of Gender, Social Inequities, and Mental Health at Simon Fraser University is at the forefront of developing research and sharing knowledge on intersections between gender, social inequities, and mental health. The centre's primary goal is to eliminate social inequities in mental health through innovative research, knowledge exchange, and training initiatives aimed at developing programs, policies, and interventions that will ultimately improve the mental health of men and women in Canada and the international community.

Women's Health Contribution Program

http://www.hc-sc.gc.ca/hl-vs/gender-genre/contribution/index-eng.php

Canada's Centres of Excellence for Women's Health are funded through Health Canada's Women's Health Contribution Program (WHCP). The centres were established in 1996 as part of the federal women's health strategy. Currently, four centres conduct and/or facilitate research on the determinants of women's health and engage in translating research into policy and accessible health information. Over the years, several working groups have also been important parts of the Women's Health Contribution Program. Women and Health Care Reform and Women and Health Protection each focused on specific areas of knowledge and action in women's health: issues related to health services and health care reform, and issues of health protection. The Canadian Women's Health Network—a voluntary national organization dedicated to improving the health and lives of girls and women in Canada by collecting, producing, distributing, and sharing information and providing networking opportunities—is another pillar of the WHCP. The Réseau québécois d'action pour la santé des femmes (RQASF) also receives some support from the WHCP.

- Atlantic Centre of Excellence for Women's Health (www.acewh.dal.ca)
- British Columbia Centre of Excellence for Women's Health (www.bccewh.bc.ca)
- Canadian Women's Health Network (www.cwhn.ca)
- National Network on Environments and Women's Health (www.yorku.ca/nnewh)
- Prairie Centre of Excellence for Women's Health (www.pwhce.ca)
- Réseau québécois d'action pour la santé des femmes (http://rqasf.qc.ca/presentation)
- Women and Health Care Reform (www.womenandhealthcarereform.ca)
- Women and Health Protection (www.whp-apsf.ca)
- Women's Health Contribution Program (http://www.hc-sc.gc.ca/hl-vs/gender-genre/contribution/index-eng.php)

Women's Health Research Network

http://www.whrn.ca/

The Women's Health Research Network (WHRN) was designed to be a catalyst for bringing together innovative groupings of gender and women's health researchers and research collaborations drawn from academic, health service, policy, and community settings. It sought to foster the generation, application, and mainstreaming of new knowledge, dedicated to increasing the understanding of and capacity for sex- and gender-based analyses, and for integrating women's health concerns into other areas of health research. A major activity undertaken by the WHRN was the publication of training manuals for researchers interested in women's health, intersectionality, the determinants of health, and community-based research. These downloadable research primers can be accessed through the WHRN website:

- Benoit, C. & Shumka, L. (2009). *Gendering the health determinants framework: Why girls' and women's health matters.* Vancouver: Women's Health Research Network.
- Hankivsky, O., Cormier, R., with De Merich, D. (2009). *Intersectionality: Moving women's health research and policy forward.* Vancouver: Women's Health Research Network.
- Johnson, J., Greaves, L. & Repta, R. (2007). *Better science with sex and gender.* Vancouver: Women's Health Research Network.
- Reid, C., Brief, E. & LeDrew, R. (2009). *Our common ground: Cultivating women's health through community-based research.* Vancouver: Women's Health Research Network.

CHAPTER 5

Building and Implementing Ecological Health Promotion Interventions

Lucie Richard and Lise Gauvin

Introduction

This chapter provides examples of innovative, contemporary health promotion programs that effectively translate social ecological conceptions into tangible health promotion interventions. The ecological approach is currently generating much enthusiasm among theorists, planners, and practitioners in health promotion and public health. As an innovation, this approach offers a vision and models congruent with the new public health and thus an increased potential of translating interventions into gains in terms of population health. However, despite this high level of interest, proponents continue to lament its poor level of integration into programming efforts. In most fields of professional practice, there is often a lag between the emergence of an innovation and its integration into professional actions. This could be the case in health promotion, where professionals have not been in a position to fully adopt and implement ecological health promotion practices. In an effort to contribute to the integration of the ecological approach into practice, the aim of this chapter is therefore to describe programs deemed as exemplary in their degree of integration of the ecological approach. Accordingly, after having briefly described the ecological approach and the historical context of its emergence in public health, we illustrate some applications by describing three highly ecological health promotion initiatives from Canada. Finally, we identify some emerging challenges to the design, implementation, and evaluation of such innovative initiatives.

The Ecological Approach

Derived from ecology, a subfield of biology, the ecological approach offers a research and action framework that emphasizes the complex interactions between people, groups, and their environments. Contrary to traditional ecology, which highlighted the physical features of environment, the ecological approach used in health promotion is more social-ecological in nature and focuses more centrally on the social, organizational, and cultural components of the environment. Within such a vision, planners and practitioners are urged to design interventions and programs that will integrate people-focused efforts to modify health behaviours with interventions that will enhance the numerous dimensions of the environment: physical, social, and cultural. Such complex intervention packages are touted as having the potential for greater success than traditional individual-focused health education interventions (Jackson et al., 2007; Richard, Gauvin & Raine, 2011; Sallis, Owen & Fisher, 2008; Smedley & Syme, 2000).

The Rise of the Ecological Perspective

Ecological thinking has a long history in disciplines such as biology and psychology. An emphasis on socio-environmental determinants of health was also at the root of public health at the turn of the nineteenth century. However, the ecological discourse re-emerged only recently in public health with the World Health Organization's European Regional Office (World Health Organization, 1984) presenting its new conceptualization of health issues as recently as the mid-1980s. This conceptualization reiterated the importance of environmental determinants of health and ecological approaches in promoting population health. Besides the WHO, several Canadian organizations played a leadership role in the emergence of the ecological approach and of the health promotion discourse (Epp, 1986; Kickbusch, 1994, 2003; World Health Organization, Health and Welfare Canada & the Canadian Public Health Association, 1986).

Oddly enough, because of its emphasis on complexity and wide-scale system influences, the ecological approach has often been seen as intimidating and difficult to operationalize (Green, Richard & Potvin, 1996). One way to address this problem has been to stratify the environment as, for example, psychologists have done: Bronfenbrenner (1979) stratified the environment into micro-, meso-, exo-, and macrosystems, whereas Moos (1979) proposed a four-strata classification revolving around physical settings, organizational factors, human aggregate factors, and social climate. Similar efforts have been undertaken in health promotion (see McLeroy, Bibeau, Steckler & Glanz, 1988; Simons-Morton, Simons-Morton, Parcel & Bunker, 1988; Stokols, 1992).

More contemporary ecological models in health promotion depart from earlier contributions in that they integrate new analytic dimensions or provide increased emphasis on conceptualizations emanating from other disciplines. For example, Stokols, Grzywacz, McMahan, and Phillips (2003) supplemented Stokols's earlier notion of a health-supportive environment by emphasizing the concept of community capacity for health improvement. Similarly, Best et al. (2003) proposed an overarching framework integrating not only a community partnering axis but also a temporal dimension highlighting the centrality of life-course processes. Other theoretical approaches draw upon concepts from the field of behaviour analysis (Hovell, Wahlgren & Adams, 2009) or sociology and anthropology (Burke, Joseph, Pasick & Barker, 2009) in order to shed light on processes through which environmental influences result in behaviour adoption and maintenance. Besides these theoretical contributions, application of the ecological approach for intervention planning was undertaken by Stokols (1996), Green and Kreuter (2005), and Bartholomew, Parcel, Kok, and Gottlieb (2006). The availability of these theoretical and planning models has paved the way for applications of the approach to a wide variety of health and disease problems (see Richard et al., 2011).

Despite these efforts, a low level of integration of the ecological approach in health promotion practice still persists (Beaglehole & Bonita, 2004; Richard, Gauvin, Ducharme, Trudel & Leblanc, 2010; Smedley & Syme, 2000). Yet, the health promotion literature, reports from the field, and testimonials of dozens of planners and practitioners indicate that descriptions of innovative programs aimed at a variety of health determinants are available as exemplars. In order to promote greater integration of the ecological approach into professional practices, we describe selected examples of successful Canadian applications of the ecological approach in health promotion programs. The selection was strategic, covering a variety of target populations, intervention areas, and geographical regions. We now turn to a description of these three success stories.

Three Examples of Programs

Promoting Healthy Living and Health Supportive Environments: Inception of a "Possibility Framework" through the PATH Project

Promoting Action toward Health (PATH) was a five-year, federally funded health promotion research project. It was implemented in a relatively disadvantaged area of a medium-sized city in western Canada. It involved a partnership between a community centre, a regional health authority, and a university. PATH was initially aimed at preventing Type 2 diabetes among middle-aged adults (35–64 years) of the target area. However, in acknowledging that many medical and non-medical causes of diabetes (e.g., obesity, poverty) are also at the root of several other chronic diseases, the need to include other age groups and to adopt a population health approach were recognized (Chappell, Funk, Carson, MacKenzie & Stanwick, 2006). It was also evident at the start of the project that involvement of the broader community would be desirable for the project to facilitate community development and health goals (Carson, Chappell & Knight, 2007). Gradually, a stronger emphasis on reducing social inequalities in health became apparent:

> PATH's goal is to support healthy living through addressing social determinants; that is, the focus is on barriers and obstacles, and making the healthy choices the easy choices. Recognizing the difficulties if not impossibility of changing root socioeconomic conditions in a time-limited research project, PATH seeks to promote healthy living and health supportive environments via initiatives at multiple levels that identify and respond to resident concerns. (Chappell et al., 2006, p. 4)

In line with the ecological approach that the promoters explicitly adopted as a theoretical underpinning (Chappell et al., 2006), a central criterion guiding the choice of initiatives for the project was the capacity to address one or more determinants of health and to effect change at multiple levels. To help ensure this multi-level focus, a planning tool allowing for the charting of project activities by level of change was used. Labelled the "Possibility Framework" (see Table 5.1), this tool "lists specific initiatives in the project by their current level of focus, and includes 'possible' examples of initiatives and activities at other levels of intervention" (Chappell et al., 2006, p. 11). Obviously, the list of initiatives shown in Table 5.1 is not exhaustive (non-listed initiatives such as health fairs, community gardens, and history and heritage activities are also mentioned by Chappell et al.), but the information illustrates the strong ecological breadth of the PATH project.

TABLE 5.1: Multi-level "Possibility Framework" for Initiatives

	Individual Level	Group Level	Organizational Level	Community Level	Macro/Policy Level
Community kitchens	Kitchen participants learn low-cost, healthy food-preparation skills	Friendships and social activities are promoted among those in support groups	Health authority becomes involved in providing training and education for kitchen participants	Kitchen group promotes sense of community via holding cooking events, publishing recipes	Potential for food-costing training, which can influence policy development around food issues
Facilitating interorganizational networks and linkages	Enhanced individual willingness to work with individuals from other organizations with different perspectives	New relationships and trust formed among those facing similar challenges in their work roles	Enhanced organizational capacity to work with one another for mutual benefit	Community capacity is enhanced through increased organizational networking	Possibility of coordinated, more powerful, co-operative interorganizational efforts to change policy affecting local residents
Community arts centre	Arts centre participants gain increased self-esteem, creative development, artistic skills, and knowledge	Promoting group bookings and events, encouraging social support and sharing of artistic ideas and experiences	School capacity for delivering art programs is enhanced	A sense of community is promoted through community art shows, outreach programs, and neighbourhood beautification through art	School board policies may become more flexible to alternate space uses and partnering with community groups for mutual benefit
Participation in city's greenways Initiative	Participants in related mapping events gain renewed appreciation of local green spaces	Formation of new groups in the area to protect local green spaces; meeting people with similar interests	Capacity of existing organizations may be strengthened, i.e., with increased resources and information	Improved neighbourhoods through creation of green spaces enhance community life	Local groups gain increased public support and effectiveness regarding local land-use policies

Note: Adapted from Chappell, N., Funk, L., Carson, A., Mackenzie, P. & Stanwick, R. (2006). Multilevel community health promotion: How can we make it work? *Community Development Journal.*

As seen in Table 5.1, initiatives implemented had potential for reaching the target popula-tion in a variety of settings—at an arts centre or community kitchens, for example. PATH also included a variety of intervention targets and strategies. At the organizational level, interorganizational networks and linkages were established "to enhance collaboration among organizations and across sectors" (Chappell et al., 2006, p. 355). For instance, community kitchens that were developed in partnership with a local community centre also involved professionals from the health authority to provide education to participants. Such a network-ing of two organizations not only facilitated the implementation of the community kitchens, but it also contributed to creating community capacity in that this new partnership bore the potential of developing additional community and advocacy initiatives. Other PATH strat-egies were aimed at developing and reinforcing personal competencies. For example, among its objectives, the Community Arts Centre explicitly aimed to enhance personal competen-cies, including participants' self-esteem, creative development, artistic skills, and knowledge.

A final strength of the PATH project pertains to the strong emphasis directed toward com-munity participation (Carson et al., 2007; Chappell et al., 2006). For example, consistent with a community activation strategy, community residents and local organizations were involved in planning, design, and management of activities. Accordingly, it was believed that initiatives ought to come from residents rather than professionals and researchers. For this reason, the project started at the individual level; "this strategy [...] helped avoid a potential paralysis of action due to multiple simultaneous commitments" (Chappell et al., 2006, p. 4). As discussed below, there is often a tension between the comprehensive focus of an ecological approach and the ideal of participation inherent in health promotion (Chappell et al., 2006; Stokols, 1996). The PATH project is a good demonstration of how such a large-scale approach can thrive with an agenda involving community participation and capacity-building.

Getting Kids on the Move and Eating Well: Stunning Impact of the Annapolis Valley Health Promoting Schools Project

Another interesting example of the application of the ecological approach is found in the Annapolis Valley Health Promoting Schools project (AVHPSP, 2010; see also PHAC Best Practices Portal: http://cbpp-pcpe.phac-aspc.gc.ca/intervention/291/view-eng.html). It is one of the few initiatives that have been evaluated in terms of behaviour and health outcomes (Veugelers & Fitzgerald, 2005).

Similar to the PATH project, the AVHPSP revolved around the theme of making the healthy choice the easy choice, but focused more specifically on promoting healthy eating and daily physical activity to fight overweight and obesity among elementary school children in Nova Scotia. Program promoters believed that "multiple strategies occurring simultan-eously to promote healthy eating and physical activity enhances the acceptance and ability to deliver the programmes at the school, school board, and community level. These strategies include policy, education, awareness, leadership development, programme development, pro-gramme implementation, and advocacy (AVHPSP, 2010). Activities were organized in six sets. First, the project aimed at shifting the focus from a "profit" framework toward a "prophet" framework by mobilizing people around the idea of changing environments and policies to effect change. This was achieved by identifying a program champion, creating links with the community, and developing leadership among school staff. The second set of activities involved conducting school surveys. This was done by developing an evaluation framework and developing different data collection activities, including a student preference survey, activity logs, and school physical activity and menu snapshots. A plan was also developed to share school-specific information with schools. A third set of activities consisted of developing a business plan for healthy food and physical activity in each participating school that are directly in line with an ecological approach. The fourth aimed at implementing a healthy eating strategy: changes were made in food offerings as well as in presentation of new types of food. The fifth strategy was the implementation of physical activity on a daily basis through noncompetitive running, playground games, "kids teaching kids" coaching clinics, equipment loan, etc. The final strategy included creating links between schools and the community by building partnerships with local stakeholders.

An effectiveness evaluation of the AVHPSP showed that children attending intervention schools had significantly lower rates of obesity and overweight, had healthier diets, and reported more physical activities (Veugelers & Fitzgerald, 2005). The AVHPSP is an example where successful integration of ecological principles led to measurable changes in indicators of population health. In addition to demonstrating effectiveness, it is noteworthy to mention that the project has been maintained and blended in with other federal (i.e., Canada Get Active) and provincial initiatives (i.e., Strive for 5) programs aimed at improving eating and activity practices among children and youth.

Moving toward Tobacco Control: Shaping the Web of Environmental Determinants in a Quebec Regional Public Health Department

A third example is the tobacco control program of one regional public health department (Breton, Richard, Lehoux, Labrie & Léonard, 2004; Richard et al., 2004). In 1994, the Quebec Ministry of Health and Social Services launched an ambitious action plan to tackle the high prevalence and incidence of smoking in the province (Ministère de la santé et des services sociaux, 1994). Supported by a budget of $20 million, this plan included four components—prevention, health protection, cessation, and surveillance/evaluation—and targeted youth and low-income populations. In addition to encouraging collaboration with community partners in the development and implementation of interventions, the plan also called for the adoption of a global ecological approach to tobacco control, including action on a variety of environmental and personal determinants of smoking initiation and maintenance. The ministry mandated the regional public health departments to implement the plan. In line with the ministerial plan, one specific public health department included a variety of initiatives (see Box 5.1) covering a variety of intervention settings and targets.

As shown in Table 5.2, four types of settings emerged as most dominant in the program: schools, health organizations, the community, and society. A variety of intervention targets were also included. Organizational elements were by far the most frequently targeted by the

---

BOX 5.1:

Selected Examples of Initiatives Identified in the Tobacco-Control Programming of a Regional Public Health Directorate

- Sensitization and training of health and school personnel in the territory with regard to the new tobacco-control law
- Implementation of a strategic committee reuniting key players from various public health organizations
- Training of physicians
- Implementation of tobacco-control policy in schools
- Development and support of a tobacco-control network among local community health centres
- Diffusion of a self-help smoking-cessation guide
- Publication of papers in a medical journal
- Implementation of tobacco-control committees in high schools
- Training of effect multipliers in community groups

Source: Richard, L., Lehoux, P., Denis, J.L., Potvin, L., Breton, E., Labrie, L. et al. (1999). Implantation de l'approche écologique dans les programmes de réduction du tabagisme de deux directions de santé publique : étude de cas. GRIS Research report (no. R99-09). Montréal: Université de Montréal, GRIS.

interventions like, for instance, the enforcement of school tobacco-control policies (i.e., the set of rules governing tobacco use on the school premises). A second example pertains to activities aimed at reinforcing the tobacco-control skills of key actors in organizations (e.g., physicians, nurses, teachers, administrators). Organizational targets were also involved in strategies aimed at networking organizations. An example here is the creation and maintenance of a network of local public health organizations involved in tobacco control in various organizations in their territory.

There were three other types of targets. For example, one initiative ("La Gang Allumée"— "The Enlightened Gang") involved networking of various actors interested in tobacco control in high school settings, including student representatives seen as key players in the interpersonal environment of the target population. A self-help cessation guide was distributed in the population through various channels; in this example, the individual is the direct target of the intervention. Finally, one initiative aimed at a political target. At the same time that these local and regional activities took place, the Quebec tobacco-control community was actively working toward the adoption of a new provincial law (Breton, Richard, Gagnon, Jacques & Bergeron, 2008); thus, many of the regional activists were also provincially involved in a strategic coalition aimed at advocating with elected officials (i.e., a political target).

This tobacco program for youth is an excellent example of an ecological intervention (Richard, Potvin, Kishchuk, Prlic & Green, 1996). First, it integrated environmental and individual targets across a variety of settings. Second, these targets translated into a diversity of strategies of which at least one was aimed directly toward the target population itself and others at the environment. It is noteworthy to mention that smoking was among the

TABLE 5.2: Frequency of Initiatives (N = 14) According to Different Types of Intervention Settings and Targets

Settings	
Schools	4
Health organizations	3
Communities	3
Society (the province)	3
Workplace organizations	2
Leisure organizations	1
Community organizations for First Nations peoples	1
Targets	
The client as a direct target	1
Interpersonal environment	1
Organizational environment	14
Community	0
Political environment	1

Note: Because an initiative may include many settings/targets, the total frequency exceeds 14.

Source: Adapted from Breton, E., Richard, L., Lehoux, P., Labrie, L. & Léonard, C. (2004). Analyser le degré d'intégration de l'approche écologique dans les programmes de promotion de la santé: Le cas des programmations de réduction du tabagisme de deux directions de la santé publique québécoises. *The Canadian Journal of Program Evaluation, 19*, 97-123.

first contemporary public health issues to be redefined from a broader social perspective that extended well beyond personal behaviour, thus calling for a comprehensive, ecological response from the public health community (Brownson, Eriksen, Davis & Warner, 1997). The tobacco-control programming described above is a good example of such a response.

Where to from Here?

We view the ecological approach as a contemporary and practicable framework within which to orient health promotion interventions. However, we also note several challenges that threaten the reach it might have for future practice and research.

The first challenge is conceptual and pertains to the role of community participation in the development and implementation of programs. Although we highlighted the fact that ecological health promotion programming is founded on a broad conception of health determinants, we also note that less emphasis has been devoted to the role of community participation even though it is seen as pivotal in health promotion and population health (Butterfoss & Kegler, 2009; Rootman, Goodstadt, Potvin & Springett, 2001). A first explanation pertains to the inherent challenge of conciliating objectives related to multi-level community outcomes and maximizing community participation, which is often fuelled by more proximal preoccupations. For example, Chappell et al. (2006) indicate that "residents may be seen to want their kitchens to remain at the individual and group level of intervention, whereas PATH may seek expansion to more macro levels. This demonstrates potential conflicting priorities for PATH facilitators between being responsive to community desires on the one hand while on the other hand seeking changes at broader levels" (p. 13).

A second explanation relates to ecological models, which have traditionally emphasized the notions of environmental determinants and their interaction with behaviour and health at the expense of other key dimensions of the ecological approach. In a recent analysis of contributions emanating from community psychologists (e.g., Trickett, 2009; Kelly, 2006), Richard et al. (2011) recalled that central to the ecological approach are features pertaining to the building of community capacity and resources. Although these concepts have always ranked high among core orientations and central concepts of health promotion, particularly in planning models (Green & Kreuter, 2005; Bartholomew et al., 2006), they still remain to be fully integrated in ecological models as they are disseminated in public health in general and health promotion in particular. In their review of contemporary ecological models in health promotion, Richard et al. (2011) have indeed noted that among such models, a limited number have included a dimension related to community capacity or participation, with models recently proposed by Stokols et al. (2003) and Best et al. (2003) being two exceptions. There is still a need to further develop a community capacity dimension thus rendering work conducted on the ecological approach more integrated with the health promotion vision.

A second challenge pertains to the apparent unwillingness of practitioners to advocate for legislative and policy changes partly because they find themselves in the awkward position of trying to influence the very people who employ them. Similarly, they are in the difficult position of interfering with the daily business of very powerful corporations (e.g., the tobacco or fast-food industries). As a result, existing health promotion programs understandably display timid efforts toward influencing the political sphere. Nevertheless, as described above, actions at the political level have been successfully undertaken. At the regional public health department referred to above, one way of facilitating political action was to support coalitions and other collaborative networks that then acted as leaders in political action and advocacy (Breton et al., 2008). Similarly, in the "Possibility Framework" of the PATH project, activities were aimed at co-operative interorganizational efforts to change policy affecting local residents. Finally, although not directly related to the AVHPSP, there have been recent efforts aimed at the development of practical tools that might facilitate advocacy and political action on physical activity. For example, the Toronto Charter for Physical Activity (Bull et al., 2010) outlines four actions based on nine guiding principles to promote health-enhancing physical activity at the population level. Significant results in health promotion programming are likely to be achieved only if practitioners, in addition to working at the individual level, are able to influence political targets (O'Neill, 1989; O'Neill, Gosselin & Boyer, 1997).

A third challenge pertains to the evaluation of the complex and multi-level health promotion programs that integrate the ecological approach. First, there is a need for appropriate methods to establish the efficacy and effectiveness of interventions. We note that AVHPSP promoters deployed unusual efforts to produce evidence of the impact of the program in preventing obesity and changing eating and activity patterns (Veugelers & Fitzgerald, 2005). As noted by several authors, though, randomized clinical trials, which still represent the gold standard for evidence, are difficult to apply in evaluating complex community programs (Victora, Habicht & Bryce, 2004) and numerous interesting alternatives exist: clustered randomized trials, quasi-experimentation, and case studies (see also Shadish & Cook, 2009). Yet, efficacy/effectiveness is not the only focus of evaluation as health promotion efforts must also address reach, adoption, implementation, and maintenance (e.g., Glasgow, Klesges, Dzewaltowski, Bull & Estabrooks, 2004). Given that the current interest in both knowledge transfer and exchange (Green, Ottoson, Garcia & Hiatt, 2009), as well as evidence-based practice (Brownson, Fielding & Maylahn, 2009) and the fact that practitioners are getting more involved in stimulating community participation and political action, we can anticipate that the complexity of conducting evaluations will likely increase.

A final challenge pertains to resources. Implementing large-scale programs and multipronged interventions requires a high level of material, financial, and time resources. Studies have indeed confirmed that the presence of plentiful resources was a critical factor in helping regional public health organizations to successfully implement ecological health promotion programs (Richard et al., 2004, 2008). It is crucial that health promotion planners and practitioners access the resources required to achieve their ambitions.

Conclusions

As shown above, integrating ecological principles in practice is possible. We anticipate that further advances will occur at an accelerated pace if researchers and practitioners devote continued efforts to comprehensive evaluation of ecological programs and to knowledge transfer and exchange activities. Research on the identification of factors associated with greater levels of integration of the ecological approach in real-world programming is also a promising avenue for future efforts.

References

AVHPSP. (2010). *Annapolis Valley health promoting schools project: Making the healthy choice the easy choice.* See: http://www.avrsb.ca/content/annapolis-valley-health-promoting-schools-program; http://cbpp-pcpe.phac-aspc.gc.ca/intervention/291/view-eng.html

Bartholomew, K.L., Parcel, G.S., Kok, G. & Gottlieb, N.H. (2006). *Planning health promotion programs: An intervention mapping approach* (2nd ed.). San Francisco: Jossey-Bass.

Beaglehole, R. & Bonita, R. (2004). *Public health at the crossroads: Achievements and prospects* (2nd ed.). Cambridge: Cambridge University Press.

Best, A., Stokols, D., Green, L.W., Leischow, S., Holmes, B. & Buchholz, K. (2003). An integrative framework for community partnering to translate theory into effective health promotion strategy. *American Journal of Health Promotion, 18,* 168–176.

Breton, E., Richard, L., Gagnon, F., Jacques, M. & Bergeron, P. (2008). Health promotion research and practice require sound policy analysis models: The case of Quebec's Tobacco Act. *Social Science and Medicine, 67,* 1679–1689.

Breton, E., Richard, L., Lehoux, P., Labrie, L. & Léonard, C. (2004). Analyser le degré d'intégration de l'approche écologique dans les programmes de promotion de la santé: Le cas des programmations de réduction du tabagisme de deux directions de santé publique québécoises [An analysis of the level of integration of the ecological approach in health promotion programmes: The tobacco-control programming of two Quebec public health directorates]. *Canadian Journal of Program Evaluation, 19*(1), 97–123.

Bronfenbrenner, U. (1979). *The ecology of human development: Experiments by nature and design.* Cambridge: Harvard University Press.

Brownson, R.C., Eriksen, M.P., Davis, R.M. & Warner, K.A. (1997). Environmental tobacco smoke: Health effects and policies to reduce exposure. *Annual Review of Public Health, 18,* 163–185.

Brownson, R.C., Fielding, J.E. & Maylahn, C.M. (2009). Evidence-based public health: A fundamental concept for public health practice. *Annual Review of Public Health, 30,* 175–201.

Bull, F.C., Gauvin, L., Bauman, A., Shilton, T., Kohl, H.W. & Salmon, A. (2010). The Toronto Charter for Physical Activity: A global call for action. *Journal of Physical Activity and Health, 7,* 421–422.

Burke, N.J., Joseph, G., Pasick, R.J. & Barker, J.C. (2009). Theorizing social context: Rethinking behavioral theory. *Health Education and Behavior, 36,* 55S–70S.

Butterfoss, F.D. & Kegler, M.C. (2009). The community coalition action theory. In R.J. DiClemente, R.A. Crosby & M.C. Kegler (Eds.), *Emerging theories in health promotion practice and research* (pp. 237–276). San Francisco: Jossey-Bass.

Carson, A., Chappell, N.L. & Knight, C.J. (2007). Promoting health and innovative health promotion practice through a community arts centre. *Health Promotion Practice, 8*(4), 366–374.

Chappell, N., Funk, L., Carson, A., MacKenzie, P. & Stanwick, R. (2006). Multilevel community health promotion: How can we make it work? *Community Development Journal, 41*(3), 352–366.

Epp, J. (1986). *Achieving health for all: A framework for health promotion.* Ottawa: Health and Welfare Canada.

Glasgow, R.E., Klesges, L.M., Dzewaltowski, D.A., Bull, S.S. & Estabrooks, P. (2004). The future of health behavior change research: What is needed to improve translation of research into health promotion practice? *Annals of Behavioral Medicine, 27,* 3–12.

Green, L.W. & Kreuter, M.W. (2005). *Health program planning: An educational and ecological approach.* New York: McGraw-Hill.

Green, L.W., Ottoson, J.M., Garcia, C. & Hiatt, R.A. (2009). Diffusion theory and knowledge dissemination, utilization, and integration in public health. *Annual Review of Public Health, 30,* 151–174.

Green, L.W., Richard, L. & Potvin, L. (1996). Ecological foundation of health promotion. *American Journal of Health Promotion, 10*(4), 270–281.

Hovell, M., Wahlgren, D. & Adams, M. (2009). The logical and empirical basis for the behavioral ecological model. In R.J. DiClemente, R.A. Crosby & M.C. Kegler (Eds.), *Emerging theories in health promotion practice and research* (pp. 415–449). San Francisco: Jossey-Bass.

Jackson, S.F., Perkins, F., Khandor, E., Cordwell, L., Hamann, S. & Buasai, S. (2007). Integrated health promotion strategies: A contribution to tackling current and future health challenges. *Health Promotion International, 21*(S1), 71–83.

Kelly, J.G. (2006). *Becoming ecological: An expedition into community psychology.* New York: Oxford University Press.

Kickbusch, I. (1994). Introduction: Tell me a story. In A. Pederson, M. O'Neill & I. Rootman (Eds.), *Health promotion in Canada: Provincial, national & international perspectives* (pp. 8–17). Toronto: W.B. Saunders Canada.

Kickbusch, I. (2003). The contribution of the World Health Organization to a new public health and health promotion. *American Journal of Public Health, 93*(3), 383–387.

McLeroy, K.R., Bibeau, D., Steckler, A. & Glanz, K. (1988). An ecological perspective on health promotion programs. *Health Education Quarterly, 15*(4), 351–377.

Ministère de la santé et des services sociaux. (1994). *Plan d'action de lutte au tabagisme* [Anti-tobacco action plan]. Quebec: Gouvernement du Québec.

Moos, R.H. (1979). Social-ecological perspectives on health. In G. Stone, F. Cohen & N. Alder (Eds.), *Health psychology—a handbook: Theories, applications, and challenges of a psychological approach to the health care system* (pp. 523–547). San Francisco: Jossey-Bass.

O'Neill, M. (1989). The political dimension of health promotion work. In C. Martin & D.V. McQueen (Eds.), *Readings for a new public health* (pp. 222–234). Edinburgh: Edinburgh University Press.

O'Neill, M., Gosselin, P. & Boyer, M. (1997). *La santé politique: Petit manuel d'analyse et d'intervention politique dans le domaine de la santé* (Monographie du Centre québécois collaborateur de l'OMS pour le développement de Villes et villages en santé). Beauport: Réseau québécois des villes et villages en santé.

Richard, L., Gauvin, L., Ducharme, F., Trudel, M. & Leblanc, M.E. (2010). Influencing the degree of integration of the ecological approach in disease prevention and health promotion programs for older adults: An exercise in navigating the headwinds. *Journal of Applied Gerontology.* Advance online publication. doi: 10.1177/0733464810382526

Richard, L., Gauvin, L., Gosselin, C., Ducharme, F., Sapinski, J.P. & Trudel, M. (2008). Integrating the ecological approach in health promotion for older adults: A survey of programmes aimed at elder abuse prevention, falls prevention, and appropriate medication use. *International Journal of Public Health, 53*, 46–56.

Richard, L., Gauvin, L. & Raine, K. (2011) Ecological models revisited: Their uses and evolution in health promotion over two decades. *Annual Review of Public Health, 32*, 307–326.

Richard, L., Lehoux, P., Breton, E., Denis, J.L., Labrie, L. & Léonard, C. (2004). Implementing the ecological approach in tobacco control programs: Results of a case study. *Evaluation and Program Planning, 27*, 409–421.

Richard, L., Potvin, L., Kishchuk, N., Prlic, H. & Green, L.W. (1996). Assessment of the integration of the ecological approach in health promotion programs. *American Journal of Health Promotion, 10*(4), 318–328.

Rootman, I., Goodstadt, M., Potvin, L. & Springett, J. (2001). A framework for health promotion evaluation. In I. Rootman, M. Goodstadt, B. Hyndman, D.V. McQueen, L. Potvin, J. Springett & E. Ziglio (Eds.), *Evaluation in health promotion: Principles and perspectives* (pp. 7–38). Copenhagen: World Health Organization.

Sallis, J.F., Owen, N. & Fisher, E.B. (2008). Ecological models of health behaviors. In K. Glanz, B.K. Rimer & K. Viswanath (Eds.), *Health behavior and health education: Theory, research, and practice* (pp. 465–485). San Francisco: Jossey-Bass.

Shadish, W.R. & Cook, T.D. (2009). The renaissance of field experimentation in evaluating interventions. *Annual Review of Psychology, 60*, 607–629.

Simons-Morton, D.-G., Simons-Morton, B.G., Parcel, G.S. & Bunker, J.F. (1988). Influencing personal and environmental conditions for community health: A multilevel intervention model. *Family and Community Health, 11*(2), 25–35.

Smedley, B.D. & Syme, S.L. (Eds.). (2000). *Promoting health: Intervention strategies from social and behavioral research*. Washington: National Academy Press.

Stokols, D. (1992). Establishing and maintaining healthy environments: Toward a social ecology of health promotion. *American Psychologist, 47*(1), 6–22.

Stokols, D. (1996). Translating social ecological theory into guidelines for community health promotion. *American Journal of Health Promotion, 10*, 282–298.

Stokols, D., Grzywacz, J.G., McMahan, S. & Phillips, K. (2003). Increasing the health promotive capacity of human environments. *American Journal of Health Promotion, 18*(1), 4–13.

Trickett, E.J. (2009). Community psychology: Individuals and interventions in community context. *Annual Review of Psychology, 60,* 395–419.

Veugelers, P.J. & Fitzgerald, A.L. (2005). Effectiveness of school programs in preventing childhood obesity: A multilevel comparison. *American Journal of Public Health, 95*(3), 432–435.

Victora, C.G., Habicht, J.P. & Bryce, J. (2004). Evidence-based public health: Moving beyond randomized trials. *American Journal of Public Health, 94,* 400–405.

World Health Organization. (1984). *Health promotion: A discussion document on the concept and principles.* Copenhagen: World Health Organization, Regional Office for Europe.

World Health Organization, Health and Welfare Canada & the Canadian Public Health Association. (1986). Ottawa Charter for Health Promotion. *Canadian Journal of Public Health, 77,* 425–430.

Critical Thinking Questions

1. How can the ideal of increased community participation in the health promotion process be reconciled with ecological intervention in health promotion?
2. How can public health interventionists further integrate advocacy and legislative action into their repertoire of action?
3. What are the most appropriate research designs for evaluating health promotion interventions that are ecological?
4. Why is the ecological approach often qualified as intimidating and difficult to operationalize? What would facilitate its integration into programs?
5. What are other examples of programs and interventions that have successfully integrated the ecological approach?

Resources

Further Readings

Bauman, A. (2005). The physical environment and physical activity: Moving from ecological associations to intervention evidence. *Journal of Epidemiology and Community Health, 59,* 535–536.

This editorial provides a provocative view on how evidence can be translated into interventions.

Kelly, J.G. (2006). *Becoming ecological: An expedition into community psychology.* New York: Oxford University Press.

A collection of landmark papers by J.G. Kelly, a founder of community psychology. Kelly formulated the "ecological metaphor," which transposes principles from biological ecology to the investigation of relationships between individuals and their environment. The ecological perspective in community psychology has inspired research and action in many disciplines.

McLaren, L. & Hawe, P. (2005). Ecological perspectives in health research. *Journal of Epidemiology and Community Health, 59,* 6–14.

A glossary of terms pertaining to an ecological approach in health research.

Smedley, B.D. & Syme, S.L. (Eds.). (2000). *Promoting health: Intervention strategies from social and behavioral research.* Washington: National Academy Press.

A landmark report from the Institute of Medicine Committee on Capitalizing on Social Science and Behavioural Research to Improve the Public Health, which emphasizes the role of social and behavioural factors in influencing health and disease throughout the lifespan. Many chapters are devoted to public health interventions.

Relevant Websites

Health Nexus

http://www.healthnexus.ca/services/index.htm

Health Nexus (formerly Ontario Prevention Clearinghouse) offers consultations, referrals, opportunities for networking, educational events like workshops and conferences, and resources (both electronic and print) on health promotion priorities.

Health Promotion Clearinghouse (Nova Scotia)

www.hpclearinghouse.ca

An online resource to find out more about what's happening in health promotion in Nova Scotia.

Institut national de santé publique du Québec

www.inspq.qc.ca/english

The mandate of the Institut is to support the minister and regional agencies in fulfilling their public health mission. The Institut's mission includes development, updating, dissemination, and implementation of knowledge. The website provides information and resources related to a variety of health issues and interventions.

Ontario Healthy Communities Consortium

http://www.ohcc-ccso.ca/en/healthy-communities-consortium

Supports community groups, organizations, and partnerships working toward building healthy communities throughout Ontario. The consortium draws on and engages the products, services, and resources of all members of the (former) Ontario Health Promotion Resource System.

Public Health Agency of Canada

www.phac-aspc.gc.ca

With the mandate of promoting and protecting the health of Canadians, the agency is involved in various activities such as program delivery, research and knowledge development, and public and professional education. Its website includes information and resources related to key health issues and interventions in Canada.

RE-AIM

www.re-aim.org

RE-AIM provides a framework to systematically evaluate health behaviour interventions. RE-AIM stands for Reach, Efficacy/Effectiveness, Adoption, Implementation, and Maintenance. The website provides links to several resources useful for researchers and interventionists.

CHAPTER 6

Promoting Health in a Globalized World:
The Biggest Challenge of All?

Ronald Labonté

Introduction

Much has changed since the first edition of this book appeared in 1994. Most of us writing about health promotion then were concerned with the persisting tensions in practice: unhealthy lifestyles/living conditions; top-down/bottom-up programming; individual change/collective mobilization; professional knowledge/community wisdom. Our locus for grappling with these tensions was the community, and our major challenge was scaling up to those policy reaches that condition and constrain health opportunities. The limited geography of our terrain was not parochial. It was merely a product of its time. These health promotion tensions and challenges still define the territory for most practitioners—the important "ordinary" of our work that needs to be celebrated, extended, and sustained into the future. But, though necessary, health promotion's empowering localism—even nationalism—is no longer sufficient. As the 2005 *Bangkok Charter for Health Promotion* states: "Health promotion must become an integral part of domestic and foreign policy and international relations" (World Health Organization, 2005). What changed?

From the International to the Global

The most obvious intrusion into national health complacency was the SARS episode of 2003, which claimed the lives of 774 people worldwide within a matter of months (World Health Organization, 2004). This figure is dwarfed by the death rates from most other infectious diseases, and is a fraction of the 35,000 estimated heat deaths that afflicted Europe in the summer of 2003 (NewScientist.com, 2003). But SARS warned the sanitized and immunized in rich nations that new and re-emerging infectious diseases were on a global rise and less than 24 hours' air travel from almost anywhere. Curbing the incidence of disease in other countries was now as much a matter of self-interest as of international largesse. This point was reinforced by more recent scares over H5N1 (avian) and H1N1 (swine) influenza pandemics, which also revealed the messy politics and economics that lay behind the rapid scale-up of responses (good), but with the greatest benefit going to rich countries' drug companies, which are making the vaccines, and the least benefit to those poorer and more crowded parts of the world, which are most likely to be epicentres of new outbreaks (bad).

Working to promote the health of others in distant lands is nothing new. Canadians have long enjoyed a reputation for being internationalists in most things, including health. Our contributions run from the medical heroism of Norman Bethune in pre-Communist China and the (usually anonymous) volunteers with Médecins Sans Frontières (Doctors without Borders), to public health efforts to prevent the spread of HIV/AIDS or slow down the advancing double burden of chronic disease in poorer countries. This is still the mainstay of what we might call international health promotion. But a series of world events over the past three decades require us to consider a global health promotion, one that recognizes that the causes and consequences of disease are no longer confined within national boundaries.

A first glimpse of the inherently global reality of our lives came with the lunar landing of 1969 and its compelling images of a lonely planet adrift in a massive universe. The physicality of being one world (and, by extension, one people) became more prominent, and arguably more powerful, than the cosmopolitan idea. The political significance of this event, which had more to do with altering consciousness than behaviour, was quickly eclipsed by another, less visible force of interconnectedness—the global recession of the early 1970s. This recession was partly caused by two major oil crises (shortages combined with cartels) that saw prices increase sharply. Many developing countries borrowed heavily from wealthier nation lenders to sustain their oil-dependent growth. When lending nations dramatically raised interest rates to control inflation within their own borders, this spike in the cost of servicing existing debts combined with a fall in the value of borrowing countries' currencies to create a developing world debt crisis that threatened—through default on loan payments—to collapse the global financial system. Financial markets had become globally entwined, a lesson even those in the rich world learned sharply and suddenly in the great (and, as of 2011, ongoing) global economic crisis of 2008.

The World Bank and International Monetary Fund (IMF), originally set up to rebuild what World War II had destroyed and to prevent economic crises from precipitating a World War III, subsequently morphed into "watchdog[s] for developing countries, to keep them on a policy track that would help them repay most of their debts and to open their markets for international investors" (Junne, 2001, p. 206). Their chosen policy track of structural adjustment, a term used to describe the economic policies developing countries had to follow to qualify for emergency loans or grants, embodied the neo-liberal ("free market") economic beliefs of the wealthier countries that (still) dominate decisions in both institutions: liberalization, privatization, welfare minimalism, cost recovery, and making the country attractive to foreign investors (Milward, 2000). This economic orthodoxy (often described as "neo-liberalism") became global gospel with the 1989 fall of the Berlin Wall, which created a normative vacuum for countries wishing to experiment with "third way" blends of state centralism and market capitalism. The result was not a fair one: rich countries—the home of foreign investors—became hugely wealthier, while poorer nations became stuck in health-debilitating poverty (Figure 6.1).

Mapping the New Territory:
The Drivers of Contemporary Globalization

The concept that has come to define the political transformation of the past two decades is globalization. Kelley Lee, a UK scholar and one of the early thinkers on the globalization/ health linkage, considers it broadly as a function of technology, culture, and economics

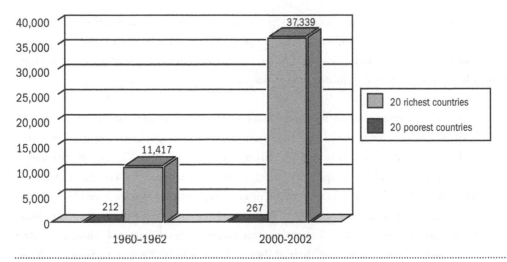

FIGURE 6.1: GDP Per Capita US$, 20 Poorest/Richest Countries

Source: World Bank (2003) *World Development Indicators* Washington: World Bank. Available at:http://www-wds.worldbank.org/external/
default/WDSContentServer/IW3P/IB/2003/05/30/000094946_03051504051563/Rendered/PDF/multi0page.pdf

---

BOX 6.1:

From Structural Adjustment to an HIV Pandemic

To make these abstract global forces real, consider Chileshe, a Zambian woman who is dying of
AIDS. She was infected by her now-dead husband, who once worked in a textile plant, but lost his
job when Zambia was forced to open its borders to cheap clothing imports. He moved to the city
as a street vendor, selling cast-offs from wealthier countries. He would get drunk and trade money
for sex, often with women whose own husbands were somewhere else, working or dead, and who
themselves desperately needed money for their children. Chileshe is a fictional character, but her
experience is not. In 1992, as part of a structural adjustment program, Zambia opened its borders
to textile imports, including second-hand clothing. Its domestic clothing manufacturers, inefficient
by wealthier nation standards, could not compete, especially since used clothing has no production
costs. Within eight years, most of Zambia's textile mills closed and 30,000 jobs disappeared.
For conventional economists, this was a textbook example of how and why liberalization works:
consumers got cheaper goods—at least for a while—and inefficient producers were driven out of
business. But many Zambians paid a heavy price for that inefficiency. Previously employed workers
came to rely on the informal, ill-paid, and untaxed underground economy. Privatization of state
enterprises, another requirement of structural adjustment, eliminated a further source of revenues
that might have been used to support education and health care. Instead, and again at the request
of the international financial institutions, Zambia imposed user fees, cut health staff, and reduced
the salaries of those who remained. All of this came at a time when the AIDS epidemic was surging
out of control (Labonté, Schrecker & Sen Gupta, 2005).

---

leading to a compression of time (everything is faster), space (geographic boundaries begin
to blur), and cognition (awareness of the world as a whole) (Lee, 2003). This is undoubtedly
true, although these have been societal qualities for as long as there have been written records
of societies. The qualitative shift lies in the intensity of these changes. Others have argued

(convincingly) that "economic globalization has been the driving force behind the overall process of globalization" (Woodward et al., 2001, p. 876). Changes in our global economy are the source of contemporary globalization's intensification, bringing with it new challenges to health and its promotion. Among these changes are:

1. *The scale of international private financial flows resulting from capital market liberalization:*
    Daily foreign currency exchanges (representing primarily speculative trading in financial markets) were worth over $3.6 trillion in 2009 (Leading Group on Innovative Financing to Fund Development, 2010), a doubling since 2004 estimates (Kahn & Yardley, 2004) "despite the fact that the intervening period has witnessed the most serious financial crisis in living memory" (Leading Group on Innovative Financing to Fund Development, 2010, p. 22). These amounts dwarf the total foreign exchange reserves of all governments, reducing their ability to intervene in foreign exchange markets to stabilize their currencies when speculative investors decide to shift their holdings, thereby precipitating a currency crisis. Each country experiencing such a crisis has seen increased poverty and inequality, and decreased health and social spending (O'Brien, 2002). The global financial crisis of 2008 differed somewhat in origin, but not in effect. Unregulated investment bankers made extensive loans to people unable to repay them (primarily mortgages in the US) and then sold the debt as investment assets. The amounts involved were trillions (some even speculate quadrillions) of dollars. When the US and other countries' real estate bubbles burst, the massive "toxic debts" carried by financial investment firms risked worldwide banking failures. The bailouts and public stimulus spending that followed has transferred much of this private banking debt into public government debt, leading in turn to dramatic cuts in health and social spending in much of the developed world. Yet the worst of the economic (and subsequent health) effects are being experienced by poorer people in poorer countries, whose livelihoods under globalization has become increasingly tied to high levels of debt-financed consumption by people in wealthier countries (World Bank, 2009; Marmot & Bell, 2009; International Labour Organization, 2009; Overseas Development Institute, 2009).

2. *The establishment of binding trade rules, primarily through the World Trade Organization (WTO):*
    With the birth of the WTO in 1995, trade agreements became more than simply lowering border barriers. They began to limit the policy flexibilities of national governments in ways that could imperil public health, a problem now aggravated by the precipitous rise in bilateral investment treaties (which give corporations the right to sue foreign governments if regulations impede their investment "takings") and so-called WTO-plus bilateral and regional trade agreements (Labonté, Blouin & Forman, 2010).

3. *The reorganization of production across national borders:*
    Multinational enterprises (MNEs) are central to this third and perhaps most significant trend. The emergence of global production or commodity chains allows MNEs to

locate labour-intensive operations in low-wage countries (often in exclusive export-processing zones, most of which lack health, safety, or labour rights), carry out research and development in countries with high levels of publicly funded education and public investment in research, and declare most of their profits in low-tax countries. Good for business; bad for public health.

4. *The crisis of climate change:*
    Climate change is undoubtedly the most urgent global health issue. The scientific consensus is that we will experience some form of profound climatic change over the next two decades—with annual death tolls of 150,000 predicted to double within a matter of years—even assuming we achieve and move well beyond the Kyoto requirements during that time (Plumb, 2003). The apocryphal tale is that of the Easter islanders, whose ideological enslavement to a belief in the ancients led to the erection of huge stone monuments, whose movement required skids of timber, which, as competition among the families for more and bigger monuments accelerated, denuded the island of every last tree (Wright, 2004). No trees, no birds, no insects, no mammals, no fresh water, no food. And by the time the Europeans bumped into the island, almost no people. The tragedy is that they likely knew what would happen even as they cut the last tree. Just as we know what will likely happen as we continue to fish our oceans to extinction, eliminate our carbon sinks and biodiversity, contaminate our sources of fresh water, grow our supposedly healthy economies with a continued addiction to toxic fossil fuels, and blind ourselves to the consequences with an ideological enslavement to growth as the only marker of progress.

Globalization and Health: Disputed Territory

If our aim is improving global health—with a particular emphasis on the poorer half of humanity facing the greatest burden of disease—we must attend to how contemporary globalization posits its health beneficent effects. These distill to a few key claims and counterclaims:

*   *Rapid diffusion of new health technologies and innovation:* This refers back to the impressive role played by several low-cost interventions (such as immunization and antibiotics) in raising life expectancies in many poor countries (World Bank, 1993). The problem is that collapsing health systems in many poor countries can no longer deliver old technologies (immunization coverage globally is declining, and rapidly so in Africa), much less new ones. And those countries that did achieve high health gains in the past did so by also providing potable water, sanitation, women's education, state subsidization of necessities (such as food), and equitable taxation and income redistribution—interventions that are now beyond the fiscal means of many of the world's poorest nations. Finally, the growth in intellectual property rights constrains considerably the diffusion of such important global public goods for health.

*   *Gender empowerment through increased employment opportunities for women:* There is some evidence supporting this, although such work is frequently in unhealthy export-processing

zones. Women's earnings are often channelled back to the control of male family members, and many women's domestic responsibilities remain unchanged, creating a double burden of work (Durano, 2002).

- *The growth-health-growth virtuous circle, which is the mainstay globalization-is-good-for-health argument:* Its proponents hold that liberalization (the removal of border barriers on the flow of goods and capital) increases trade, which increases growth that decreases poverty; and any decline in poverty is good for people's health (Dollar, 2001). Economic growth also provides revenue for investments in health care, education, women's empowerment programs, and so on. Improved health increases economic growth (World Health Organization Commission on Macroeconomics and Health, 2001) and the circle closes virtuously upon itself. But the counterclaims are many. Trade and financial liberalization does not inevitably lead to increased trade or economic growth (Rodriguez & Rodrik, 2000). Those countries where liberalization led to growth (primarily Southeast Asia and China) did so by protecting their domestic industries and financial markets while subsidizing their exports (the same way today's wealthy nations became so), and not by following the World Bank/IMF conditions and free trade rules (Chang, 2002). While their growth did lift many people out of poverty at the abject less than $1 per day level (an imperfect measure used by the World Bank), it did not lift them very far. Poverty at the less than $2 per day level increased by almost the same amount over the same period (Wade, 2004).[1] For the rest of the world, declines in poverty in some regions were more than offset by even greater increases elsewhere. Economic growth has also given rise to escalating income inequalities within most nations, especially those that have grown the fastest (Cornia & Court, 2001), while trade liberalization has led to the increased marketing and adoption of unhealthy Western lifestyles by larger numbers of people, globalizing new pandemics of tobacco-related diseases, obesity, and diabetes.

Healthy Global Public Policy: A Modest Agenda

The recent global economic changes recounted in this chapter did not just happen. They required policy decisions by governments around the world, decisions from which most affected citizens were often excluded. During the 1990s, the breadth and depth of that exclusion generated a new global social movement that was, if not actively hostile to the present form of globalization, at least profoundly skeptical about the "rising tide lifting all boats" claims made by its cheerleaders. This movement received considerable media attention as a result of protests during meetings of the WTO, the G8,[2] the World Bank and IMF, and the World Economic Forum. The social justice and environmental sustainability concerns of this global movement have long shaped grassroots campaigns in low- and middle-income countries, and the quality of its research and advocacy have compelled acceptance of such campaigns' legitimacy and even many of their conclusions. These conclusions—the leverage points for change presented below—focus on globalization's key economic drivers and counterbalances.

Fair Financing

As the new millennium dawned, the global community of countries, imperfectly constituted as the United Nations, consolidated a list of Millennium Development Goals (MDGs) that it thought must be, and could be, achieved by the year 2015 (see Box 6.2). These MDGs—all concerning health or its determinants—were endorsed by all nations, with the wealthiest declaring that the poorest should not lack for the resources necessary to attain them. The rhetoric has not been matched by action. Official development assistance (ODA or simply "aid") is the principal form of public wealth transfers from rich to poor countries. For over 20 years, most of the world's wealthier donor nations have pledged to contribute at least 0.7 percent of their GDP to ODA. Very few have. Recent promises to increase ODA are welcome; the European Union countries have pledged to reach the 0.7 percent target by 2015; the US, Japan, and Canada (the only donor country to post consistent budget surpluses in the first

---

BOX 6.2:

The Millennium Development Goals

- Eradicate extreme poverty and hunger
- Achieve universal primary education
- Promote gender equality and empower women
- Reduce child mortality
- Improve maternal health
- Combat HIV/AIDS, malaria, and other diseases
- Ensure environmental sustainability
- Develop a global partnership for development

Source: United Nations. (2005). *The United Nations millennium development goals.* Retrieved from: www.un.org/millenniumgoals

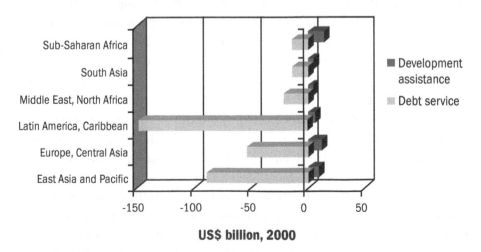

US$ billion, 2000

FIGURE 6.2: How debt service obligations dwarf development assistance

Source: Labonte et al, 2005.

five years of the new millennium) have not. Canadian aid levels are stuck at just over 0.32 percent, and in 2008 Canada ranked a dismal sixteenth place among the top donor countries (OECD Development Assistance Committee, 2009).

Fulfilling aid commitments is one essential financing plank for global health promotion. But it is insufficient in itself partly because, with the recent exception of sub-Saharan Africa, developing countries actually send to wealthy nations far more money in debt repayments than they receive in aid (see Figure 6.2). Wealthy countries began a program of debt relief in 1998 for some of the world's poorest and most indebted countries, which has freed up some funding for health and education services. But the program has been inadequate and, even with more generous debt cancellation announced at the G8 summit in the UK in 2005, will keep most developing countries trapped in a downward spiral of debt. It also requires countries receiving debt cancellation to follow the structural adjustment rules laid out by the IMF and World Bank, essentially placing their economies in the hands (and interests) of the lending nations (Labonté & Schrecker, 2006). Effective cancellation of poor countries' debts without economic strings attached (though perhaps requiring good public accountability for how the freed-up funds are used to improve health equity within a country's borders) becomes another key element of fair financing for health, as does cancellation of odious debts, which under international law are loans made when creditors know that there is no public knowledge or consent or no benefit to recipients. This often implies that the funds are used for corrupt, militaristic, or other suppressive purposes (New Economics Foundation, 2006).

Inherently global health problems, however, demand inherently global solutions. Four solutions have been suggested. The first urges greater funding for global public goods for health, such as cures for disease, control of air and water pollution, new health research, and curbing epidemics. Because such goods directly or indirectly benefit all, funding them should be based on ability to pay. The establishment of the Global Fund to Fight AIDS, Tuberculosis, and Malaria in 2000 is one example of such a good. As with aid, however, support to the fund by those countries with the ability to pay has never matched estimates of demand for its resources: in 2009 the fund cut project funding by 10 percent, delayed the next round of applications for new funding, and expressed uncertainty about future donor pledges (Anderson, 2009).

The second solution—a more radical one—urges new forms of global taxation to fund health and human development on a global scale (Leading Group on Innovative Financing to Fund Development, 2010). Such taxes include small levies on currency exchange, arms trade, carbon emissions, and international travel/jet fuel, the latter already being implemented by 29 countries and raising around $500 million annually for scaling up treatment for HIV/AIDS, tuberculosis, and malaria. The technically easiest tax (on foreign currency exchanges), sometimes called the Tobin tax, could raise over $35 billion annually at the very low rate of 0.05 percent (5 cents on every $1,000) (Leading Group on Innovative Financing to Fund Development, 2010) and considerably more at slightly higher but almost market-negligible rates. Wealthier individuals or institutions paying these taxes would scarcely notice the extra charge, while the redistributive impacts on health in poorer countries would be substantial.

The third solution calls for closure of tax-haven countries. Many of these tax havens operate under UK or US protectorate status, and are increasingly being used by MNEs and their highly paid executives to hold their wealth exempt from taxation. Between $8 trillion and $13 trillion sit in such tax havens (the low estimate comes from the IMF; the high estimate from the international Tax Justice Network). Using the low estimate and assuming a 5 percent return, taxed at 40 percent, this would raise $160 billion a year (UNRISD, 2000)—about the estimated amount required in extra financing for developing countries to reach the MDG targets. Slow progress has been made on this issue since the 2008 crisis, but nothing conclusive had been achieved yet.

The fourth solution calls for full transparency in global economic transactions. Much is made of how, despite receiving large amounts of aid, many developing countries (especially those in Africa and Haiti) continue to perform below expectations. What is not often discussed is that far more capital (wealth) flows out of such countries illicitly than flows into these countries legally. In 2006 (the most recent year for which estimates have been made) around $1 trillion fled developing countries illegally (Kar & Cartwright-Smith, 2008), about 5 percent attributed to corruption, another 31 percent to criminal activities, but fully 64 percent due to commercial pricing practices and use of tax havens (Eurodad, n.d.).

Fair Trade

Economics, while dominating global policy in a particularly selfish form during "the greediest decade in history," as Nobel Prize winner and former World Bank chief economist, Joseph Stiglitz, subtitled his book *The Roaring Nineties* (Stiglitz, 2003), is nonetheless important to global health. Trade will remain a key component. At issue are the ecological and equity implications of the current terms of global trade. Developing country mobilizations—particularly among the African nations—together with civil society analyses and campaigns, helped to reveal the hypocrisy of the early generation of WTO agreements: the slow removal of rich world subsidies to economic sectors where developing countries might have an advantage (such as agriculture); the introduction of protectionism (in the form of the TRIPS agreement), which runs counter to the notion of free trade; the preponderance of rich world delegates who dominate WTO negotiations (given the ability of wealthier nations to afford to do so); and enforcement rules (trade sanctions) that poorer countries cannot afford to use, even if they win a trade dispute (a form of cash penalty would be of much greater benefit) (Jawara & Kwa, 2003). Fair trade rules require changes in all of these areas.

But an even greater requirement is that poorer countries be extended exemptions to trade rules until they are as comparatively developed as the already wealthy players. Equal rules for unequal players only produce unequal results. There are some exemptions to WTO agreements for developing countries, referred to as "special and differential treatment." Despite repeated promises and commitments to strengthen these in trade agreements, wealthier WTO member nations—including Canada—have not supported actions to do so. Moreover, as talks stalemate in the multilateral WTO, wealthier nations (notably the US, the EU as a bloc, and even Canada) are negotiating bilateral (country to country) and regional trade treaties with small (and politically and economically weaker) developing nations, requiring more extensive forms of liberalization and intellectual property rights protection than those found in WTO agreements (Labonté, Blouin & Forman, 2010).

Fair Governance

All this imbalance demands new forms of global governance. Global governance does not imply global government. The difficulties of even modest reform at the United Nations and the significant unilateralism of the United States, even in the Obama age, makes global government, for a foreseeable future, an impossible dream (or nightmare, depending on one's point of view). But global governance, a term describing the occasional confluence of private, public, and civil society interests shaping collective actions at a global level, is now occurring. Some of the structures for this governance already exist in the WTO, the World Bank, and the IMF, but they are not yet fair or transparent. The WTO is nominally the most democratic (one country, one vote) and is becoming more transparent, although in practice the sheer economic weight of the wealthier nations still predominates. The World Bank and IMF are notorious for the secrecy of their decision-making and their undemocratic governance, in which the donor nations (those contributing to the institutions' funding) have voting privileges commensurate to the amount they give. A key reform plank long advocated by developing countries and civil society groups has been to shift the balance of power within these institutions toward developing countries, which is only now beginning (slightly) to occur in the wake of the 2008 global financial crisis.

Other governance efforts are controversial, such as the increase in "global public-private-partnerships," in which large MNEs participate in policy-making at the UN or its agencies alongside member nations. The driving force behind these "3-Ps"—which also exist and confound public policy-making within national borders—is the simple need for more money to deliver programs, although, as seen above, fairer forms of taxation could also meet this need without ceding increased influence or authority to the private sector (Deacon, 2003). The gradual incursion of peak civil society groups within these global policy circles holds some hope for more balanced discussions, though the risk that these groups become another form of elites far removed from the lives of those they claim to better is real and not unfamiliar to health promoters well versed in the dynamics of local community organizing.

There have been some successes in fair global health governance, in which Canadians can take legitimate pride. One of these was the creation of the *Framework Convention on Tobacco Control*, described as the world's first global public health treaty. The convention is now in force, and requires countries to adopt a number of measures on advertising, marketing, warning labels, and smoking restrictions. The idea was instigated by Canadians at the World Health Assembly, and strongly supported by Canadian health activists during its lengthy negotiating phase (Lencucha, Labonté & Rouse, 2010). It is weaker than activists wanted (the convention, for example, does not explicitly state that its protocols would trump trade rules)—and there are concerns over how it might be enforced (Fidler, 2002). Whether the experience of the convention can generalize to other global health governance issues is debatable, but it does show that it is possible.

That possibility, in many ways, was created by and fuels the new global social movements for health. I argued in 1994 that health promotion (then) was an embodiment of and response to the knowledge challenges of (then) progressive social movements (Labonté, 1994). The nascent practice of global health promotion is similarly a product of new civil society configurations:

- the World Social Forum, the populist and immensely popular alternative to the elite World Economic Forum
- a multiplicity of international groups that have long campaigned on specific issues, such as Health Action International and its anti-drug-monopoly work, the Infant Feeding Action Coalition and its boycott of companies violating an internationally agreed marketing code for infant formula, and MSF's Access to Essential Medicines Campaign
- a new, integrating group: the People's Health Movement (PHM), a growing global coalition of health activists supporting each other in national and international campaigns. The PHM, in its first five years, has convened two global assemblies, created and lobbied several declarations and charters, worked with the World Health Organization and its 2005–2008 Commission on the Social Determinants of Health, helped to produce *Global Health Watch 2005–2006* and *Global Health Watch 2,* equity-oriented and activist-motivated "alternative world health reports," and launched a global "right to health campaign" in 2005 (see Box 6.3)

In sum, there is no absence of opportunity for global health promotion activism.

BOX 6.3:

The Right to Health

The human right to health is embodied in a variety of international declarations, covenants, and plans of action. Most notably, Article 12 of the *International Covenant on Economic, Social, and Cultural Rights* (ICESCR) proclaims "the right of everyone to the enjoyment of the highest attainable standard of physical and mental health," and specifically obligates states parties to ensure "provision for the reduction of the stillbirth-rate and of infant mortality and for the healthy development of the child; the improvement of all aspects of environmental and industrial hygiene; the prevention, treatment and control of epidemic, endemic, occupational and other diseases; and the creation of conditions which would assure to all medical service and medical attention in the event of sickness." One hundred and fifty countries, including Canada, are states parties to the covenant. Although state obligations are limited to the "progressive realization" of this right in view of available resources, all states must show measurable progress toward its full realization. States parties to the ICESCR must also "respect" the right to health in other countries, partly by ensuring that other agreements into which they enter "do not adversely impact upon the right to health" (para. 39). They are also obliged to "protect" against infringements of this right by third parties such as corporations, and to "fulfill" the right in other countries through international assistance and co-operation (para. 38–41).

Source: Office of the United Nations High Commissioner for Human Rights. (1966). *The international covenant on economic, social, and cultural rights.* Retrieved from: www2.ohchr.org/english/law/cescr.htm

---

BOX 6.4:
_____

Canada's Global Health Promotion Contributions Past and Future

Canada has played a formative role in many of the civil society actions that are improving global health. A coalition of Canadian groups helped block the unpopular *Multilateral Agreement on Investment* in the 1990s, sparking a global movement critical of the form of contemporary trade agreements. Canada has helped to nurture public health associations around the world, strengthening their ability to engage in healthy public policy. We were leaders in the *Framework Convention on Tobacco Control* and also created another new global convention on national autonomy to protect cultural diversity. More recently, we became strong financial supporters of the World Health Organization's Commission on Social Determinants of Health, whose "knowledge network" on globalization was based at the University of Ottawa. But our foreign policy for health is still weak on several counts:

1. In the decade since the first edition of this book, Canada's aid contributions experienced the steepest decline among all donor countries. It's now starting to rise again, but there is no fiscal reason why we cannot immediately move to the 0.7 percent of GNI target. Doing so would cost only one-third to one-sixth of the value of the tax cuts promised in the 2003 budget (Canada Department of Finance, 2003; OECD Development Assistance Committee, 2005). Canada more recently led the G8 in pledging new financial support to maternal health (the so-called Muskoka Initiative, named after the 2010 G8 Summit hosted by Canada). But the aid monies Canada committed to this initiative (up to $1 billion over several years) will come at the cost of other development assistance programs since the federal government also announced that the aid budget will be frozen at 2010 levels for the next several years.

2. Even as we work to prevent tobacco use in Canada, we are still inviting Canadian tobacco farmers and industries to join Team Canada and Team Ontario trade missions to developing countries. End this hypocrisy.

3. Our federal government years ago passed a resolution supporting the currency transaction tax, useful for funding global health initiatives and dampening speculative foreign investments that can damage national economies. But Canada never acted upon it. Now is a good time, as international support for such a tax is rising.

4. While we have given better market access to products from the world's least developed countries, we haven't supported strengthening their exemptions from trade rules until they become economically stronger. Fair trade is not the same as free trade.

5. The IMF requires poor indebted countries to keep their public sector spending within a tight limit to maintain "macroeconomic equilibrium." This policy is forcing many of their health professionals to leave and risks preventing these countries from accepting the global funds needed to cope with HIV and other pandemic diseases. Canada can become an outspoken advocate against these and other health-damaging economic policies.

Conclusions

But there are also only so many hours in a day, and a seemingly intractable morass of global health problems. It would be nice to offer a simple prescription for transforming what is toxic in contemporary globalization, allowing its healthful potential (the idealization of the global village) to flourish. But there are no easy remedies, despite the abundance of policy options and entry points. The perennial difficulty is creating that ephemeral beast called "political will." For better or worse, this "will" remains locked behind borders. A curious irony in creating fairer forms of global governance is that it relies upon the choices of individual nation-states. This irony nonetheless opens an opportunity for lobbying and activism by health promoters within their own countries, adopting actions or utilizing strategies with which they are not unfamiliar. For instance:

- We can align ourselves with the local chapter or organizations of the larger global social movements for health and justice. Just as our advocacy has helped to push local health issues into local political arenas, it can help to prod global health issues into national ones, but not if we attempt it alone.

- We can build empowering health promotion partnerships that link poorer nations with wealthier ones. Many of these already exist, partly through the funding mechanism of ODA, or through the new proliferation of international public-private partnerships for health, such as the Global Fund. Many of these new initiatives suffer the same "top-down" problem of early health promotion, with a focus on specific diseases, treatments, or behaviour change without sufficient attention to the social and economic determinants of these diseases. Many health promoters are skilled in good "bottom-up" and more empowering development approaches that can be diffused through these global partnerships. Look for opportunities, and seize them.

- We can enter the growing debates over how globalization enhances or imperils global health equity. We might do this as individuals, or by joining global social movements, or by ensuring our professional associations take strong, evidence-based positions on how globalization should change to improve health outcomes. Health promotion has developed some useful tools over the past years that can be harnessed to issues central to contemporary globalization, such as applying the techniques of health impact assessment to trade or ODA policies, using capacity-building forms of evaluation to health projects funded through ODA or the new global health partnerships, or working with our national health ministries to promote more international health "laws" like the *Framework Convention on Tobacco Control* (the obesity pandemic is a good next target).

- We need to inject this work with the idealism that made the early days of the healthy cities/healthy communities programs so compelling. Envisioning how we want to live is as important as analyzing why we are not yet doing so. We are not living in "the best of all possible worlds." TINA—There Is No Alternative—is simply disempowering propaganda. It is not "the end of history" in which Western economic liberalism settles in for an unmovable eternity (which, given its environmental appetite, will not last long anyway). We need to rekindle an ethical social imaginary.

As health promoters in a new millennium, the most disturbing implication of globalization may be that it forces us to confront the fundamental fallacy of our field: promoting the physical and mental health of individuals whose well-being rests, in part, on economic practices that are today's equivalent of logging the last Easter Island tree is morally unacceptable and, from an intergenerational health vantage, indefensible.

What are we to say and to do about that?

Notes

1. In recent years these figures have been revised to $1.25 and $2.50 per day to reflect the increased cost of consumer goods around the world. The adjectives of abject, and near-abject, poverty, however, are still cogent.
2. The group of eight leading industrialized nations: Canada, France, Germany, Italy, Japan, Russia, the US, and the UK (with special participation from the European Union). The G8 holds annual summits that formalize economic policies among themselves; by virtue of their combined economic size and dominance in multilateral organizations, these essentially become global economic policies for the rest of the world.

References

Anderson, T. (27 February 2009). Charities hedge their bets on funding. *The Guardian Weekly*, p. 45.

Canada Department of Finance. (2003). *The Budget Plan 2003*, Table A1.9. Ottawa: Department of Finance.

Chang, H.J. (2002). *Kicking away the ladder: Development strategy in historical perspective*. London: Anthem Press.

Cornia, G.A. (Ed.). (2004). *Inequality, growth, and poverty in the era of liberalization and globalization*. Oxford: Oxford University Press.

Cornia, G.A. & Court, J. (2001). *Inequality, growth and poverty in the era of liberalization and globalization*. Wider Policy Brief no. 4. Retrieved from: http://www.wider.unu.edu/publications/policy-briefs/en_GB/pb4/

Deacon, B. (2003). Global social governance reform: From institutions and policies to networks, projects, and partnerships. In B. Deacon, E. Ollila, M. Koivusalo & P. Stubbs (Eds.), *Global social governance: Themes and prospects* (pp. 11–35). Helsinki: Globalism and Social Policy Programme.

Dollar, D. (2001). *Globalization, inequality, and poverty since 1980*. Washington: World Bank.

Durano, M. (2002). *Foreign direct investment and its impact on gender relations: Women in development Europe*. WIDE Information Sheet. Retrieved from: http://www.wide-network.org/index.jsp?id=365.

Eurodad. (n.d.). *Capital flight diverts development finance*. Retrieved from: http://www.eurodad.org/uploadedFiles/Whats_New/Reports/factsheet_capitalflight08.pdf

Fidler, D. (2002). *Global health governance: Overview of the role of international law in protecting and promoting global public health*. WHO Global Health Governance Discussion paper no. 3. Geneva: World Health Organization.

International Labour Organization. (2009). *Global employment trends 2009*. Geneva: ILO.

Jawara, F. & Kwa, E. (2003). *Behind the scenes at the WTO: The real world of international trade negotiations*. London: Zed Books.

Junne, G.C.A. (2001). International organizations in a period of globalization: New (problems of) legitimacy. In J.M. Coicaud & V. Heiskanen (Eds.), *The legitimacy of international organizations* (pp. 189–220). Tokyo: United Nations University Press.

Kahn, J. & Yardley, J. (2004, August 1). Amid China's boom, no helping hand for young Qingming. *New York Times* late edition, p. 1.

Kar, D. & Cartwright-Smith, D. (2008). *Illicit financial flows from developing countries 2002–2006*. Global Financial Integrity. Retrieved from: http://ec.europa.eu/development/services/events/tax_development/docs/td_gfi.pdf

Labonté, R. (1994). Death of program, birth of metaphor: The development of health promotion in Canada. In A. Pederson, M. O'Neill & I. Rootman (Eds.), *Health promotion in Canada* (pp. 72–90). Toronto: W.B. Saunders.

Labonté, R., Blouin, C. & Forman, L. (2010). *Trade, growth, and population health: An introductory review*. Ottawa: Collection d'études transdisciplinaires en santé des populations/Transdisciplinary Studies in Population Health Series. 2010. ISSN 1922-1398. Retrieved from: http://www.iph.uottawa.ca/eng/transdis/files/trade-health.pdf

Labonté, R. & Schrecker, T. (2006). The G8 and global health: What now? What next? *Canadian Journal of Public Health, 97*(1), 32–34.

Labonté, R., Schrecker, T. & Sen Gupta, A. (2005). *Health for some: Death, disease, and disparity in a globalizing era.* Toronto: CSJ Research and Education.

Leading Group on Innovative Financing to Fund Development. (2010). *Globalizing solidarity: The case for financial levies.* Paris: Taskforce on International Financial Transactions for Development. Retrieved from: http://www.leadinggroup.org/IMG/pdf_Financement_innovants_web_def.pdf

Lee, K. (2003). *Globalization and health: An introduction.* London: Palgrave Macmillan.

Lencucha, R., Labonté, R. & Rouse, M. (2010). Beyond idealism and realism: Canadian NGO/government relations during the negotiation of the FCTC. *Journal of Public Health Policy 31*(1), 74–87.

Marmot, M. & Bell, R. (2009). How will the financial crisis affect health? *BMJ, 338,* 858–860.

Milward, B. (2000). What is structural adjustment? In G. Mohan, E. Brown, B. Milward & A.B. Zack-Williams (Eds.), *Structural adjustment: Theory, practice, and impacts* (pp. 24–38). London & New York: Routledge.

New Economics Foundation. (2006). *Odious lending: Debt relief as if morals mattered.* Retrieved from http://www.neweconomics.org/sites/neweconomics.org/files/Odious_Lending.pdf

NewScientist.com. (2003). *European heatwave caused 35,000 deaths.* Retrieved from: www.heatisonline.org/contentserver/objecthandlers/index.cfm?id=4485&method=full

O'Brien, R. (2002). Organizational politics, multilateral economic organizations, and social policy. *Global Social Policy, 2,* 141–162.

OECD Development Assistance Committee. (2005). Development co-operation 2004 report. *DAC Journal, 6*(1).

OECD Development Assistance Committee. (2009). *Development aid at its highest level ever in 2008.* Retrieved from: http://www.oecd.org/dataoecd/47/52/42458612.pdf

Overseas Development Institute. (2009). *Children in times of economic crisis: Past lessons, future policies.* Background Note, March. London: ODI.

Plumb, C. (2003). Climate change death toll put at 150,000. December 11, 2003: Reuters. Retrieved from: www.commondreams.org/headlines03/1211-13.htm

Rodriguez, F. & Rodrik, D. (2000). Trade policy and economic growth: A skeptic's guide to the cross-national evidence. Discussion paper no. 2143. London: Centre for Economic Policy Research.

Stiglitz, J. (2003). *The roaring nineties.* New York: Penguin Books.

UNRISD. (2000). *Visible hands: Taking responsibility for social development.* Geneva: United Nations Research Institute for Social Development.

Wade, R.H. (2004). Is globalization reducing poverty and inequality? *World Development, 32*(4), 567–589.

Woodward, D., Drager, N., Beaglehole, R. & Lipson, D. (2001). Globalization and health: A framework for analysis and action. *Bulletin of the World Health Organization, 79,* 875–881.

World Bank. (1993). *World development report 1993: Investing in health.* New York: Oxford University Press.

World Bank. (2009). *The global economic crisis: Assessing vulnerability with a poverty lens.* Washington: The World Bank.

World Health Organization. (2004). *Summary of probable SARS cases with onset of illness from November 1, 2002 to July 31, 2003.* Retrieved from: www.who.int/csr/sars/country/table2004_04_21/en/index.html

World Health Organization. (2005). *The Bangkok Charter for health promotion.* Retrieved from: www.who.int/healthpromotion/conferences/6gchp/bangkok_charter/en/index.html

World Health Organization Commission on Macroeconomics and Health. (2001). *Macroeconomics and health: Investing in health for economic development.* Geneva: World Health Organization. Retrieved from: http://www.cid.harvard.edu/archive/cmh/

Wright, R. (2004). *A short history of progress.* Toronto: House of Anansi Press.

Critical Thinking Questions

1. What are some of the ways in which contemporary globalization might affect your own health?
2. Is a return to nationalism (a retreat from globalization) something that will be healthier for people?
3. Should we develop global rules for multinational enterprises—and the smaller companies from which they source their materials—to ensure healthier and fairer working conditions? Or are voluntary codes enough?
4. How can we promote the idea of global health equity?
5. Are there other steps Canadian health promoters can take to reduce global inequalities in health?

Resources

Further Readings

Labonté, R., Schrecker, T., Packer, C. & Runnels, V. (Eds.). (2009). *Globalization and health: Pathways, evidence, and policy.* London: Routledge.

This book is a consolidation of 12 extensive background papers and a final report on various aspects of globalization as a health determinant, prepared by the Globalization Knowledge Network of the World Health Organization's Commission on Social Determinants of Health. Half of the book's chapters are now free online at www.globalhealthequity.ca, where a link also takes one to all of the background research papers. The site also has links to numerous other articles and reports on global health.

Labonté, R., Schrecker, T. & Sen Gupta, A. (2005). *Health for some: Death, disease, and disparity in a globalizing era.* Toronto: Centre for Social Justice.

This short book uses the stories of four people's lives from around the world to unpack how contemporary globalization creates both health risks and opportunities. It concludes with a discussion of viable policy options for a healthier globalization. Available online at: www.socialjustice.org.

Lee, K. (2003). *Globalization and health: An introduction.* London: Palgrave Macmillan.

As the title suggests, this short text provides an introductory overview of globalization and health. It is particularly useful for its focus, global health policy.

People's Health Movement, Medact, Global Equity Gauge Alliance, UNISA Press & Zed Books. (2005). *Global health watch 2005–2006: An alternative world health report.* London: Zed Books and *Global Health Watch 2* (2008).

The product of hundreds of health activists and organizations around the world, these two volumes examine health in a globalizing world, with foci on health systems and vulnerable populations, development assistance and migration, and global health governance. An entire multi-chapter section is devoted to holding countries and multinational institutions accountable for improving global health. Available online at: www.ghwatch.org.

UNDP Human Development Report 2005. (2005). *International cooperation at a crossroads: Aid, trade, and security in an unequal world.* New York: Oxford University Press.

Each year the UNDP issues its annual report, with its landmark *Human Development Index.* Its 2005 report became another landmark by focusing on the major economic problems that create barriers to human (and hence health) development and what can be done about them. The report also includes up-to-date global statistics on health and its many determinants.

Relevant Websites

Canadian Coalition on Global Health Research

www.ccghr.ca

Research is only one of many pathways to improving global health, but it is an important one. The Canadian Coalition was formed on the fateful day of 9/11 (quite by chance) and is committed to harnessing global health research evidence to policy action.

Canadian Society for International Health

www.csih.org

The CSIH is a non-governmental organization that undertakes international health promotion activities and other health development projects around the world. It also hosts an annual international health conference in the fall, one of the best ways for health promoters interested in global health to learn and network.

Global Health Watch

www.ghwatch.org

This site provides up-to-date information on global health campaigns, solicits inputs for future Global Health Watches, and offers useful advice and materials for global health promoting campaigners.

Globalization and Health

www.globalizationandhealth.com

This open access journal publishes important, peer-reviewed research and commentary.

People's Health Movement

www.phmovement.org

The PHM is an activist group dedicated to the cause of "health for all" through a combination of national actions and international mobilizations. Its *People's Charter for Health* is the most widely publicized, translated, and endorsed statement on international health since the *Alma-Ata Declaration on Primary Health Care.*

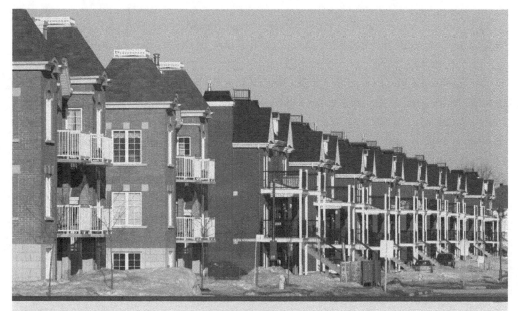

PART II

Addressing Issues, Populations, and Settings through Health Promotion

The second section of the book includes five chapters and looks at health promotion practice using three of the classical entry points used to develop interventions in the field: issues, populations, and settings. In Chapter 7, which opens the section, Frohlich, Poland, and Shareck revisit a chapter of the second edition that influenced the editors' decision to centre the third one on practice. Making a critique of how each of these entry points has its strengths but also its shortcomings, the chapter helps to realize the types of assumptions, often taken for granted, on which most interventions are based. They also offer a proposal, with their concept of "collective lifestyle," to go one step further and develop practices in an innovative way.

This chapter provided the editors with a framework to look at concrete practices in Canadian health promotion. They thus selected, for each entry point, a set of topics that seemed to represent the state of the art of current practice in the country. They then selected contributors for each topic, trying as much as was feasible to have teams representing the anglophone and francophone experiences, as well as diverse perspectives. These teams were asked to produce short contributions, including the overall situation of the interventions on that topic and providing at least one example of a "promising practice." The four other chapters of the section, which were written specifically for this third edition, thus provide a very significant sample of how health promotion is currently practised in Canada.

In Chapter 8, coordinated by Rootman, key *issues* are addressed. Stachenko and Riley first look at how chronic disease, which accounts for most of the burden of disease in Canada, can be approached using a health promoting perspective. Ardiles and Provencher then look at how mental health promotion can deal with one of the most alarming health-related issues in modern societies. After that, Gillis and Kaszap take up health literacy, a recent but increasingly popular issue in the field, and present how it can be best addressed to promote the health of people. Finally, in our era of global warming and other preoccupying ecological issues, Hancock discusses how sustainable development and health promotion can be allies not only at the global, national, or provincial levels, but also at the local level, which is easier to work at for most practitioners.

Chapter 9, coordinated by Pederson, looks at various populations frequently targeted by health promotion programs. The first contribution describes an innovative research program supported by the Mental Health Commission of Canada. Frankish and colleagues argue that the "housing first" approach, exemplified in the At Home-Chez Soi program, supports individuals with mental illness to stabilize by dealing with issues of shelter first and using that as a base for linking to other services to manage their illness, income, employment, and other needs. Edwards and Plouffe address the importance of health promotion among older adults and provide a current example of a global and Canadian initiative called "age-friendly cities," which, using health promotion principles, attempts to make cities and rural communities more supportive of seniors and of active and healthy aging. In the context of Canadian multiculturalism, where the impact of immigration always gets more and more significant, how to promote health appropriately in increasingly diverse ethnocultural populations is discussed by Vissandjée and colleagues to demonstrate the value of targeting and tailoring approaches to health promotion within migrant communities. They identify two promising practices that address both structural and individual determinants of health in ways that recognize the distinctiveness of specific migrant communities and their experiences. The final contribution, by Nancy Poole and Tatiana Fraser, describes the model of programming offered through groups affiliated with the Girls Action Foundation network. The model that frames their programs is explicitly feminist and empowering; it starts where girls are and offers them support in developing leadership skills and media literacy while addressing health issues such as sexual health and gendered violence. Together, these four contributions illustrate the importance of working with a deeply contextualized understanding of a particular population in order to support their agency in identifying and addressing their own health promotion priorities while simultaneously working on the factors that constrain their capacity to address systemic barriers to change.

In Chapter 10, Reading and Reading outline an Aboriginal approach to health promotion to complement the Western approach that dominates in Canada and illustrate it in action through four promising initiatives grounded in the distinct cultural concepts, contexts, and approaches of their respective Aboriginal communities. These are: a diabetes prevention program in Kahnawake; a cross-jurisdictional collaboration between five First Nation communities as well as local health authorities and Dalhousie University to create an Indigenous model of primary health care; a food initiative in northern Canada that includes a food mail program and a community freezer program; and a Saskatchewan stroke-related outreach and services intervention to health care providers in Aboriginal communities. According to Reading and Reading, Aboriginal health promotion entails "two-eyed seeing"—that is, recognizing and addressing the differences in Indigenous and Western approaches to health promotion and understanding the importance of the political, social, cultural, and historical determinants of Aboriginal peoples' health.

Chapter 11, coordinated by O'Neill, looks at *settings*, the third entry point proposed by Frohlich and her colleagues. The first set of locations for which the settings approach to health promotion were developed in the mid-1980s—municipal entities, be it a city, a village, or even a community—is discussed by Simard, Sasseville, Mucha, Losier, and McCue. Following this, the school as a setting is taken up by McCall, Deschesnes, and Laitch, who show how the settings approach has thoroughly transformed traditional school health programs in a more comprehensive healthy schools strategy. Lagarde and Hancock then discuss how another type of setting, the *health care facility* (especially the hospital), has taken up the challenge to become health promoting. Health promotion at the workplace is then analyzed by Pelletier and Shain, and, in the last section, Stirling and Niquette look at a new but increasingly important set of settings in people's lives: the Internet and other virtual venues.

At the end of this second section, the reader should have a good idea of how the practice of health promotion is currently organized in Canada, as well as of the positive but also problematic sides of such a situation. The numerous "promising practices" described should also have provided inspiring ideas and examples to eventually develop or modify one's specific interventions.

CHAPTER 7

Contrasting Entry Points for Intervention in Health Promotion Practice:

Situating and Working with Context

Katherine L. Frohlich, Blake Poland, and Martine Shareck

Introduction

Historically there have been three main entry points for intervention in health promotion practice: (1) issues, (2) specific population groups, and (3) settings. Each approach reflects different assumptions about what shapes health, what is most important, and what can most feasibly be changed. Concomitantly, each has singled out different aspects of analysis and intervention. In all three approaches the social context has some relevance and importance to what they do, yet in different ways.

We begin by giving a brief description of each of the three traditional approaches to intervention. We then briefly outline how each of these approaches has grappled with the notion of the social context, discussing their strengths and weaknesses. We conclude with a suggestion of a fourth potential entry point for health promotion research and practice.

Issues, Specific Population Groups, and Settings as Points of Health Promotion Intervention

Issues

The *Ottawa Charter for Health Promotion* (World Health Organization, 1986) set the stage for health promotion practice as we understand it today. The scope of the *Ottawa Charter* was broad, covering five large areas of action and multiple conditions and resources for health. Progressives within the movement lauded the expanded focus and attention to prerequisites to health, foundational social determinants, and community involvement. Nevertheless, for reasons (of perceived feasibility, political expediency, vested interests, etc.) that remain poorly articulated, the emerging personal wellness industry, large bureaucracies oriented to health education, and (in the main) the North American public, were not so easily dissuaded from a deep cultural and institutional commitment to individualism. As a result, "developing personal skills" was one of the areas identified in the *Charter* that continued to receive the lion's share of funding, research, and public attention in the decades that followed its release. Within the *Charter*, developing personal skills was described as being possible through "providing information, education for health, and enhancing life skills. By so doing, it increases the options available to people to exercise more control over their own health and their environments, and to make choices conducive to health" (World Health Organization, 1986, p. 3).

Prior to the *Ottawa Charter*, and definitively since then, health promotion practice has been dedicated to developing these personal skills in three major ways: (1) by focusing on a reduction in the prevalence and incidence of those diseases seen to be burdening the population the most (cardiovascular disease, diabetes, and HIV/AIDS); (2) by focusing on the reduction of *risk factors*, especially health behaviours linked to prevalent health problems facing the population (such as smoking, poor eating habits, lack of exercise, lack of condom use); and (3) by reducing *risk conditions* such as homelessness, which is neither a disease nor a health behaviour. Even so, the overwhelming focus since the *Ottawa Charter* has continued to be on the reduction of health lifestyle habits such as smoking, poor diet, lack of exercise, and risky sexual behaviour through information and education programs. A larger focus on increasing the options available to people to exercise more control over their own health and their environments in order to reduce disease prevalence, incidence, and risk conditions has been, for the most part, more evident in rhetoric than in practice.

The focus on risk factors in health promotion interventions has a protracted history stemming from health promotion's historical roots in epidemiology and health education, as well as the influence of the Lalonde Report (Lalonde 1974). It is well known that what we measure (and how) at the problem identification and needs assessment stage has a profound impact on subsequent phases of program development, implementation, and evaluation. Tannahill (1992) describes the fundamental role that epidemiology plays for health promotion in identifying and prioritizing prevalent health problems and their causes. First, and most obviously, programs and interventions are oriented to address the problems highlighted in epidemiological studies. So, for instance, the focus on cardiovascular disease, diabetes, or HIV/AIDS, driven by epidemiologic studies, has created great impetus for health promotion programs to address these issues. Second, epidemiologists derive categories of risk factors associated with these health problems, which, if prevented, are presumed to reduce illness and death (Frohlich & Potvin, 1999). These risk factors are then often directly translated into health promotion programs. Because many of these risk factors (high blood pressure, overweight, and risky sexual behaviour) are seen to be modifiable through behaviours (dietary changes, exercise, condom use), the focus of health promotion has often been more on the proximal (those factors most directly related to the health outcome in question), and supposedly most modifiable, individual-level risk factors.

Lalonde's contribution to the framing of health promotion interventions is also significant (Lalonde, 1974). Lalonde's report recommended that public health interventions focus attention on the segment of the population with the highest level of risk exposure as indicated by health risk behaviours (e.g., smoking, alcohol consumption) or biological markers (e.g., body mass index, blood pressure). In this way, interventions became focused on what were termed populations "at risk" or groups showing elevated risk for some disease.

As a result of both epidemiology's and Lalonde's focus on individual-level risk factor reduction, health promotion drew on individual-level theories to guide the creation of its intervention programs. These understandings come largely from models of social psychology such as the health belief model (Becker, 1974), Bandura's social cognitive theory (Bandura, 1986), and Ajzen and Fishbein's theory of reasoned action (1980). All focused attention on the major biomedical and behavioural risk factors for developing the major health problems of concern at the time. Underlying these models is the assumption that population prevalence of adverse risk conditions are modifiable by providing education and behaviour-change tools to individuals to help them achieve lifestyle changes (Barnett et al., 2005).

Specific Population Groups

A second major entry point of intervention in health promotion, focusing on specific population groups, has largely sought to target particular groups thought to share certain key characteristics. These characteristics are frequently thought to predispose certain groups to be at greater risk for "suboptimal" health outcomes.

The main advantage of this approach is that it provides an opportunity to see how behaviours cluster within populations. This approach also fits structurally with how many organizations (governmental and non-governmental) and funding bodies are organized, with separate structures for Aboriginal health, organizations working with the homeless, the elderly, etc.

To illustrate interventions by populations, we draw on the example of Aboriginal peoples in Canada (Adelson, 2005; Frohlich et al., 2006). Aboriginal peoples are a diverse group of many tribes, languages, and cultures, but they all share a common experience of colonization and all that this has entailed (forced resettlement, residential schools, removal of ancestral lands, violations of treaty rights, rights to minimum services defined according to governmental arbitration of who qualifies as status or non-status Indians, and so forth). The resultant cultural upheaval, family and community breakdown, sedentarization, disrupted connection to the land, etc., has had severe consequences in terms of community and individual mental, social, spiritual, and physical health (examples of the outcomes include issues of addiction, diabetes, suicide and HIV/AIDS). Aboriginal leaders have long fought against the dominant Western cultural paradigm's tendency to blame the victim (labelling Aboriginal peoples as lazy, stupid, backwards, or uneducated) and to advocate instead for an understanding that places current community health problems in their proper historical context (as impacts of colonization, institutional racism, etc.).

Settings

Settings where people live, work, and play are a third entry point for intervention in health promotion practice (Poland, Green & Rootman, 2000). Settings can be defined as "the place or social context in which people engage in daily activities in which environmental, organizational and personal factors interact to affect health and well-being" (Nutbeam, 1998, p. 14). We describe two conceptualizations of settings. The first views them as physically bounded entities with a given organizational structure and within which "captive" target populations (for health promotion intervention) can be found. In practice, this conceptualization of settings has been associated with individually focused health promotion activities such as mass media campaigns, health education, and personal skills development aiming to directly change people's behaviours (Richard et al., 1996; Whitelaw et al., 2001; Dooris, 2004). Examples include stress reduction programming in the workplace or nutrition education programs in schools to promote healthy eating among pupils. It is not difficult to see the administrative appeal of using settings in this way to reach conveniently "captive" audiences for intervention (Whitelaw et al., 2001), negotiating entry through organizational leaders (rather than the messier dynamics of outreach in community settings).

A second conceptualization of settings sees them as open and dynamic systems (Dooris, 2004, 2009) and has three main characteristics. First, it is based on an ecological model of health (Figure 7.1), which assumes that differences in levels of health are influenced by an interaction between personal, interpersonal, organizational, community, and policy factors, an interaction that unfolds over the life course of individuals, families, and communities (McLeroy et al., 1988; Stokols, 1996; Smedley & Syme, 2000; see also Chapter 5).

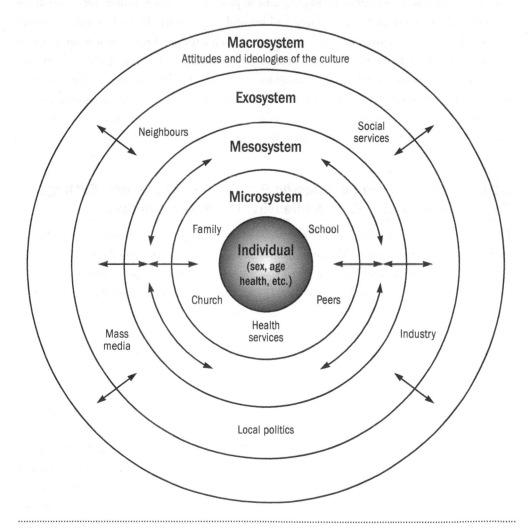

Figure 7.1: Adaptation of Bronfenbrenner's Ecological Model

Source: Adapted by McLaren, L. & Hawe, P. (2005). Ecological perspectives in health research. *Journal of Epidemiology and Community Health, 59,* 6–14.

Second, it involves a systems perspective that implies settings are comprised of multiple components (individuals and structures) that constantly interact with one another, creating a whole that is more complex than the sum of its parts (Dooris, 2006; Dooris et al., 2007). Third, this perspective involves a whole system development and change approach. This means that focus must be on changing the whole setting's organization and structure, as opposed to changing only the individuals found within it (St. Leger, 1997; Dooris, 2006, 2009). Viewing settings as systems also implies that the experiences of individuals inside a given setting (e.g., a school) are influenced by their experiences in other settings (e.g., the household or community) (Dooris, 2004).

A major advantage of this systems perspective is that interventions focus not so much on the individuals changing their behaviour but on changing the setting itself to be more health-enhancing. This includes policies and programs to provide the opportunities for populations to change their practices, but it extends well beyond this as well. To build on the example presented above, promoting healthy eating not only requires nutritional education, but also policies to improve access to affordable healthy foods. Similarly, increasing physical activity requires access to playgrounds, parks, and green spaces. In addition, by altering the structural and social conditions that shape individual health behaviours, interventions on settings viewed as systems assist not only in reducing the risk for those currently at risk, but simultaneously reduce the risk of future generations (Smedley & Syme, 2000).

Why Focusing on Issues, Specific Population Groups, and Settings Can Come up Short When Addressing the Social Context

Thus far we have documented three traditional main entry points of intervention in health promotion practice. We have addressed some of their successes and described some of the ways in which each of these addresses the social context. However, the premise of this chapter is that in their own ways each comes up short when it comes to addressing social context. In this section we explore and illustrate how that might be the case and we offer some suggestions for how this could be more fully addressed.

Issues and Social Context: Some Limitations

With regard to an issue-based approach, one of the most substantiated critiques of the "developing personal skills" approach to health promotion practice has been that individually based models of behaviour change have often yielded disappointing results. For example, in the Multiple Risk Factor Intervention Trial (MRFIT), 6,000 men, all of whom were in the top 10–15 percent risk group in the United States due to their high rates of cigarette smoking, hypertension, and hyper-cholesterol levels, were enrolled in a six-year intervention program. The intervention was state-of-the-art: well funded, well staffed, and used the best behaviour-change techniques available. Even so, the results were disappointing: 62 percent of the men were still smoking after the six-year period, 50 percent still had hypertension, and few men had changed their dietary patterns (Multiple Risk Factor Intervention Trial Research Group, 1981, 1982).[1]

Among the many reflections on the MRFIT experience, one has been that the gains are short-lived because new smokers are continually being recruited into lifelong addiction by a combination of tobacco industry tactics, media, and structural conditions of poverty and hardship. The underlying problem with the high-risk behaviour modification approach, if one is truly interested in sustained population change, is that it does not address what has been termed the "fundamental causes" (Link & Phelan, 1995). The concept of fundamental causes posits that one has to understand the factors, as well as the mechanisms, that put people at risk in the first place (that is, the social context), and not just focus on risk factors alone.

Specific Population Groups and Social Context: Some Limitations

An important critique of interventions concerned with specific populations is that they focus on the higher exposure of these populations to a specific risk factor or disease outcome, thus dealing only with one risk factor or disease at a time. But groups at higher risk of some diseases are typically at higher risk of others also. At issue are not just the specific risk factor exposures for a single disease, but the *patterning* of exposure across many factors that predispose some groups to be routinely more vulnerable than others. In other words, the question to be asked is: Why are these groups more at risk for a wide range of risk factors and diseases than others?

To address this, it has been suggested that interventions be developed using the heuristic of "vulnerable" populations (Frohlich & Potvin, 2008). "Vulnerable" populations differ from specific population groups in that, due to their position in the social strata, they are commonly exposed to contextual conditions that distinguish them from the rest of the population. As such, what defines vulnerable populations are shared social characteristics generated by non-random distributions of material and social conditions. These characteristics have their roots in power relations structured in society to create cleavages along race, class, and gendered lines (Grabb, 2002) as key enduring features of the social context (Poland et al., 2006, 2008). This involves the structured relationships between what Saul Alinsky (1971) would call the "haves" and the "have-nots" and involves the power that operates through control over material, ideological, and human resources (Grabb, 2002). In this sense, the label of "vulnerability" may be inappropriate as it could be seen to be blaming the victim (vulnerability is understood as a property of those so labelled), whereas the term "marginalized" more clearly names the issue of marginalization (shifts the implied blame to those responsible for marginalization).

Settings and Social Context: Some Limitations

In relation to interventions focused on settings, a major limitation of those based on the first conceptualization of settings resides in their targeting individual health issues (such as diabetes or healthy eating) in one setting at a time (such as the school or workplace), and promoting individual behaviour change without attending to healthfulness of the setting itself (Poland et al., 2000). This can lead to "blaming the victim" or to interventions that potentially aggravate the situation of the worst off (Frohlich et al., 2010). In fact, it is increasingly acknowledged that behaviour change needs to be supported by environmental conditions that favour its emergence and maintenance. If a setting's structures are not modified to accommodate change, it may be difficult for individuals to sustain behaviour change once they are outside the targeted setting (Dooris, 2004). A systems perspective on settings may contribute to overcoming this limitation by harnessing the social context defined through both a setting's structure and the individuals found within it (Poland, Frohlich & Cargo, 2008). This more complex conceptualization of settings and related interventions is more challenging to translate in practice. More importantly, action on settings, even action that seeks to make settings themselves more health-enhancing, is rarely informed by a deeper social analysis of the intersectionality of race/class/gender/ableism, the myriad ways in which inequity is sustained and reproduced in and through interpersonal and institutional practices, as well as extra-local policy and practice (see Chapter 4).

A number of established theoretical approaches offer potentially useful insights into these issues. For example, *complexity theory* can contribute to our understanding of the settings' complex nature and provide us with change theories that go beyond those of planned and structured change by considering complex systems' emerging properties (Norman, 2009; Holman, 2010). Complexity's central object of inquiry is the complex adaptive system (CAS)—"a collection of individual agents with freedom to act in ways that are not always totally predictable, and whose actions are interconnected so that one agent's actions change the context for other agents" (Plsek & Greenhalgh, 2001, p. 625). A CAS is thus a complex, non-linear, and interactive system within which "semi-autonomous agents ... adapt by changing their rules and, hence, behaviour, as they gain experience" (Zimmerman, Lindberg & Plsek, 2001, p. 263). Complexity theory draws on new discoveries in the biological and social/organizational sciences; empirical examples of the failure of central planning (e.g., strategic planning exercises that produce little change); and the power of groundswell, organic innovation from the margins. It is a perspective that emphasizes the power of distributed (as opposed to centralized) control, relationships, the co-evolution of systems in embedded environments, and the interplay of micro and macro. It shows us that outcomes are inherently slippery, potentially resistant, and ultimately not always open to influence using traditional top-down change strategies. It suggests that the key to the kind of adaptive innovation required in a changing and fast-paced world is the identification of new ways to harness the creativity and knowledge of frontline staff by stimulating and supporting "communities of practice" (Brown & Duguid, 1991; Wenger & Snyder, 2000; Westley, Zimmerman & Patton, 2006).

Similarly, by focusing on interactions between individuals and structures, *critical realism* can help us unpack and understand the social context of settings-related interventions. Critical realism is a logic of inquiry, drawing on the work of Bhaskar (1979), whose central premise is that constant conjunction (empirical co-occurrence) is an insufficient basis for inferring causality, and that what is required is the identification of generative mechanisms whose causal properties may or may not be activated, depending on circumstance (Connelly, 2001; Julnes, Mark & Henry, 1998; Stame, 2004; Williams, 2003). Mechanisms can coincide under real-world conditions to produce *emergent properties* contingent in time and space (Sayer, 2000). Thus, from a critical realist perspective, context is not an undifferentiated social ether in which programs and phenomena "float," but a series of generative mechanisms in constant interaction with complex and contingent combinations of events and actors. The notion of contingency contrasts with positivist notions of universal logical necessity (natural laws, generalizable truths) by highlighting the uncertain nature of phenomena (i.e., that propositions may hold true only under certain circumstances). Weiss (1997) argues for developing sound program theory, specifying the interrelated sequence of events expected to occur and how they relate to each other in space and time, thereby making transparent the underlying logic and assumptions of a given intervention. Critical realism encourages us to uncover *how* interventions work and through what *mechanisms,* rather than solely focusing on whether or not interventions have an *effect* (Porter, 1993; Poland et al., 2008; Kontos & Poland, 2009). The potential that both of these theories offer to a settings approach to health promotion are discussed in Dooris et al. (2007) and Poland et al. (2008), but see also Holman (2010) for an excellent understanding of engaging emergence.

Shortcomings: A Summary

In the main, all three main entry points for health promotion intervention have largely, in practice, fallen short in taking into account the social context of risk factors and interventions. We suggest that to improve the situation, we need to know, more specifically, how social inequities in health are (re)produced, and thus, what it is about the social environment that contributes to ill health; not only *which* factors are important, but *how* and *why* they are important. We are fully cognizant, however, that even in the face of the growing recognition of the importance of addressing inequities in health, it is enormously difficult to change institutional practices and that most public health practitioners' room to innovate is significantly limited by questions of funding, politics, and human resources. Despite institutional limitations, we make the plea that what is desperately needed is an understanding of how individuals, their behaviours, and their social circumstances interact to bring about the health problems faced by health promotion today. We maintain that this knowledge can help us intervene more appropriately.

What Can Be Done Differently?

The Structure/Agency Debate

Studies of the social context of health behaviours and outcomes bring us inevitably to a critical discussion as old as Western philosophy—that of individual free will versus structural determinism, or what is today referred to as the structure/agency debate. Proponents of structural explanations emphasize the power of structural conditions in shaping individual behaviour (Cockerham, 2005). So, for instance, if one were to take a structural position to understanding tobacco consumption, one might be particularly concerned with the role of social class (which is one instantiation of the social structure) in shaping smoking. Advocates of agency, on the other hand, accentuate the capacity of individual actors to choose and influence their behaviour regardless of structural influences.

This structure/agency dichotomy was also defined in terms of "life chances" and "life choices" by Max Weber (1922), who was, coincidentally, the first theorist to discuss the term "lifestyle." Weber viewed life chances as the opportunities that people encounter due to their social situation (their position within the social structure). Choices, on the other hand, are the decisions people make. So, whereas health-related choices are (more or less) voluntary, life chances either enable or constrain choices as choices and chances interact to shape behavioural outcomes. What Weber highlighted, then, is that both chances and choices are socially determined, and thus choices cannot simply be individually controlled. In so doing, Weber also underscored the collective nature of behaviours by associating lifestyles with status groups, and not solely with individuals; that is, choices are shaped by one's position within the social hierarchy. What Weber witnessed was that people from different social classes tended to share certain behaviours and practices.

French sociologist Pierre Bourdieu goes further in arguing that "choices" are an expression of a *habitus* that itself is a dynamic, evolving inculcation of structuring structures (or "chances," to use Weber's term) (Bourdieu, 1980, 1992). The *habitus*, according to Bourdieu, is produced by the objective conditions of existence combined with positions in the social structure, and it generates practices and tastes that together result in a lifestyle. While there is an element of choice with regard to one's lifestyle, people are seen to be predisposed by their habitus toward a certain choice of lifestyle. Bourdieu therefore viewed it as being entirely misleading to separate, analytically, "choices" and "chances" (see Chapter 3).

Collective Lifestyles as a Useful Heuristic Device to Address Social Context Issues in Health Promotion

Considerations of the role of lifestyle are far from new in health promotion practice. Green and Kreuter (1999), for instance, pay particular attention to the important role that lifestyle has played in permitting health promotion to move away from its earlier emphasis on health behaviour alone. While these authors were mindful of the collective aspect to lifestyles, they tend to consider them more in terms of practice and behavioural patterns, rather than situating these practices within the broader social structure as Weber and Bourdieu do.

We maintain that a theory-based sociological approach to understanding "collective lifestyles" (Frohlich et al., 2002), building on the ideas of Weber and Bourdieu, has the potential to offer more to health promotion practice than simply a synonym for patterns of individual risk behaviours and packages of variables. Instead it takes into account both behaviours and social circumstances (Abel, Cockerham & Niemann, 2000). Collective lifestyles comprise interacting patterns of health-related behaviours, orientations, and resources adopted by groups of individuals in response to their social, cultural, and economic environment (Abel et al., 2000, p. 63). Viewed in this way, collective lifestyles are akin to the social environmental approach in that they take into consideration the social, cultural, and economic environments in which people live, get sick, and die. There are a number of important differences, however, between these two approaches that make the collective lifestyle option increasingly palatable to a health promotion hungry for change.

First, the collective lifestyles framework develops further the issue of choices and chances by adopting current sociological language. Within this framework, therefore, we speak of *social* practices (Bourdieu, 1980, 1992; Giddens, 1984) (or behaviours) and *social* structure (or social conditions). Social practices are routinized and socialized behaviours common to groups. Social structure is defined as the way in which society is organized, involving norms, resources, policy, and institutional practices. Similarly to choices, social practices are understood as emerging from the structure, and thus the relationship between structure and practices is always explicit and recursive. In this way, an individual behaviour, or social practice, is never divorced from its position within the social structure. Further, this rela-tionship is not unidirectional; the structure is seen to shape people's social practices, but in turn, people's social practices are understood to influence the structure by both reproducing and transforming it. So, social practices are embedded within the social structure, but have a critical role in transforming it.

Second, social practices are not considered purely in terms of health behaviours. If tak-ing a collective lifestyles approach to obesity prevention, for instance, one would examine not only what people eat and whether they exercise or not, but also people's other activities, in various settings, that might have a bearing on obesity. Examples might be examinations of the constraints on physical activity such as lack of time, neighbourhood walkability, car dependence, or the replacement of physical activity by video games. One would seek to fur-ther understand the reasons behind the uneven social distribution of these activities, such as the roles of race, gender, and class in structuring health experiences, life opportunities, etc.

A third component of the collective lifestyle framework, in contrast to past perspectives, is a focus on the constraints on individual capacity (agency) and what the implications of the constraints are for true empowerment to take place. People's position within the social structure clearly shapes their agency. Approaches that focus on changing health behaviours give attention to agency, but what is often missing is a well-developed analysis of the struc-tural constraints to individual agency; that is, a direct link established between structure and agency. While the *Ottawa Charter* initially suggested focusing on increasing the options avail-able to people to exercise more control over their health, in practice this has been addressed mostly through environmental change; that is, changing the conditions rather than focusing on how these changes might increase individual control. The collective lifestyle framework suggests that one has to understand people's agency in relation to the social context of the health problem of concern. Using again the example of obesity, certain groups of people may not have the ability to exercise given lack of money and familial constraints. While they may have the knowledge and desire to exercise, their agency is reduced due to economic and other constraints. Knowledge of this barrier to agency would enable health promotion interventions to address it in order to more successfully reach some of these hard-to-reach populations.

Fourth, an implicit but underdeveloped aspect to the collective lifestyle framework is the issue of power. Power relations are central to shaping the uneven social distribution of health behaviours and disease outcomes among groups and ultimately in creating and sustaining the social structure. A focus on power relations draws attention to the ways in which the social patterning of health behaviours and disease outcomes mirrors the patterning of other processes of marginalization and disadvantage through both the social structure and social practices. A focus on power further invites us to consider our role, within health promotion practice, as active actors within systems of power and relative privilege or marginality. We are, of course, active participants in the social context of health promotion as we influence, through our research and interventions, the way disease, health, and behaviours are understood. Reflections and action on such issues are vital for a true focus on social context to be realized (Frohlich et al., 2010).

An important aspect of a collective lifestyle framework for understanding the social context is therefore reflexivity with respect to the social location of health promotion as a field (see also Chapter 12). By reflexivity we mean the maintenance of a self-critical attitude and a questioning of the taken-for-granted assumptions regarding the political nature of our work and its intended and unintended effects, as well as the social distribution of these effects (Caplan, 1993; Poland et al., 2006). More concretely this could include: (1) attention to the tacit knowledge and perspectives that practitioners bring to their work (see Chapter 16); (2) an openness to being transformed by the experience of engaging with individuals who may question the practice of health promotion; (3) a questioning of "received knowledge" (what we hold to be self-evident and true); (4) a curiosity about and openness toward other perspectives and ways of seeing; and (5) an awareness of power relations and one's own social location and positionality (how we fit into class and gender relations and how this affects the work we do individually and as a group performing health promotion) (Poland et al., 2006).

Conclusions

Health promotion has come a long way since the *Ottawa Charter* in its position on where the entry points of intervention in health promotion practice could and should be. We have learned much in health promotion practice and research by focusing on issues, specific population groups, and settings. As we have seen, however, each falls short in addressing the full complexity and social embeddedness of health determinants and the recursive relationship of structure and agency.

We offer an approach to addressing social context as a potential fourth point of intervention using the collective lifestyles framework, as well as issues relating to power and reflexivity. In so doing, we address a number of the critiques discussed throughout this chapter.

First, by focusing on social practices and their relationship to the social structure, one would no longer focus only on high-risk behaviours, but also the conditions that structure, and are structured, by behaviours. Second, because the focus of collective lifestyles is on conditions and behaviours, one would address the issue of high-risk individuals replacing those who are no longer at risk as the conditions are addressed, not just the behaviour alone. Third, a collective lifestyles approach focuses on group influences and thus potentially addresses how to change population patterns of disease and behaviours. Lastly, a collective lifestyles approach focuses specifically on why groups of people engage in the (social) practices that they do, and thus a purposive focus is given to ensuring that issues of equity are addressed.

Note

1. Although a 38 percent quit rate would be phenomenal if generalized to the entire population, focused "best practice" intervention trials are typically so resource-intensive that the costs of doing so would be prohibitive (and would compete politically with other determinants of health, programs, and service priorities).

References

Abel, T., Cockerham, W.C. & Niemann, S. (2000). A critical approach to lifestyle and health. In J. Watson & S. Platt (Eds.), *Researching health promotion* (pp. 54–77). London: Routledge.

Adelson, N. (2005). The embodiment of inequity: Health disparities in Aboriginal Canada. *Canadian Journal of Public Health, 96,* S45–S61.

Ajzen, I. & Fishbein, M. (1980). *Understanding attitudes and predicting social behaviour.* Englewood Cliffs: Prentice-Hall.

Alinsky, S.D. (1971). *Rules for radicals: A realistic primer for realistic radicals.* New York: Random House.

Bandura, A. (1986). *Social foundations of thought and action: A social cognitive theory.* Englewood Cliffs: Prentice-Hall.

Barnett, E., Anderson, T., Blosnich, J., Halverson, J. & Novak, J. (2005). Promoting cardiovascular health: From environmental goals to social environmental change. *American Journal of Preventive Medicine, 29,* 107–112.

Becker, M.H. (1974). The health belief model and personal health behaviour. *Health Education Monographs, 2,* 324–508.

Bhaskar, R. (1979). *The possibility of naturalism.* Atlantic Heights: Humanities Press.

Bourdieu, P. (1980). *Le sens pratique.* Paris: Les Éditions de Minuit.

Bourdieu, P. (1992). *Réponses: Pour une anthropologie réflexive.* Paris: Éditions du Seuil.

Brown, J.S. & Duguid, P. (1991). Organizational learning and communities of practice: Towards a unified view of working, learning, and innovation. *Organization Science, 2,* 40–57.

Caplan, R. (1993). The importance of social theory for health promotion: From description to reflexivity. *Health Promotion International, 8,* 147–157.

Cockerham, W. (2005). Health lifestyle theory and the convergence of agency and structure. *Journal of Health and Social Behavior, 46,* 51–67.

Connelly, J. (2001). Critical realism and health promotion: Effective practice needs an effective theory. *Health Education Research, 16,* 115–120.

Dooris, M. (2004). Joining up settings for health: A valuable investment for strategic partnerships? *Critical Public Health, 14*(1), 49–61.

Dooris, M. (2006). Health promoting settings: Future directions. *Promotion and Education 23*(2), 1–4.

Dooris, M. (2009). Holistic and sustainable health improvement: The contribution of the settings-based approach to health promotion. *Perspectives in Public Health, 129*(1), 29–36.

Dooris, M., Poland, B., Kolbe, L., de Leeuw, E., McCall, D. & Wharf-Higgins, J. (2007). Healthy settings: Building evidence for the effectiveness of whole systems health promotion—challenges and future directions. In D.V. McQueen & C.M. Jones (Eds.), *Global perspectives on health promotion effectiveness* (pp. 327–352). New York: Springer.

Frohlich, K.L., Corin, E. & Potvin, L. (2002). A theoretical proposal for the relationship between context and disease. *Sociology of Health and Illness, 23,* 776–797.

Frohlich, K.L. & Potvin, L. (2008). The inequality paradox: The population approach and vulnerable populations. *American Journal of Public Health, 98,* 216–221.

Frohlich, K.L., Poland, B. Mykhalovskiy, E., Alexander, S. & Maule, C. (2010). Tobacco control and the inequitable socio-economic distribution of smoking: Smokers' discourse and implications for tobacco control. *Critical Public Health, 20*, 35–46.

Frohlich, K.L. & Potvin, L. (1999). Health promotion through the lens of population health: Toward a salutogenic setting. *Critical Public Health, 9*(3), 211–222.

Frohlich, K.L., Ross, N. & Richmond, C. (2006). Health disparities in Canada today: Evidence and pathways. *Health Policy, 79*, 132–143.

Giddens, A. (1984). *The constitution of society.* Cambridge: Polity Press.

Grabb, E.G. (2002). *Theories of social inequality: Classical and contemporary perspectives* (4th ed.). Toronto: Harcourt Brace.

Green, L.W. & Kreuter, M.W. (1999). *Health promotion planning: An educational and ecological approach* (3rd ed.). Mountain View: Mayfield Publishing Company.

Holman, P. (2010). *Engaging emergence: Turning upheaval into opportunity.* San Francisco: Berret-Koehler.

Julnes, G., Mark, M. & Henry, G. (1998). Promoting realism in evaluation: Realistic evaluation and the broader context. *Evaluation, 4*, 483–504.

Kontos, P.C. & Poland, B.D. (2009). Mapping new theoretical and methodological terrain for knowledge translation: Contributions from critical realism and the arts. *Implementation Science 4*(1). 1–10.

Lalonde, M. (1974). *A new perspective on the health of Canadians.* Ottawa: Government of Canada. Retrieved from: http://www.phac-aspc.gc.ca/ph-sp/pdf/perspect-eng.pdf

Link, B.G. & Phelan, J. (1995). Social conditions as fundamental causes of disease. *Journal of Health and Social Behavior,* Extra Issue, 80–94.

McLaren, L. & Hawe, P. (2005). Ecological perspectives in health research. *Journal of Epidemiology and Community Health, 59*, 6–14.

McLeroy, K.R., Bibeau, D., Steckler, A. & Glanz, K. (1988). An ecological perspective on health promotion programs. *Health Education Quarterly, 15*, 351–377.

Multiple Risk Factor Intervention Trial Research Group. (1981). Multiple Risk Factor Intervention Trial. *Preventive Medicine, 10*, 387–553.

Multiple Risk Factor Intervention Trial Research Group. (1982). Multiple Risk Factor Intervention Trial: Risk factor changes and mortality results. *Journal of the American Medical Association, 24*, 1465–1476.

Norman, C.D. (2009). Health promotion as a systems science and practice. *Journal of Evaluation in Clinical Practice, 15*(5), 868–872.

Nutbeam, D. (1998). Health promotion glossary. *Health Promotion International, 13*(4), 349–364.

Plsek, P.E. & Greenhalgh, T. (2001). The challenge of complexity in healthcare. *British Medical Journal, 323*, 625–628.

Poland, B., Frohlich, K.L. & Cargo, M. (2008). Context as a fundamental dimension of health promotion program evaluation. In L. Potvin & D.V. McQueen (Eds.), *Health promotion evaluation practices in the Americas values and research* (pp. 299–317). New York: Springer.

Poland, B., Frohlich, K.L., Haines, R.J., Mykhalovskiy, E., Rock, M. & Sparks, R. (2006). The social context of smoking: The next frontier in tobacco control? *Tobacco Control, 15*(1), 59–63.

Poland, B.D., Green, L.W. & Rootman, I. (Eds.). (2000). *Settings for health promotion: Linking theory and practice.* Thousand Oaks: Sage Publications.

Porter, S. (1993). Critical realist ethnography: The case of racism and professionalism in a medical setting. *Sociology, 27*(4), 591–665.

Richard, L., Potvin, L., Kishchuk, N., Prlic, H. & Green, L.W. (1996). Assessment of the integration of the ecological approach in health promotion programs. *American Journal of Health Promotion, 10*(4), 318–328.

Sayer, A. (2000). *Realism and social science.* London: Sage.

Smedley, B.D. & Syme, S.L. (Eds.). (2000). *Promoting health: Intervention strategies from social and behavioral research*. Washington: National Academy Press.

Stame, N. (2004). Theory-based evaluation and types of complexity. *Evaluation, 10*, 58–76.

St. Leger, L. (1997). Health promoting settings: From Ottawa to Jakarta. *Health Promotion International, 12*(3), 99–101.

Stokols, D. (1996). Translating social ecological theory into guidelines for community health promotion. *American Journal of Health Promotion, 10*, 282–298.

Tannahill, A. (1992). Epidemiology and health promotion: A common understanding. In R. Bunton & G. Macdonald (Eds.), *Health promotion: Disciplines and diversity* (pp. 42–65). London: Routledge.

Weber, M. (1922). *Wirschaft und Gesellschaft (Economy and society)*. Tübingen: Mohr Siebeck.

Weiss, C.H. (1997). Theory-based evaluation: Past, present, and future. *New Directions for Evaluation, 76*, 41–56.

Wenger, E. & Snyder, W. (2000). Communities of practice: The organizational frontier. *Harvard Business Review*, (January–February), 139–145.

Westley, F., Zimmerman, B. & Patton, M. (2006). *Getting to maybe: How the world is changed*. Toronto: Random House.

Whitelaw, S., Baxendale, A., Bryce, C., Machardy, L., Young, I. & Witney, E. (2001). Settings' based health promotion: A review. *Health Promotion International, 16*(4), 339–353.

Williams, G.H. (2003). The determinants of health: Structure, context, and agency. *Sociology of Health & Illness, 25*(3), 131–154.

World Health Organization. (1986). *Ottawa Charter for Health Promotion*. Ottawa: Canadian Public Health Association.

Zimmerman, B., Lindberg, C. & Plsek, P. (2001). *Edgeware: Insights from complexity science for health care leaders* (2nd ed.). Irving: VHA Inc.

Critical Thinking Questions

1. What are the advantages and disadvantages to the points of intervention discussed in this chapter?
2. Are there other ways in which we could intervene in health promotion that would better take into account the social context?
3. Do current interventions in health promotion stand to be improved and, if yes, why?
4. Is there a danger of increasing inequalities in health by intervening in health promotion?
5. What theories can we draw on to help improve our interventions in health promotion?

Resources

Further Readings

Emmons, K.M. (2000). Health behaviors in a social context. In L.F. Berkman & I. Kawachi (Eds.), *Social epidemiology* (pp. 242–266). New York: Oxford University Press.

This chapter reviews data on risk factor change and examines some of the factors that help to explain the relatively low rate of long-term change produced by most health promotion interventions.

Frohlich, K.L., Corin, E. & Potvin, L. (2002). A theoretical proposal for the relationship between context and disease. *Sociology of Health and Illness, 23*, 776–797.

This article develops the notion of collective lifestyles drawing on the work of Pierre Bourdieu, Anthony Giddens, and Amartya Sen.

Poland, B., Frohlich, K.L., Haines, R.J., Mykhalovskiy, E., Rock, M. & Sparks, R. (2006). The social context of smoking: The next frontier in tobacco control? *Tobacco Control, 15,* 59–63.

This article moves beyond the discussion developed in this chapter to include the exploration of social context through the sociology of the body as it relates to smoking, collective patterns of consumption, the construction and maintenance of social identity, the ways in which desire and pleasure are implicated in these latter two dimensions in particular, and smoking as a social activity rooted in place.

Poland, B.D., Green, L.W. & Rootman, I. (Eds.). (2000). *Settings for health promotion: Linking theory and practice.* Thousand Oaks: Sage Publications.

This book outlines the history, content, and utility of the settings approach in health promotion interventions.

Williams, G. (2003). The determinants of health: Structure, context, and agency. *Sociology of Health and Illness, 25,* 131–154.

Williams reviews the ways in which the concept of social structure has been deployed within medical sociology, paying particular attention to its role in the debate over health inequalities and the role of the social context in shaping these inequalities.

Relevant Websites

A critique of the settings approach,
hosted by University of New South Wales School of Public Health

www.ldb.org/setting.htm

Health promotion recognizes the idea that people live in social, cultural, political, economic, and environmental contexts. This acknowledgement may have been new for public health; however, sociologists and social psychologists have been aware of the embeddedness of behaviour into larger contexts for a longer period of time. However, the acknowledgement by public health practitioners that health is developed in the context of everyday life, which itself is structured by its related social system, has not led to a fundamental reconsideration of the social science basis of public health concepts and its incorporation into planning and activity.

Health Promotion and Education Online

http://rhpeo.net/newfrontpage.html

RHP&EO is the electronic journal of the International Union for Health Promotion and Education (IUHPE). The journal published an editorial response to the previous article, arguing about the conceptualization of "settings" employed in the earlier piece.

World Health Organization—Settings Approach

http://www.who.int/healthy_settings/en/

This multilingual site describes the history of the WHO Settings for Health approach. Specifically, Settings for Health emphasizes practical networks and projects to create healthy environments such as healthy schools, health-promoting hospitals, healthy workplaces, and healthy cities. Settings for Health builds on the premise that there is a health development potential in practically every organization and/or community.

CHAPTER 8

Issues as a Point of Entry into Health Promotion

Irving Rootman, Sylvie Stachenko, Barbara Riley, Paola Ardiles, Hélène Provencher, Doris Gillis, Margot Kaszap, and Trevor Hancock

Introduction

Irving Rootman

As noted by the authors of Chapter 7, "issues" have frequently been used as a point of entry in health promotion. To date, most of the issues that have been used in this way have been defined in terms of behaviours that have had undesirable consequences. These include smoking, use of alcohol or other drugs, unhealthy consumption of foods, physical inactivity, and unsafe sexual activity. One reason why health promoters have focused on such issues is that they are of concern to society because of their actual and potential negative health, economic, or other consequences. Another is that they appear to be matters that can be addressed relatively easily using existing technologies and approaches, such as information and education programs, although often this proves not to be the case. A third is that many of the relatively well-developed and tested theories that have guided health promotion to date have been focused on individuals' behavioural changes.

Although many critics of health promotion, including several represented in this book, have criticized this approach as "blaming the victim" and as drawing attention away from the powerful structural and "contextual" causes of destructive health behaviour, it is likely that for the reasons just noted, "issues" will continue to be used as an entry point for health promotion by many agencies and people working in the field for the foreseeable future. However, the framing of issues can be broadened beyond this individualistic ideology to better reflect the complexities of contemporary life that impact on health and the multiple layers of health promotion practice. Fortunately, there are a growing number of examples of sophisticated initiatives using "issues" as a point of intervention that take the social and environmental determinants of health and contextual factors seriously into account in their development and execution, and are consistent with the basic principles and values of health promotion such as "empowerment" and "participation." Several such examples will be presented and discussed in this chapter.

Specifically, it will consider recent Canadian examples of initiatives that focus on four important issues, namely, chronic disease, mental health, health literacy, and sustainable development. These issues were chosen because they have a much broader focus than trying to simply change behaviours and because they illustrate the value of a comprehensive approach to addressing health issues from a health promotion perspective. Each of the authors was chosen because of his or her intimate knowledge and experience with the issue and ability to identify "promising practices" that emerge around the issue at stake. The lessons learned will be summarized and discussed in the concluding section of the chapter, which is followed by some questions to stimulate critical thinking about the examples and the strategy of adopting an initial focus on a particular issue as a point of entry into practice.

Chronic Disease

Sylvie Stachenko and Barbara Riley

Background

Chronic diseases (CDs) such as diabetes are associated with 60 percent of all deaths and 46 percent of the burden of disease worldwide (WHO, 2005). Recent reports and studies describe CDs as threatening health systems and economic stability around the world (World Economic Forum, 2008), partly because the human and economic toll associated with them is expected to increase substantially over the years to come (WHO, 2006). In Canada, the total cost of illness, disability, and death due to CDs is estimated to be over $80 billion annually (Health Council of Canada, 2006). Chronic disease experts have long maintained that dealing effectively with CDs, individually or collectively, requires multifaceted approaches involving multiple strategies and sectors.

The World Health Organization (WHO) and others call for comprehensive, integrated, and strategic approaches in dealing with CDs (WHO & Government of Canada, 2005; Pan-American Health Organization, 2007; WHO, 2008a). Such approaches can also be applied to single diseases or risk factors. In Canada, an integrated approach to a single disease was first realized through the Canadian Heart Health Initiative (CHHI) (Riley, Stachenko, Wilson et al., 2009), which implemented community-based cardiovascular disease (CVD) prevention programs for 20 years from 1986 with co-funding from provincial and federal governments. Since then, a next generation of integrated approaches has emerged, which includes broader intersectoral action, a key feature of large-scale health promotion programs.

One such example is ActNowBC, launched in 2005 in British Columbia. In its first six years, ActNowBC illustrated an intersectoral approach to CD prevention in Canada, building on lessons from the CHHI. A recent case study of ActNowBC helps to illustrate some emerging ingredients for successful intersectoral action (Public Health Agency of Canada, 2009). Following a brief overview of ActNowBC, we describe some early lessons related to political leadership, targets, and accountability, and the role of non-governmental organizations (NGOs).

Overview of ActNowBC

ActNowBC was conceived as a cross-government and multi-year health promotion initiative launched in 2005 to improve the health of British Columbians through integrated action to simultaneously target multiple risk factors and reduce chronic disease. The initial goals were:

1. to make British Columbia the healthiest jurisdiction to host the Olympic and Paralympic Winter Games
2. to improve the health of British Columbians by encouraging them to be more active, eat healthy foods, live tobacco-free, and make healthy choices during pregnancy
3. to build community capacity to create healthier, more sustainable, and economically viable communities
4. to reduce demand on the health care system

Political Leadership

ActNowBC enjoyed high-level political leadership by the BC premier during its developmental phase as a whole-of-government initiative. Although the Ministry of Health had the initial responsibility for ActNowBC, it was clear that it would grow to become a cross-government initiative. Leadership and shared governance structures were used to give the ActNowBC initiative an intersectoral vision and direction. In 2006, the premier also appointed a minister of state under the Ministry of Tourism, Sports, and Arts for ActNowBC who, with the Cabinet, provided strategic facilitation and coordination and used transformational incentives (e.g., holdbacks from deputy ministers for not achieving targets set out in their service plans).

Targets and Accountability

One important mechanism that ActNowBC used to increase coordination across government was the establishment of goals and targets (Van Herten & Gunning-Shepers, 2000). ActNowBC set five targets and developed an accountability framework, consistent with the need for all stakeholders to have a clear understanding of their roles and responsibilities. Otherwise, accountability would have been weakened, and achieving organizational objectives potentially would have been less likely (Wilkins, 2002). Nonetheless, defining clear accountability frameworks can be difficult when devising whole-of-government strategies,

---

BOX 8.1:

ActNowBC TARGETS

The five ActNowBC targets by 2010 were:
* Physical activity: Increase the percentage of the BC population that is physically active by 20 percent.
* Healthy eating: Increase the percentage of BC adults who eat at least five servings of fruits and vegetables daily by 20 percent.
* Overweight/obesity: Reduce the percentage of BC adults who are overweight or obese by 20 percent.
* Tobacco use: Reduce tobacco use by 10 percent.
* Healthy choices in pregnancy: Increase the number of women who receive counselling about the dangers of alcohol and tobacco use during pregnancy by 50 percent.

Source: Government of British Columbia. (2006). *Measuring our success: Baseline document.* Victoria: Government of British Columbia. Retrieved from: http://www.actnowbc.ca/media/ActNow-BC-Measuring-our-Success-Baseline-Document-2006-11.pdf

since co-operation across sectors inevitably blurs the traditional boundaries of budget alloca-
tion, dispersal, accounting, authority, and responsibility (Hunt, 2005).

The Role of Non-governmental Organizations: The BC Healthy Living Alliance

After the launch of ActNowBC, there was a consensus among Ministry of Health officials
that the support and contribution of individuals and organizations outside of government was
needed to achieve the ActNowBC goals. The BC Healthy Living Alliance (BCHLA), a coalition of nine civil society organizations formed in 2003, was a natural partner for ActNowBC
(Public Health Agency of Canada, 2009). In March 2005, the BCHLA submitted to the BC
government "The Winning Legacy: A Plan for Improving the Health of British Columbians,"
which included a number of recommendations that paralleled ActNowBC. The following
year, the province invested $30 million in the non-governmental sector, with $25.2 million
to the BCHLA.

The BCHLA identified community capacity-building as a critical element to effectively
address the wide range of risk factors for CDs (BCHLA, 2010). Consequently, the Alliance
has been especially active in communities with significant barriers to healthy living, including
rural, remote, and Aboriginal communities.

The BCHLA initiatives demonstrated that using a community development approach was
a highly effective way to implement successful and sustainable healthy living programming.
The Alliance helped to create healthier environments; for example, introducing salad bars into
schools and eliminating sugar-sweetened beverages. Initiatives provided skills to individuals
who needed to learn how to cook, how to quit smoking, or how to get active, and brought
communities together to plan for a healthier future with accessible facilities, bike routes,
walking trails, and outdoor hockey rinks.

There is a growing body of literature about the significant roles that NGOs can play in
supporting intersectoral action for health (Barrett, 2003). While their role is well documented, there is less evidence about the partnership and funding models between government
authorities and NGOs that are effective in the field of health promotion for the longer term.

Recent Developments

Following the 2010 Olympics, ActNowBC funding was substantially reduced, and the political leadership and intersectoral action have diminished. While sustainability of the whole-
of-government approach is uncertain, planning for sustainability was built into the BCHLA
initiatives so that successes would endure beyond the one-time grant.

Conclusion

While the principle of intersectoral action for health is widely accepted as an important health
promotion strategy, it takes innovative, pragmatic approaches like ActNowBC to make it
more real. ActNowBC illustrates that intersectoral action is possible, and can be sustained
over a number of years. It also highlights some ingredients for initial success, including:
high-level political commitment, shared leadership, publicly stated goals and targets (hence,

accountability), and engaging civil society organizations. ActNowBC also raises important and challenging questions about health promotion practice: What interplay of factors influences the vulnerability, lifespan, and evolution of whole-of-government approaches in dynamic socio-political environments? How does a bold (if time-limited) initiative like ActNowBC influence future investments in health promotion and disease prevention in BC and other jurisdictions? Ongoing systematic and context-sensitive analysis will reveal rich lessons on which to build the next generation of intersectoral approaches to health promotion.

Mental Health

Paola Ardiles and Hélène Provencher

Mental Health and Well-being

Mental health (MH) is an integral component and important determinant of overall health. MH is more than the absence of mental illness, it is:

> … the capacity of each and all of us to feel, think and act in ways that enhance our ability to enjoy life and deal with the challenges we face. It is a positive sense of emotional and spiritual well-being that respects the importance of culture, equity, social justice, interconnections, and personal dignity. (Centre for Health Promotion, 1997, p. 1.)

Although this chapter section will use the concept of positive mental health and mental well-being interchangeably, many other terms can be found to refer to positive aspects of mental health, such as mental capital, psychological resilience, flourishing, mental wellness, etc.

Mental health influences a very wide range of outcomes for individuals and communities, including healthier lifestyles; better physical health; improved recovery from illness; fewer limitations in daily living; higher educational attainment; greater productivity, employment, and earnings; better interpersonal relationships; more social cohesion, engagement, and improved quality of life; reduction in crime rates; and decreased harms associated with substance use (Friedli, 2009). Growing evidence reveals that these wide range of outcomes are not just a result of the absence of mental illness, but are linked to the presence of positive mental health, sometimes referred to as mental "well-being" (Freidli, 2009; Cooke et al., 2011). The key factors that influence mental well-being include emotional resources, cognitive resources, social skills, and meaning and purpose (see Figure 8.1) (Cooke et al., 2011).

The reciprocal relationship between positive mental health (PMH), physical health, and illness has been well documented (Canadian Institute for Health Information, 2009), and this understanding is critical to a more effective and holistic approach to health promotion. Empirical evidence supports the Complete Model of Mental Health (see Figure 8.2) and demonstrates that one's mental health can be enhanced regardless of a mental illness diagnosis (Keyes, 2007, 2010). For instance, research demonstrates that a high level of PMH among adults free of mental illness is associated with:

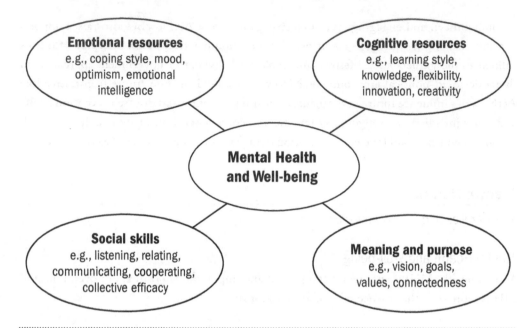

FIGURE 8.1: Dimensions of Mental Well-being

Source: Lynne Friedli from Cooke, A., Friedli, L., Coggins, T., Edmonds, N., Michaelson, J., O'Hara, K., Snowden, L., Stansfield, J., Steuer, N. & Scott-Samuel, A. (2011). *Mental well-being impact assessment: A toolkit for well-being* (3rd ed.). London: National MWIA Collaborative. Retrieved from: http://www.apho.org.uk/resource/item.aspx?RID=95836

- higher levels of self-rated physical and mental health
- the fewest chronic physical conditions
- the lowest rates of cardiovascular disease and health limitations of activities of daily living
- lower levels of mental illness
- the highest level of psychosocial functioning (e.g., perceived control in life)
- the lowest health care use (e.g., medical visits and medications)
- the fewest workdays missed
- fewer reduced activity days than people with moderate or low levels of positive mental health (CIHI, 2009; Keyes, 2007)

In addition, among individuals with at least one of the four mental disorders (i.e., major depressive episode, panic, generalized anxiety, and alcohol dependence), those who were flourishing (showing the highest level of positive mental health) functioned better than those who were languishing (lower levels of positive mental health). Thus, levels of positive mental health differentiate levels of impairment and disability even among adults who have had a mental illness in the past year (Keyes, 2007).

PMH has been recognized as a key resource for population well-being and the social and economic prosperity of society (Barry, 2009), and contributes to an individual's ability to recognize the importance of behaviours that support physical health, and take actions to manage physical illness (Keleher & Armstrong, 2006).

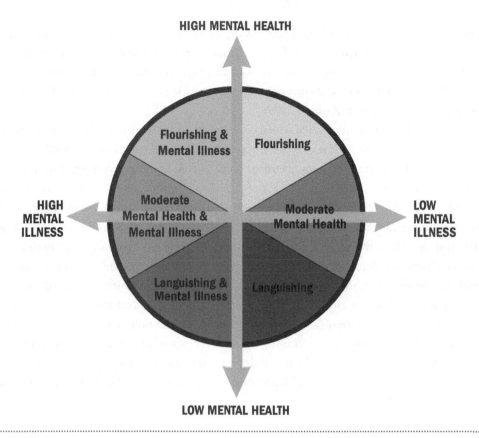

FIGURE 8.2: Keyes's Model of Complete Mental Health

Source: Keyes, C.L.M. (2010). The next step in the promotion and protection of mental health. *Canadian Journal of Nursing Research,* 42(3), 21

Mental Health Promotion

Mental health promotion (MHP) and mental illness prevention both aim to increase protective factors and decrease risk factors in order to build individual skills that support MH. However, a unique and essential component of MHP is to build and sustain environments that reinforce PMH at the population level (Barry, 2009; Keleher & Armstrong, 2006). Therefore, MHP is applicable for all and includes strategies for individuals and populations at risk of developing mental illness (Albee, 1993; Barry, 2009).

MHP can also address the needs of those recovering from mental illness and striving for the achievement of pleasant and fulfilling roles and activities despite enduring symptoms or illness-related deficits. Based on the model of complete MH (Keyes, 2007), "recovery" is conceived as two complementary processes and outcomes—restoration from mental illness and optimization of PMH—and is promoted through the use of individual and community-oriented interventions (Provencher & Keyes, 2011).

Several key principles guide MHP initiatives such as: (1) a positive conceptualization of MH; (2) emphasis on meaningful engagement, participatory and empowerment-oriented approaches that enable individuals, groups, and communities to achieve and maintain their health; (3) special focus on building upon existing strengths, assets, and capacities rather than a focus on problems or deficits; (4) collaborative action on the determinants of MH; (5) multiple interventions across a wide range of sectors, policies, programs, settings, and environments; (6) approaches that are tailored and culturally appropriate; and (7) actions informed by evidence and practice (GermAnn & Ardiles, 2009).

Multi-level MHP strategies are necessary to allow individuals, families, communities, and societies to flourish. At the individual level, the optimal development of PMH includes the building of resilience and empowerment skills, as well as those promoting psychological and social well-being dimensions (see above). At the community level, actions are oriented toward the creation of supportive environments that foster social capital, social participation, and civic engagement (e.g., in workplaces, school settings). At the societal level, MHP strategies aim to address the determinants of MH, and reduce health and social inequities (e.g., poverty, discrimination, violence) through improved access to economic resources, employment, education, affordable housing, as well as increased opportunities for social inclusion (e.g., supportive family relationships, participatory structures in community organizations) (Raphael, 2009). These strategies require multi-level interventions across a wide number of sectors, programs, settings, and environments, such as collaborative strategies among physical health, MH, and social services for improving policies, making organizational change, fostering community development, and supporting local initiatives (Keleher & Armstrong, 2006; Cooke et al., 2011).

Promising MHP Canadian Practice

Originally developed in Australia, the Triple P—Positive Parenting Program—has been globally recognized as a leading public health initiative. It consists of a multi-level system of parenting support and intervention designed to improve the quality of parenting advice available to parents (Sanders, 1999, 2008). The program recognizes the importance of the community assets and family atmosphere in children's development, and promotes parental self-care. In Canada, the Government of Manitoba, through the Healthy Child Manitoba Office, is playing a leading role in MHP by implementing this program across various urban and rural settings.

The success of the Triple P program to date is largely due to the cross-government commitment to promoting well-being at a population level, as well as the ownership across multiple levels of intervention and settings. Triple P continuously strives for delivery of culturally appropriate resources and services by actively involving stakeholders from across the province, including francophone, rural, and Aboriginal community members and practitioners. Triple P program core components have been adapted for a telephone helpline to reach remote and rural areas, and have also been translated into French. In addition, a national Aboriginal advisory group was created to aid with the development of tools tailored to meet the needs of Aboriginal communities.

"Mental health can flourish in environments that are safe, just and equitable, and that foster quality connections" (CIHI, 2009, p. 16). The Triple P is an exemplary program in Canada that aims to promote MH by applying all key MHP principles (identified above), while striving to meet diverse needs of Canadians. Investing in MH is a priority that holds a universal benefit (WHO, 2003). Promoting MH is beyond the scope of health services and necessarily involves individual and collective efforts across various sectors and settings.

Health Literacy

Doris Gillis and Margot Kaszap

The Issue

Although literacy is a well-recognized determinant of population health (Ronson & Rootman, 2004), as noted in Chapter 2, health literacy has only recently appeared as an issue of concern in Canada. Growing evidence points to the effect of health literacy on health outcomes and health disparities in Canada. In 2008, the Canadian Council on Learning (CCL) reported that 60 percent of Canadian adults do not have the health literacy skills to adequately manage their health and health care needs, such as finding appropriate health services or understanding information, such as instructions on medication or food products. Findings on the health literacy performance of Canadian adults was based on analysis of data from the 2003 International Adult Literacy and Skills Survey (IALSS) using a health literacy scale derived from the survey tools (CCL, 2007). Striking differences were seen in levels of health literacy across regions and various population groups. The report concluded that "differences in health status that are associated with differences in health–literacy are large enough to imply that significant improvement in overall levels of population health might be realized if a way could be found to raise adult health–literacy levels" (CCL, 2008, p. 29), and that such improvement offers potential not only for the improved health of citizens but also for health care savings and contributions to national productivity. In 2008, the Canadian Expert Panel on Health Literacy concluded that "Low health literacy is a serious and costly problem that will likely grow as the population ages and the incidence of chronic disease increases" (Rootman & Gordon-El-Bihbety, 2008, p. 11).

In response to the growing concern about health literacy, the Expert Panel called for a pan-Canadian strategy to address health literacy in Canada. Health literacy was defined as *"The ability to access, understand, evaluate and communicate information as a way to promote, maintain and improve health in a variety of settings across the life-course"* (Rootman & Gordon-El-Bihbety, 2008, p. 11). This definition takes into account people's ability as well as the demands for health literacy imposed by various health contexts. It implies that health literacy is mediated by *"education, culture and language, by the communication skills of professionals, by the nature of materials and messages, and by the settings in which health-related supports are provided"* (Rootman & Gordon-El-Bihbety, 2008, p. 11). Informed by health promotion thinking, this view emphasizes shared responsibility for addressing health literacy in ways that extend beyond the health care system to the multiple contexts in which people engage with information in making decisions pertinent to their health.

It has been argued both by Nutbeam (2000, p. 261,263) and Rootman, Frankish, and Kaszap (2007, p.62) that health literacy is a key outcome of health promotion and by the latter authors that that it is an outcome that the field could legitimately be held accountable for (Rootman et al., 2007, p.62). Moreover, Rootman and colleagues have suggested that the concept of health literacy has potential to revitalize health promotion thinking and change the way practitioners approach their work. Although health literacy is a robust field of study (Rudd, Anderson, Oppenheimer & Nath, 2007), the conceptualization of health literacy within the health promotion field and critical examination of the complexities and practicalities of health literacy as applied within varied contexts and settings require more attention (Peerson & Saunders, 2009). Research is needed to shed more light on what health literacy interventions in Canada actually look like and the mechanisms through health literacy improvement can influence the capacity of individuals and systems to achieve positive health outcomes.

Looking for Promising Practices

As mentioned above, it is only relatively recently that health literacy has emerged as a concept and an issue of concern in Canada. Many practitioners are reportedly not aware of its implications for their practice (Rootman & Gordon-El-Bihbety, 2008). One barrier to incorporating health literacy into practice may indeed be the lack of a single or shared definition. Definitions of health literacy have emanated from different fields of practice and various contexts in which practitioners interact with issues relevant to literacy and health. Whereas most definitions of *literacy* have centred on the fundamental need for individuals to have command over use of the written word, more recent views recognize health literacy as composed of many facets with implications for both the users and the providers of information in contexts both inside and outside the health care system. It is notable that interventions tend to reflect the varied conceptualizations of health literacy and it is only recently that a "created in Canada" definition of health literacy has appeared.

Not surprisingly, few Canadian health literacy interventions have been rigorously evaluated (King 2007). Initiatives have tended to be short-term and lacking in funding to sustain efforts or evaluate outcomes. The Expert Panel pointed to a lack of evidence-based practice from which practitioners can draw lessons. However, they also suggested that community-based and participatory approaches offer promise (Rootman & Gordon El-Bihbety, 2008). Such approaches characteristically highlight the importance of understanding and taking into account the context and varied situations in which people confront health literacy demands. By building on principles of community-based development, adult education, and participatory evaluation, one demonstration project funded by the Public Health Agency of Canada aims to draw lessons to inform health literacy practice in Canada. The design, pilot testing, and evaluation of embedded learning approaches to improve health literacy outcomes of specific populations known to face barriers to health literacy is the central thrust of the Learning for Health: Health Literacy Embedded Learning project.[1] Three population groups in three regions of Canada are involved: (1) adults in a retirement program in Manitoba; (2) families in a rural Nova Scotia family resource centre; and (3) new immigrants and government-assisted refugees in a new Canadians' centre in Newfoundland. The variety of interventions undertaken at each of these sites reflects the diversity of participants and the contexts in which they engage with information for their health.

The issue of health literacy appears to be capturing the interest of Canadian practitioners. A recent scan of Canadian health literacy initiatives identified a wide variety of interventions, including health literacy materials, protocols, and local initiatives. Notably, authors pointed to the need for an overarching body to take responsibility for disseminating such resources and supporting a health literacy approach within public health in Canada (Frankish et al., 2011). Although there is not as yet one national mechanism to connect Canadian practitioners interested in health literacy practice, networks are forming. For example, a coalition of organizations and individuals interested in health literacy has recently been established in British Columbia, and in Quebec there is the Centre for Documentation on Adult Learning and the Condition of Women (CDÉACF). There is also the Canadian Federation for French Literacy (FCAF), which supports health literacy efforts through COMPAS, a repository for research reports[2] and CORAL, a network that includes academics, practitioners, administrators, and learners.[3] In 2008, the rationale and core principles of health literacy curricula development and evaluation relevant to grade K–12 students, adult learners, and health care workers/students were created by practitioners and researchers attending an institute organized in Calgary by the Centre for Literacy in Quebec.[4] Known as the *Calgary Charter on Health Literacy*, it highlights the importance of professional development as an intervention for improving health literacy at the health system level.

Summary and Conclusion

A view of health literacy that highlights the varied settings and contexts in which people face diverse demands for accessing, understanding, evaluating, and communicating information relevant to their health is in keeping with the evolution of health promotion in Canada. Not only has health promotion thinking contributed to how we frame health literacy as a relevant and important issue in Canada, emerging understandings of health literacy suggest new ways of approaching health promotion practice. Integrating health literacy into health promotion interventions can draw together a broad range of health and literacy practitioners to address the health concerns of marginalized groups most likely to face barriers to health due to low literacy. Lessons learned from more rigorously evaluated interventions that incorporate health literacy will inform future practices with the goal of enhancing the contribution of health promotion efforts to improving health outcomes.

[Un]sustainable Development

Trevor Hancock

Clearly, sustainability is a "larger" agenda than health promotion, as it constitutes a general principle on how we organize our societies overall. (Kickbusch, 2010, p. 11)

The Issue

There has been much emphasis in recent years on the *social* determinants of health (WHO Commission on the Social Determinants of Health [CSDH], 2008b; Mikkonen & Raphael, 2010), yet the Earth, this living planet Gaia, is the ultimate determinant of our health. Without its ecosystem, goods (natural resources such as plants, animals, minerals, etc.) and services (oxygen generation, the ozone layer, the water cycle, etc.), human life—and the existence of a myriad other species—would be impossible. History has taught us that civilizations that exhaust their ecosystems collapse and die (Diamond, 2005), yet at a global scale that is precisely what we are doing.[5]

The *Ottawa Charter for Health Promotion* (WHO, 1986) was the first WHO document to identify "a stable ecosystem" and "sustainable resources" as prerequisites for health. Anticipating the report of the Brundtland Commission on Sustainable Development (Brundtland, 1987), the *Charter* made explicit the link between health and sustainable development. The *Charter* was followed by a WHO report on health and environment (WHO, 1992) and a CPHA report on human and ecosystem health (CPHA, 1992), both of which expanded upon this link.

BOX 8.2:

CPHA REPORT ON HUMAN AND ECOSYSTEM HEALTH

The report stated:
- "Human development and the achievement of human potential requires a form of economic activity that is environmentally and socially sustainable in this and future generations" (CPHA, 1992) and went on to identify three major categories of ecosystem change that have profound implications for human health:
- Global climate and atmospheric changes, including ozone depletion, global warming, acid and toxic rain;
- Depletion of both renewable and non-renewable resources, including the loss of habitat and species extinctions;
- Ecotoxicity - the contamination of regional ecosystems and food chains (and humans) with minute quantities of persistent organic pollutants, heavy metals and other contaminants.

Source: Canadian Public Health Association. (1992). *Human and Ecosystem Health.* Ottawa: CPHA.

Today, almost 20 years later, and almost 40 years since the First UN Conference on the Environment in 1972, these ecosystem changes have, for the most part, worsened. The World Wildlife Fund's (WWF) Living Planet Index, which measures the health of three major ecosystems (marine, freshwater, and terrestrial), has declined almost 30 percent between 1970 and 2007, while the Ecological Footprint, which measures the human demand on the Earth's ecosystems, has more than doubled since 1960, and in 2007 stood at 2.7 hectares per person, compared to an estimated global bio-capacity of 1.8 hectares per person. If the whole world had the same consumption patterns as Denmark, Belgium, or the US (approximately 8 hectares per person), we would need more than four Planet Earths to meet our global demand (WWF, 2010).

Troublingly, this accords well with an analysis by Turner (2008), who looked back at the scenarios used by Meadows et al. in their famous 1972 Club of Rome report, "The Limits to Growth" and the actual record since then and concluded that "thirty years of historical data compare favorably with key features of a business-as-usual scenario called the 'standard run' scenario which results in collapse of the global system midway through the 21st century" (Turner 2008, Abstract). In fact, the late Meadows and her colleagues concluded in the most recent update of their report that because we have already exceeded the limits to growth on a finite planet, we faced two options:

> ... to bring the throughputs that support human activities down to sustainable levels through human choice, human technology and human organisation, or let nature force the decision through lack of energy, food or materials, or through an increasingly unhealthy environment. (Meadows, Randers & Meadows, 2004, p. 13)

Clearly, our civilization (by which I mean our now-global industrialized world) is faced with ecological decline at a global scale if not, in some regional and local ecosystems, complete collapse. When ecosystems and societies decline or collapse, so too does health. Hence, working to reverse our current perilous course should be one of the highest priorities for health promotion and for the public health system.

Some will say that this message of doom and gloom is disempowering, that it frightens people, turns them off, and should be avoided. I disagree; it would be like saying "Let's not tell her she has cancer—it will upset her!" But how can someone get treatment for cancer[6] and make the necessary adjustments to get better if he or she remains unaware or adopts a policy of denial? A failure to face the facts squarely is in fact unhealthy and yet, to a large extent, that is what we are doing!

So one of the key challenges facing health promotion in the twenty-first century is to make clear the links between human and ecosystem health, the depth of the problem we now face, and to work with allies to help find solutions. This has to happen at local, municipal, provincial, federal, and international levels.

Happily, we are not without knowledge of what to do (although, sadly, we have known what to do for decades, but largely have not done it); we need to make the transition to a more sustainable and healthier way of life.

Who are those allies in creating a more sustainable and healthier future? In a nutshell, the environmental movement in all its guises, including:

- those pursuing the transition to a post–fossil fuel future based on energy conservation and clean energy
- those working for food security, which includes creating an ecologically sustainable food system (e.g., Food Secure Canada and local food security groups)
- urban planners and municipal governments that are creating "green" or sustainable communities, particularly where they are linking this explicitly to the healthy communities approach.

A Few Promising Practices at the Local and National Levels

As was the case with tobacco control, climate change action, and many other challenging issues, it is not at the provincial or federal levels that we are likely to find leadership, but at the municipal level. A good example of this integrated approach to creating healthier and more sustainable communities is the work of the Public Health Department at the Region of Waterloo, Ontario.

The department adopted a "healthy community" model some years ago and has applied it particularly with respect to urban planning, growth management, and food security. A recent report prepared as a contribution to the Regional Growth Management Strategy (Region of Waterloo Public Health, 2007) examines how the built environment can contribute to health (and sustainability) in five ways: (1) increasing physical activity through urban design improvements; (2) improving food access and food intake by increasing the availability of healthy food options; (3) improving air quality by focusing on emissions from local energy and fuel consumption; (4) increasing social capital in neighbourhoods by influencing the built environment; and (5) strengthening rural health by improving local farm viability and addressing rural isolation.

A new movement that health promoters will need to relate to as they work to create healthier and more sustainable communities is the "transition towns" movement.[7] There is a growing network of transition towns in Canada[8] and health promoters should link up to their nearest group or help to start one locally!

BOX 8.3:

Transition Initiative

"A Transition Initiative ... is a community-led response to the pressures of climate change, fossil fuel depletion and increasingly, economic contraction. There are thousands of initiatives around the world starting their journey to answer this crucial question:

'for all those aspects of life that this community needs in order to sustain itself and thrive, how do we significantly rebuild resilience (to mitigate the effects of Peak Oil and economic contraction) and drastically reduce carbon emissions (to mitigate the effects of Climate Change)?'"

Source: http://www.transitionnetwork.org/support/what-transition-initiative

---

Finally, at the national level, a key resource is CoPEH–Canada (Community of Practice on Ecosystem Health), which is "an adaptive community of scholars and practitioners dedicated to the understanding, teaching and application of ecosystem approaches to address current challenges to a healthy and sustainable global future."[9] Expanding the understanding that human and ecosystem health are inextricably linked and that an ecosystem approach needs to be used in considering human health is fundamental to the future health and perhaps the very survival of our societies. It is the most important issue health promotion faces in the coming decades.

Conclusion

Irving Rootman

Although the four issues presented in this chapter are quite different, there are a number of elements common to the discussions of all, or the majority of them. First, all of the authors attempted to make a case for the importance of health promotion. In doing so, all identified serious consequences of not dealing with the issue effectively. They all referred to negative health consequences for individuals or populations and costs, and in the case of the issue of "sustainability," to the very survival of the human species. Also mentioned were the positive consequences of taking action on the issue, including the reduction of inequities, improved productivity, prosperity, and the achievement of human potential. Interestingly, two of the issues were framed using negative terms (chronic disease and unsustainable development) and the other two used positive ones (mental health and health literacy). In the case of mental health, the emphasis was on taking a positive approach emphasizing such things as meaningful engagement, building on strengths, as well as assets and capacities. This suggests that both positive and negative framing can be and is used to make the case for issues in health promotion, perhaps reflecting the possibility that framing it negatively may work better for some audiences and framing it positively better for others. For example, framing an issue in negative terms may be more likely to capture the attention of politicians as retaining their job may depend on how effectively they deal with problems. On the other hand, framing it more positively may stimulate action by communities and individuals by providing inspiration and avoiding attribution of blame.

Second, all of the discussions suggested a number of approaches that should be used in addressing issues through health promotion based on the literature as well as the examples presented. Terms that were commonly used to describe these approaches were: multifaceted, comprehensive, integrated, intersectoral, collaborative, participatory, community-based, multi-strategy, multi-sectoral, multi-level, and whole-of-government. Moreover, it was implied that several of these approaches should be used in combination with one another. All of these terms certainly go beyond a focus on the individual, which, as noted in Chapter 7, has characterized much of "issue-focused" health promotion to recognize the importance of the environment and, to some extent, the "context." The section on health literacy in fact explicitly recognizes the importance of "context" in understanding what health literacy is and how it might be approached.

Third, based on the examples of successful or potentially successful health promotion interventions, a number of promising practices were identified. They included: sharing leadership; publicly stating goals and targets; engaging civil society organizations; ensuring that stakeholders understand their roles and responsibilities; establishing an accountability framework; using tranformational incentives; developing culturally appropriate resources and services; building on community assets and using community development approaches; establishing ownership of the initiative by the stakeholders; building empowerment and resilience skills; encouraging and supporting self-care; embedding health promotion in existing initiatives; understanding and taking context into account; evaluating the initiative rigorously; and building in sustainability. Again, it was implied that using these approaches in combination would be desirable.

Finally, several of the discussions identified some key resources or prerequisites for effective health promotion action, including: high-level political commitment and leadership, existing or new networks, supportive environments, funding, and social capital. It was also suggested that using evidence to develop health promotion interventions was important.

Thus, this chapter and the examples that are cited provide some useful guidance to health promotion practitioners who are interested in addressing particular issues that are of concern to them or others. Having said that, it is clear that while a particular "issue" may be an entry point for undertaking health promotion action, it does not preclude also using a "settings" approach or a "population" approach or a "contextual" approach as a way of addressing the issue effectively. Furthermore, as suggested in Chapter 5 on ecological approaches, which gives two examples of "issue-focused" initiatives, using an ecological theoretical framework is also compatible with using an "issue" as an entry point to health promotion interventions. Given this, it is important to learn more about these approaches from the chapters that follow, other chapters in this book, and other sources. Finally, the examples in this chapter are all complex issues that draw together a number of threads of concern emerging over time. This reflects the complexity of concerns that health promotion as a field of practice needs to address today and why we need new ways of looking at our work that recognize this complexity.

Notes

1. Retrieved from: http://hpclearinghouse.net/blogs/hlel/pages/home.aspx
2. Retrieved from: http://cdeacf.ca/cdeacf
3. Retrieved from: http://www.linkedin.com/groups?mostPopular=&gid=2539106
4. Retrieved from: http://www.centreforliteracy.qc.ca/Healthlitinst/Calgary_Charter.htm
5. It is important to understand that the Earth itself is not in danger, life as a whole is not in danger—although we are undergoing a (human-induced) great extinction—nor is the human species likely in danger of extinction—we are a very resilient species. But our societies and our civilization are in danger of collapse, and we would not be the first to experience that fate.
6. I use the analogy of cancer very deliberately. From Gaia's perspective, or at least from the perspective of species facing extinction, our current industrial civilization is a cancer, growing exponentially and ultimately sickening or killing the victim—in this case, many species—but not life itself, in all likelihood.
7. Retrieved from: http://www.transitionnetwork.org/support/what-transition-initiative
8. Retrieved from: http://www.transitionnetwork.org/initiatives
9. Retrieved from: http://www.copeh-canada.org/index_en.php

References

Barrett, P. (2003). *Governance and joined-up government: Some issues and early successes.* Melbourne: Australian National Audit Office.

Barry, M.M. (2009). Addressing the determinants of positive mental health: Concepts, evidence, and practice. *International Journal of Mental Health Promotion, 11*(3), 4–17.

BC Healthy Living Alliance [BCHLA]. (2010). *Leading British Columbia towards a healthy future.* BC Healthy Living Alliance Report: Healthy Living Initiatives 2007 to 2010. October 2010. Vancouver, BC; B.C. Healthy Living Alliance.

Brundtland, G.H (1987). *Our common future.* Oxford: Oxford University Press.

Canadian Council on Learning (CCL). (2007). *Health literacy in Canada: Initial results from the International Adult Literacy and Skills Survey.* Ottawa: Canadian Council on Learning.

Canadian Council on Learning (CCL). (2008). *Health literacy in Canada: A healthy understanding.* Ottawa: Canadian Council on Learning.

Canadian Institute for Health Information (CIHI). (2009). *Improving the health of Canadians: Exploring positive mental health.* Ottawa: CIHI. Retrieved from: https://secure.cihi.ca/estore/productFamily. htm?locale=en&pf=PFC1051&lang=en&media=0

Canadian Public Health Association (CPHA). (1992). *Human and ecosystem health.* Ottawa: CPHA.

Centre for Health Promotion. (1997). *Proceedings from the International Workshop on Mental Health Promotion.* Toronto: University of Toronto. Cited on p. 16 in Joubert, N. & Raeburn (1999). Mental health promotion: People power and passion. *International Journal of Mental Health Promotion, 1,* 15–22.

Commission on the Social Determinants of Health (CSDH). (2008). *Closing the gap in a generation: Health equity through action on the social determinants of health.* Geneva: World Health Organization.

Cooke, A., Friedli, L., Coggins, T., Edmonds, N., Michaelson, J., O'Hara, K., Snowden, L., Stansfield, J., Steuer, N. & Scott-Samuel, A. (2011). *Mental well-being impact assessment: A toolkit for well-being* (3rd ed.). London: National MWIA Collaborative. Retrieved from: http://www.apho.org.uk/resource/item.aspx?RID=95836

Diamond, J. (2005). *Collapse: How societies choose to fail or succeed.* New York: Penguin.

Frankish, J., Gray, D., Soon, C. & Milligan, C.D. (2011). *Health literacy scan project.* Prepared for the Chronic Disease Interventions Division, Centre for Chronic Disease Prevention & Control, Public Health Agency of Canada. Vancouver: Centre for Population Health Promotion Research.

Friedli, L. (2009). Mental health, resilience, and inequalities. Prepared for WHO Europe. Retrieved from: http://www.euro.who.int/document/e92227.pdf

GermAnn, K. & Ardiles, P. (2009). *Toward flourishing for all.* Mental Health Promotion and Mental Illness Prevention: Policy Background Paper. Pan-Canadian Steering Committee for Mental Health Promotion and Mental Illness Prevention. Retrieved from: http://www.bcmhas.ca/Research/ TowardFlourishingForAll.htm

Government of British Columbia. (2006). *Measuring our success: Baseline document.* Victoria: Government of British Columbia. Retrieved from: http://www.actnowbc.ca/media/ActNow-BC-Measuring-our-Success-Baseline-Document-2006-11.pdf

Health Council of Canada. (2006). *Health care renewal in Canada: Clearing the road to quality.* Annual Report to Canadians—Chronic Disease. Toronto; Health Council of Canada.

Hunt, S. (2005). Whole-of-government: Does working together work? In *Policy and governance discussion paper 05-01.*Canberra: Asia Pacific School of Economics and Government.

Keleher, H. & Armstrong, R. (2006). *Evidence-based mental health promotion resource.* Melbourne: Department of Human Services. Retrieved from: www.health.vic.gov.au/healthpromotion/downloads/mental_health_resource.pdf

Keyes, C.L.M. (2007). Promoting and protecting mental health as flourishing. *American Psychologist, 62*(2), 95–108.

Keyes, C.L.M. (2010). The next step in the promotion and protection of mental health. *Canadian Journal of Nursing Research, 42*(3), 17–28.

Kickbusch, I. (2010). *Triggering debate—white paper—The food system.* Geneva: Health Promotion Switzerland.

King, J. (2007). *Environmental scan of interventions to improve health literacy: Final report.* Antigonish: National Collaborating Centre for Determinants of Health.

Masny, D. (dir.). (2009). *Lire le monde: les littératies multiples et l'éducation dans les communautés francophones.* Ottawa: les Presses de l'université d'Ottawa.

Meadows, D. et al. (1972). *The limits to growth*. White River Junction: Chelsea Green.

Meadows, D., Randers, J. & Meadows, D. (2004). Limits to growth: The 30-year update. White River Junction: Chelsea Green.

Mikkonen, J. & Raphael, D. (2010). *Social determinants of health: The Canadian facts*. Toronto: York University School of Health Policy and Management. Retrieved from: http://www.thecanadianfacts.org/

Nutbeam, D. (2000). Health literacy as a public health goal: A challenge for contemporary health education and communication strategies into the 21st century. *Health Promotion International, 15*(3), 359–367.

Pan-American Health Organization. (2007). *Regional strategy and plan of action on an integrated approach to the prevention and control of chronic diseases including diet, physical activity, and health*. Washington: Pan-American Health Organization.

Peerson, A. & Saunders, M. (2009). Health literacy revisited: What do we mean and why does it matter? *Health Promotion International, 24*, 285–296.

Provencher, H.L. & Keyes, C.L.M. (2011). Complete mental health recovery: Bridging mental illness with positive mental health. *Journal of Public Mental Health, 10*(1), 54–66.

Public Health Agency of Canada. (2006). *The human face of mental health and mental illness in Canada 2006*. Ottawa: Minister of Public Works and Government Services, Canada. Retrieved from: http://www.phac-aspc.gc.ca/publicat/human-humain06/pdf/human_face_e.pdf

Public Health Agency of Canada. (2009). *Mobilizing intersectoral action to promote health: The case of ActNowBC in British Columbia, Canada*. Cat. no. HP5–85/2009. In Herten, L. & Gunning-Shepers, L. (2000). Targets as a tool in health policy. Part II: Guidelines for application. *Health Policy, 53*, 13–23.

Raphael, D. (2009). Restructuring society in the service of mental health promotion: Are we willing to address the social determinants of mental health? *International Journal of Mental Health Promotion, 11*(3), 18–31.

Region of Waterloo Public Health. (2007). *Healthy growth: Health and the built environment in Waterloo Region*. Retrieved from: http://www.regionofwaterloo.ca/en/doingBusiness/resources/BlueprintShapingGrowth.pdf

Riley, B., Stachenko, S., Wilson, E., Harvey, D., Cameron, R., Farquharson, J., Donovan, C. & Taylor, G. (2009). Can the Canadian heart health initiative inform the Population Health Intervention Research Initiative for Canada? *Canadian Journal of Public Health, 100*(1), Suppl. i, 20–26.

Ronson, B. & Rootman, I. (2004). Literacy: One of the most important determinants of health. In D. Raphael (Ed.), *Social determinants of health: Canadian perspectives* (1st ed.) (pp. 139–169). Toronto: Canadian Scholars' Press Inc.

Rootman, I., Frankish, J. & Kaszap, M. (2007). Health literacy: A new frontier. In M. O'Neill, A. Pederson, S. Dupere & I. Rootman (Eds.), *Health promotion in Canada: Critical perspectives* (2nd ed.) (pp. 61–73). Toronto: Canadian Scholars' Press Inc.

Rootman, I. & Gordon-El-Bihbety, D. (2008). *A vision for a health literate Canada: Report of the Expert Panel on Health Literacy*. Ottawa: Canadian Public Health Association.

Rudd, R.E., Anderson, J.E., Oppenheimer, S. & Nath, C. (2007). Health literacy: An update of medical and public health literature. In J.P. Comings, B. Garner & C. Smith (Eds.), *Review of adult learning and literacy* (1st ed.) (pp. 175–203). Mahwah: Lawrence Erlbaum Associates.

Ryff, C.D. & Singer, B. (1996). Psychological well-being: Meaning, measurement, and implications for psychotherapy research. *Psychotherapy and Psychosomatics, 65*(1), 14–23.

Sanders, M.R. (1999). The Triple P—Positive Parenting Program: Towards an empirically validated multilevel parenting and family support strategy for the prevention of behavior and emotional problems in children. *Clinical Child and Family Psychology Review, 2*(2), 71–90.

Sanders, M.R. (2008). Triple P—Positive Parenting Program as a public health approach to strengthening parenting. *Journal of Family Psychology, 22*(3), 506–517.

Turner, G. (2008). *A comparison of the limits to growth with thirty years of reality*. Canberra: CSIRO.

Van Herten, L. & Gunning-Shepers, L. (2000). Targets as a tool in health policy. Part II: Guidelines for application. *Health Policy*, *53*, 13–23.

Wilkins, P. (2002). Accountability and joined-up government. *Australian Journal of Public Administration*, *61*(1), 114–119.

World Economic Forum. (2008). *Working towards wellness: The business rationale*. Geneva: World Economic Forum/Price Waterhouse Coopers. Retrieved from: www.pwc.com/gx/en/healthcare/working-towards-wellness-business-rationale.jhtml

World Health Organization (WHO). (1986). *Ottawa charter for health promotion*. Ottawa: World Health Organization, Health and Welfare Canada & Canadian Public Health Association.

World Health Organization (WHO). (1992). *Our Planet, Our Health* (Report of the WHO Commission on Health and Environment). Geneva: WHO.

World Health Organization (WHO). (2003). *Investing in mental health*. Geneva: World Health Organization. Retrieved from: http://www.who.int/mental_health/en/investing_in_mnh_final.pdf

World Health Organization (WHO). (2005). Preventing chronic diseases: A vital investment: *WHO global report*. Geneva: World Health Organization. Retrieved from: www.who.int/chp/chronic_disease_report/en/index.html

World Health Organization (WHO). (2006). *Gaining health: The European strategy for the prevention and control of non-communicable diseases*. Copenhagen: World Health Organization.

World Health Organization (WHO). (2008). *2008–2013 action plan for the global strategy for the prevention and control of non-communicable diseases*. Geneva: World Health Organization.

WHO & Government of Canada. (2005). *WHO global forum IV on chronic disease prevention and control*. Geneva & Ottawa: WHO & Health Canada.

WWF. (2010). *Living planet report 2010*. Retrieved from: http://wwf.panda.org/about_our_earth/all_publications/living_planet_report/2010_lpr/

Critical Thinking Questions

1. What are the advantages and limitations of using an "issue" as a point of entry and approach in health promotion?

2. To what extent are the issues cited in this chapter important ones for health promotion to address? Which do you think is the most important and the least important? Why? What other issues do you think are important for health promotion to address? Why?

3. What are the relative advantages and disadvantages of framing an issue in positive or negative terms? What is the value of changing the framing of an issue? How can you see this applied in practice?

4. Where does the responsibility for addressing these issues discussed in this chapter reside—with the individuals and communities, providers, systems, governments?

5. As is evident in the chapter, these "issues" require multiple approaches and partnerships. How can a health promotion practitioner promote joint ownership across sectors for an issue they are dealing with, in order to create collective action?

Resources

Further Readings

Brown, L. (2007) *Plan B 3.0: Mobilising to save civilization*. Jakarta: Yayasan Obor Indonesia.

Lester Brown founded the Worldwatch Institute in 1974. The institute is an authoritative organization that has been publishing the annual *State of the World* reports for many years. These reports, which are also worth reading, provide a combination of information on what the problems are (with a different focus each year) and what the solutions might be. Brown moved on to establish the Earth Policy Institute some years ago and this book provides his plan for how we can navigate through the present crisis to a more sustainable future.

Canadian Council on Learning. (2008). *Health literacy in Canada: A healthy understanding.* Ottawa: CCL. Retrieved from: http://www.ccl-cca.ca/CCL/Reports/HealthLiteracy/

This report examines the relationship between levels of health literacy and health outcomes (e.g., diabetes). It also outlines how certain characteristics, such as education and age, can affect health literacy. The website also contains other reports on health literacy that might be of interest to the reader.

Institut national de santé publique du Québec (INSPQ). (2008). *Avis scientifique sur les interventions efficaces en promotion de la santé mentale et en prévention des troubles mentaux.* Ottawa: Institut canadien d'information sur la santé. Retrieved from: http://www.inspq.qc.ca/pdf/publications/789_Avis_sante_mentale.pdf

This report from the Quebec National Institute of Public Health is an evidence review of mental health promotion and mental illness prevention interventions, commissioned by the provincial government.

Ontario Chronic Disease Prevention Alliance and Health Nexus. (2008). *Primer to action: Social determinants of health, Toronto, ON.* Retrieved from: http://www.healthnexus.ca/projects/primer.pdf

This is a resource for health and community workers, activists, and local residents to understand how the social determinants of health impact chronic disease and what can be done about it.

Pape, B. & Galipeault, J.P. (2002). *Mental health promotion for people with mental illness: A discussion paper.* Ottawa: Public Health Agency of Canada. Retrieved from: http://www.phac-aspc.gc.ca/publicat/mh-sm/mhp02-psm02/pdf/mh_paper_02_e.pdf

This paper explores the potential of mental health promotion for people with mental illness. In the first section it discusses related concepts and builds these into a proposed conceptual model. It then proceeds to examine mental health promotion strategies for people with mental illness: first, general strategies corresponding to identified action areas for health promotion, and then some specific examples of national or provincial programs. The paper ends with a set of recommendations for the federal government and an appendix offering specific tools and implementation methods for governments or communities to use in pursuing this issue (Pape & Galipeault, 2002, p. 1).

Rootman, I. & Gordon-El-Bihbety, D. (2008). *A vision for a health literate Canada: Report of the Expert Panel on Health Literacy.* Ottawa: Canadian Public Health Association. Retrieved from: http://www.cpha.ca/uploads/portals/h-l/report_e.pdf

This report presents the Canadian Expert Panel of Health Literacy's vision of a health literate Canada, as well as an analysis of the nature of the issue and some promising ways to address it.

Soskolne, C. & Westra, L. (Eds.). (2007). *Sustaining life on Earth: Environmental and human health through global governance.* Blue Ridge Summit: Lexington Books.

Colin Soskolne is a professor of epidemiology at the University of Alberta and has a strong interest in the links between health and (un)sustainable development. In this book, which argues that humanity has collective problems and that it is only through collective action that solutions will be found, various contributors suggest ways to move forward that would ensure health and well-being for all in both present and future generations.

World Health Organization. (2005). *Promoting mental health: Concepts, emerging evidence, practice.* Retrieved from: http://www.who.int/mental_health/evidence/MH_Promotion_Book.pdf

Promoting Mental Health: Concepts, Emerging Evidence, Practice aims to bring to life the mental health dimension of health promotion. The promotion of mental health is situated within the larger field of health promotion, and sits alongside the prevention of mental disorders and the treatment and rehabilitation of people with mental illnesses and disabilities. Like health promotion, mental health promotion involves actions that allow people to adopt and maintain healthy lifestyles and create living conditions and environments that support health. This book describes the concepts relating to promotion of mental health, the emerging evidence for effectiveness of interventions, and the public health policy and practice implications. It complements the work of another major WHO project focusing on the evidence for prevention of mental illnesses (World Health Organization, 2005, p. xii).

Relevant Websites

Canadian Public Health Association (CPHA) Health Literacy Portal

http://www.cpha.ca/en/portals/h-l.aspx

This website is a source of reports and resources relevant to health literacy in Canada.

COMPAS

http://cdeacf.ca/cdeacf

COMPAS is a francophone repository for research reports related to health literacy.

MHP Resources from the Centre for Addiction and Mental Health (CAMH), Toronto

http://knowledgex.camh.net/policy_health/mhpromotion/Pages/default.aspx

Contains resources related to mental health promotion.

MHP Resources from Victoria Health Foundation, Victoria, Australia

http://www.vichealth.vic.gov.au/en/Publications/Mental-health-promotion.aspx

Contains resources related to mental health promotion.

Qualaxia: Réseau de promotion de la santé mentale, Montreal, Quebec

http://www.qualaxia.org/

Contains resources in French related to mental health promotion.

Triple P Program Resources

http://www.pfsc.uq.edu.au/

Contains resources related to the Triple P Program.

Worldwatch Institute

http://www.worldwatch.org/

The Worldwatch Institute is an independent research organization recognized by opinion leaders around the world for its accessible, fact-based analysis of critical global issues.

CHAPTER 9

Population Approaches to Health Promotion in Canada

Ann Pederson, Jim Frankish, Catharine Hume, Michael Krausz, Michelle Patterson,
Verena Strehlau, Julian Somers, Peggy Edwards, Louise Plouffe, Bilkis Vissandjée,
Ilene Hyman, Axelle Janczur, Marjorie Villefranche, Nancy Poole, and Tatiana Fraser

A Population Approach to Health Promotion: Bringing People Back in

Ann Pederson

If we think of the three entry points identified by Frohlich and colleagues in Chapter 7 as the "what" (issues), the "who" (populations), and the "where" (settings) of health promotion practice, this chapter reflects upon the question of "who." Specifically, this chapter examines approaches to health promotion from the entry point of four demographic or socially defined groups: homeless people, older adults, immigrants, and girls.

Using the population as the entry point for planning aligns with the various diagnostic phases of Green and Kreuter's PRECEDE-PROCEED planning model in which intense analysis is directed at identifying and understanding a "target" population for health promotion interventions (see Green & Kreuter, 2004). The rationale behind programs directed at specific population groups is the assumption that the individuals within a defined population share important characteristics that predispose them to certain health risks, behavioural patterns, or living conditions *by virtue of being members of that population*. Epidemiological analyses, which commonly stratify findings by socio-demographic characteristics—such as income, age, sex, geographic location, and ethnicity or racial background—have contributed to the development of programs and policies through this lens of "populations." In fact, a population approach has long been a staple approach within public health. Consider, for example, the targeted vaccination campaigns directed at children and seniors and specific reproductive screening programs directed at women to detect cervical and breast cancer. Indeed, women and children have both been major populations of interest in health promotion because of the health problems they experience and because of their potential roles in primary prevention efforts (Daykin & Naidoo, 1995).

In this chapter, each "population" is discussed by contributors familiar with the particular population and health promotion initiatives directed at improving specific aspects of their health. Each contribution provides a commentary on particular aspects of the population group that warrant attention in the development and implementation of health promotion and provides an example to illustrate "promising" practice in Canada associated with the population group. No attempt has been made to create a unified voice among the contributors; rather, each segment maintains the distinct perspective of its authors. Following the presentation of the specific population examples, however, some unifying suggestions are made about conclusions that could be drawn from reviewing the approaches used in each case, including the benefits and limitations of a population-based approach to health promotion.

As promising practices, the particular examples described in this chapter go some of the distance toward addressing the concerns raised by Frohlich and colleagues in Chapter 7. They do this by interrogating the factors associated with the particular population of concern that contribute to the risks that these groups face and explicitly identify and address the historical, economic, and political factors that shape the lives and health of members of these population groups. Significantly, each of the interventions described here as a promising practice is considered one because it stresses the importance of context in generating both health challenges and opportunities for health improvement. All of the authors demonstrate the value of situating interventions designed to address the health issues of a particular demographic or social group within a specific historical, political, cultural, and economic context. Thus, the interventions described here have elements that are both generalizable and context-specific, reminding us that "who" we are is as much about social location as genetics or shared identity.

Homeless People and Health Promotion

Jim Frankish, Catharine Hume, Michael Krausz, Michelle Patterson, Verena Strehlau, and Julian Somers

Homelessness affects every rural or urban community in Canada. Twenty percent of Canadians have low incomes (Lee, 2000) and a growing number of Canadians have experienced periods of unstable housing and absolute homelessness (Liard, 2007). In January 2007, the Canadian Council on Social Development applied Statistics Canada's Low Income Cut-off measurement (LICO) to 2001 census data and found that "almost one-quarter of Canadian households—more than 2,700,000 households—are paying too much of their income to keep a roof over their heads. Almost 3 million households are paying more than they can afford for housing" (Canada Newswire, January 30, 2007. http://www.newswire.ca/en/story/189567/almost-3-million-households-paying-more-than-they-can-afford-for-housing).

Homeless individuals tend to have lower self-rated health and higher rates of mortality and morbidity compared to the general population (Hwang, 2001). Moreover, homelessness is associated with poly-substance use, mental illness, chronic health conditions, and difficulty in accessing services (Bashir, 2002). The homeless, as a population, are ever more complex in their physical, mental, and social needs (Hwang et al., 2005). Homeless people with mental and/or physical illness present challenges that often increase the use and costs of services (Bird, Sullivan, Wenzel et al., 2002). They also appear to experience less than optimal treatment from health and social services than others, marked by difficulty accessing and receiving integrated and continuous care (Frankish, Quantz, Stevenson & Clemmer, 2003; Frankish, Hwang & Quantz, 2005).

Increasingly, low-income, homeless citizens may be seeking out supportive housing and related services. All levels of government, the private sector, and non-governmental organizations (NGOs) are investing in supportive housing both within and outside of the health sector. The proliferation of supportive housing initiatives represents a rich but largely untapped collection of *"experiences"* that exemplify adoption of a health promotion perspective in work with vulnerable people who have experienced homelessness.

An exemplary Canadian initiative is the At Home-Chez Soi project funded by the Mental Health Commission of Canada. This research demonstration project is exploring mental health and homelessness in five Canadian cities.[1] The project is based on a "housing first" approach in which housing is addressed before other needs; an estimated 2,285 homeless people living with a mental illness will participate. The model has shown positive results in other cities where it has been implemented (Patterson, Somers, McIntosh et al., 2008; Tsemberis, Gulcur & Nakae, 2004). The rationale for this approach is that once a person is given a place to live, he or she can then, with support, better address other health and quality of life issues. The At Home-Chez Soi project is founded on the value of participant choice and autonomy, as well as providing support and needed services in a wide variety of modalities. The project aims to generate evidence about what services and systems can best help people who are living with a mental illness and are homeless. The project is one of the largest of its kind underway in the world.

The principles (and implied practices) of the *Ottawa Charter for Health Promotion* (WHO, 1986) are inherent in a housing first approach to addressing homelessness. First and foremost, the *a priori* provision of a home exemplifies the *creation of a supportive environment* for health. Second, in the At Home-Chez Soi project, the Commission is working closely with provincial and municipal levels of government, researchers, many local service providers, and individuals who have experienced homelessness and mental illness. Together, they are *strengthening community action* and developing *healthful public policy* regarding housing, health and social services, and the broader, non-medical determinants of health. This includes the *"re-orientation of health services"* toward community-based, client-guided mental and physical health resources. Lastly, the At Home-Chez Soi project emphasizes the empowerment and development of clients' *personal skills* by improving health literacy, and educational, occupational, and psychosocial skills and resources.

In sum, health is created, promoted, and lived by people within the settings of their everyday life—in their communities. At Home-Chez Soi and its housing first approach exemplifies the values, processes, and outcomes of health promotion by emphasizing that health is created by caring for oneself and others, by being able to make decisions and have control over one's life circumstances, and by ensuring that the society one lives in creates conditions that allow the attainment of health by all its members. "Housing first" approaches capture both the spirit and substance of health promotion's original definition as "the process of enabling people to increase control over, and to improve, their health" (WHO, 1986, p. 1), as well as its elaboration as "the process of enabling [individuals and communities] to increase control over [the determinants of health] and [thereby] improve their health" (Nutbeam, 1998, p. 1). These definitions have clear implications for the ways in which health promotion is practised with homeless citizens in settings such as supportive housing. Specifically, they imply that health promotion involves enabling formerly homeless people to address the factors that affect their health by increasing their "control" over these factors or "determinants." This might be accomplished through helping them obtain access to resources that they need for this purpose, or by helping them develop their personal and collective capacities for doing so. The definition also suggests that the desired outcome of health promotion is "improvement" of health and quality of life for homeless and at-risk people rather than simply its maintenance. It implies that health is a "positive" concept that formerly homeless people with serious mental illness can strive toward. Finally, the use of the terms "individuals" and "communities" as a substitute for "people" in the second definition suggests that health promotion is an enterprise or set of activities that is focused on homeless individuals, as well as the communities in which they live. This view de-medicalizes the issue of care, avoids notions of dependence, and reflects a broader cadre of services or activities with which a homeless individual may be involved beyond the receipt of treatment for illness or disease. This view suggests that people who are homeless, community partners, health professionals, policy-makers, service providers, and decision-makers should be involved in the planning, implementation, and evaluation of any new services or programs. While research is underway to evaluate the effectiveness of the housing first approach, as Sir Austin Bradford Hill (1965) said, "*incomplete scientific evidence does not give us the freedom to ignore the knowledge we already have, or to postpone the action that it demands*" (p. 300, emphasis added).

Age-Friendly Communities: A Health Promotion Intervention with Older Adults

Peggy Edwards and Louise Plouffe

As a result of the aging of the large baby boom generation, low fertility rates, and increases in life expectancy, Canada's population is aging rapidly. Within 25 years, the population aged 65 and over will grow from 4.7 million (14 percent of Canadians in 2010) to 10.3 million (25 percent in 2036) (Statistics Canada, 2010). While the majority of older Canadians live in large urban centres, some 23 percent live in rural and remote areas and small towns (Turcotte & Schellenberg, 2007). Seniors who wish to "age in place" in rural communities can face barriers to remaining healthy, active, and engaged in their communities due to limited options for housing and transportation, as well as limited access to health and social services.

While the majority of seniors living in the community view their health as good, the prevalence of chronic conditions, disabilities, and dementias tends to increase with age (Turcotte & Schellenberg, 2007). For example, the percentage of Canadians with two or three chronic conditions jumps from 23 percent among adults aged 45–64 to 41 percent among those aged 65 and over (Statistics Canada, 2008/2009). At the same time, older adults continue to make significant economic and social contributions to their families, friends, neighbours, and communities, as well as through paid and unpaid (voluntary) work (Federal, Provincial, and Territorial Committee of Officials [Seniors], 2006). Health promotion strategies directed to and developed with older adults are therefore designed to address the vulnerabilities of this population group while also building their capacity for personal well-being, mutual aid, and leadership in the community.

"Age-friendly cities" (called "age-friendly communities" or AFC in Canada) is a global health promotion strategy that addresses the importance of creating enabling physical and social environments that support the well-being and productivity of older residents. The Global Age-Friendly Cities project was developed by the World Health Organization (WHO) in 2005 in collaboration with 33 cities in 22 countries (WHO, 2007a). The goal of the project was to identify the essential characteristics of cities that promote active aging and to stimulate community development to make cities more "age-friendly." Canada used the WHO model and research framework to develop a companion guide that focuses on smaller communities and rural regions (Federal, Provincial, Territorial Ministers Responsible for Seniors, 2007). As of July 2011, more than 400 communities of all sizes in Canada have taken steps to become age-friendly, and seven provinces have developed AFC strategies.

In an age-friendly community, policies, services, settings, and structures support and enable people to age actively by:

- recognizing the wide range of capacities and resources among older people
- anticipating and responding flexibly to aging-related needs and preferences
- respecting the decisions and lifestyle choices of older adults
- protecting those older adults who are most vulnerable
- promoting the inclusion of older adults in, and contributions to, all areas of community life (WHO, 2006).

Age-friendly communities employ the health promotion principles and strategies described in the *Ottawa Charter for Health Promotion* (WHO, 1986).

1. *An enabling objective and process:* An AFC enables older individuals and communities "to take control of and improve their health" (WHO, 1986; Nutbeam, 1998) by encouraging "active aging," the process of optimizing opportunities for health, participation, and security in order to enhance quality of life as people age (WHO, 2002). Older adults are involved from the start when they are invited to identify and analyze the characteristics of the community that are salient for older people's well-being through interviews, focus groups, or surveys with older people, as well as with caregivers, service providers, and expert groups. These features then serve as the basis to develop specific standards or criteria to guide community assessment and action.

2. *Use of health promotion strategies:* Age-friendly communities use all five strategies outlined in the *Ottawa Charter*, and most clearly three: *creating supportive environments, strengthening community action*, and *developing healthy public policy*. These strategies address the needs and capacities of older residents in eight domains related to the three pillars of active aging (health, participation, and security). The domains are:
   - outdoor spaces and buildings
   - transportation
   - housing
   - social participation

- respect and social inclusion
- communication and information
- community support and health services
- civic participation and employment opportunities

Policies and programs that address these themes are multi-sectoral and incorporate all aspects of the natural, built, and social environment. They interact to foster community action and create healthier environments. For example, housing affects health and social services needs, while social and civic participation partly depend on the accessibility and safety of outdoor spaces, buildings, and transportation.

3. *Addressing inequities and the broad determinants of health:* The eight domains in the AFC model take into account the influence of the social determinants of health on healthy, active aging. The realization of active aging is determined by multiple personal, social, economic, and environmental factors affecting individuals over the life course. Functional capacities in older adulthood vary widely as a result of the combined and cumulative effects of all these factors. These determinants account for the considerable gaps in life expectancy, health status, and social well-being between older people in wealthier and poorer countries (WHO, 2002), as well as between older people from wealthy and deprived areas within an individual city or community (Plouffe & Kalache, 2010). To ensure that the needs and concerns of economically disadvantaged older adults are taken into account in community planning, the WHO age-friendly cities research design (WHO, 2007b) included respondents from middle and lower socioeconomic (SES) neighbourhoods (Plouffe & Kalache, 2010).

Age-friendly communities begin with a specific population group—older adults. However, there is much congruence between the characteristics of supportive communities identified by older people and respondents in other population groups (Alley, Liebig, Pynoos et al., 2007). For example, extended crossing times at street lights and ramps into public buildings benefit mothers with strollers and toddlers and people with disabilities, as well as seniors. AFC is, therefore, an intergenerational model that helps several population groups overcome barriers to full health, participation, and security at the community level. In the words of Bernard Issacs, founding director of the Birmingham Centre for Applied Gerontology, "Design for the young and you exclude the old; design for the old and you include the young" (Retrieved from: http://www.designinnovation.ie/why_society_sec2.html).

Age-friendly communities relates to the ecological perspective (see Chapter 5), which articulates the dynamic interplay between individual adaptation and environmental alteration to maintain optimal functioning in older age (Lawton & Nahemow, 1973). It also draws on the settings approach and in particular the concept of healthy cities/healthy communities, which emerged in the early 1980s as a key strategy in health promotion (Awofeso, 2003; Hancock, 1997). In this model, the city or community is a setting in its own right, but also includes a number of other settings, such as recreation centres, hospitals, neighbourhoods, and parks. Other influences include related but distinct concepts in urban design and in service planning for disability and for aging services, such as universal design, accessibility, livable communities, walkable communities, and aging in place (Alley et al., 2007; Keller & Kalashe, 1997).

We all are members of an aging society, old and young alike. "It is crucial that societies adjust to this human paradigm as record numbers of people live into very old age, if we are to move toward a society for all ages" (United Nations Programme on Aging, 2010).

Searching for Promising Health Promotion Practices for Immigrants: Accounting for Intersecting Determinants

Bilkis Vissandjée, Ilene Hyman, Axelle Janczur, and Marjorie Villefranche

Good health is one of the critical elements of successful immigrant integration. Ensuring the continued good health of first- and second-generation immigrants and their families remains a challenge. A number of studies have demonstrated that certain groups of immigrants experience a greater prevalence of health and mental health issues with increased time spent in Canada (Hyman & Jackson, 2011; Pottie, Ng, Switzer et al., 2008; Chui, Maheux & Tran, 2007; Hyman, 2007; Newbold, 2005). Of particular concern is the fact that addiction behaviours represent a greater risk among second-generation youth compared to first (Georgiades, Boyle & Duku, 2007; CAMH, 2005).

Yet being a migrant is not a health risk in and of itself. Nor are all immigrant groups at the same risk of transitioning to poorer health, pointing to the need to examine critical intersections with age, sex, gender, ethnicity, migratory experience, socio-economic status, and geography when designing, implementing, and evaluating health programs. Rather, it has been shown that health and well-being result from the complex interplay of determinants that operate at the macro level, the community level, and the individual level (Picot, Hou & Coulombe, 2008; McMurray, 2007; Ng et al., 2005). Failing to account for these intersections may affect the ethical obligation of the health care system to provide universal access (CSDH, 2008). A population health approach that aims to curtail health inequities among population groups may be the key to successful health promotion practices for newcomer women and men (Fawcett, Schultz, Watson-Thompson et al., 2010; Reid, Pederson & Dupéré, 2007; Spitzer, 2005).

Health promotion strategies may not apply equally well to all immigrant populations, especially more recent ones. Socio-cultural, linguistic, and economic factors, as well as informational barriers, influence the health choices of newcomers compared to women, men, and families who have had exposure to promotion and prevention for a longer time period within a host society. Evidence suggests the need to use targeted and tailored approaches in order to prevent widening socio-economic inequalities. Such inequalities have been reported in the uptake of general health screening, healthful dietary advice, smoking cessation, anti-hypertensive prescribing, and adherence to Type 2 diabetes management programs (Choudhury, Brophy, Fareedi et al., 2009; Baradaran, Knill-Jones, Wallia et al., 2006; Vissandjée, Desmeules, Cao et al., 2004).

Targeting is identifying a population subgroup to insure that the group will be exposed to the intervention, while tailoring is developing health messages and materials consistent with a group's cultural characteristics and beliefs. Cultural tailoring operates at two levels. Surface tailoring includes specific actions, such as providing information in a language and idioms that women and men can adequately understand given socio-cultural and economic pressures; it also means actively involving members of the recipient group in the design, adaptation, implementation, and evaluation of the health messages. Deep tailoring builds on cultural tailoring, but requires more systematic incorporation of cultural values and norms into health promotion messages and strategies. Health promotion strategies aimed at newcomers may therefore emphasize concepts such as interconnection, reciprocity, and spousal and filial responsibility in order to align with key cultural and social values in the community (Lawton, Ahmad, Hanna et al., 2008; Vissandjée et al., 2007).

Below are selected Canadian-based promising health promotion practices sensitive to the context of newcomers to Canada. Such approaches require concerted cross-sectoral efforts ranging from recognition of foreign credentials to access to safe environments and reductions in workplace stress.

Access Alliance Multicultural Community Health Centre
Peer Outreach Worker Program

The peer outreach worker (POW) program at the Access Alliance Multicultural Community Health Centre (AAMCHC, www.accessalliance.ca) in Toronto incorporates peer outreach workers into its core interdisciplinary team. POWs are typically contracted for three years, full-time; they are supported by a health promoter on staff. They are trained to provide language-appropriate and culturally sensitive information, referrals, and social support to newcomer families through outreach in selected communities, and they also deliver workshops or co-facilitate groups. An extensive training program allows POWs to work independently with partner agencies in areas where there are a significant number of new-comer families from priority communities such as Arabic, Tamil, Hindi, Punjabi, and Farsi-speaking families with children aged 0–6. The peer worker is often the one who identifies vulnerable families through their outreach activities.

The program aims to provide employment experience to newcomer women and to develop their knowledge and skills related to community health work; to improve access to the programs and services provided by AAMCHC and community-based agencies; and to build community partnerships and reduce the organizational barriers preventing newcomer women and their families from accessing programs and services.

The POW program directly addresses macro-level determinants of immigrant health by contributing to the identification of employment opportunities for newcomer women. AAMCHC has trained nearly 100 peer outreach workers and approximately 80 percent of the peer out-reach workers have gained employment elsewhere following their initial contract with Access Alliance (Koch & Tyrell, 2007). POWs link newcomer mothers and their families with a range of programs and services. The annual report indicates that immigrant women and men value the personal contact with someone who speaks the same language and understands the challenges of integrating into a new society. POWs themselves report that the training and work experience have transformed their lives personally and professionally (Hyman & Guruge, 2002).

Community Meets the University at Maison d'Haïti

Maison d'Haïti (www.mhaiti.org) in Montreal is dedicated to the education and integration of immigrant women, men, and their families while contributing to the reduction of health and social inequalities in the host society. It offers programs to improve the health, living conditions, and rights of Quebecers of Haitian origin and other newcomers in its geographic catchment area. A culturally adapted, peer-led diabetes self-management program is being implemented through a partnership between trained "expert" community members, front-line health care professionals, and university researchers. This program is integrated with ongoing programs addressing health literacy, economic, social, and cultural challenges for newcomers and long-term immigrants.

The Public Health Agency of Canada supports this program and a similar one based at the Access Alliance Multicultural Community Health Centre in Toronto. Interdisciplinary study teams in both Toronto and Montreal have found that the prevalence and risk of diabetes are on the rise among recent immigrants, especially women from countries in South Asia, Latin America/Caribbean, and sub-Saharan Africa. Variation in living and working circumstances, again mostly among women, was thought to contribute to diabetes risk. Self-help management sensitive to gender was identified as an important determinant to consider in the design and implementation of health promotion strategies (Hyman, Zaidi, Sivasamy et al., 2010; Vissandjée, Yared, Rabasa-Lhoret et al., 2010). These determinants of self-management operate from the level of the health system (such as commitments to reduce linguistic barriers), to neighbourhood level (such as availability of support systems), to the level of immigrant women and men themselves in regard to their capacity to manage their daily hurdles as newcomers (Lawton et al., 2008; Speller, Wimbush & Morgan, 2005; Raphael, Anstice, Raine et al., 2003; Spallek, Zeeb & Razum, 2010). The intervention's strength may lie in case-management models with interdisciplinary and intersectoral team members who are sensitive to the life context of immigrant women, men, and their families.[2]

Conclusion

These selected examples suggest the following principles as common to "promising practices" to improving newcomers' health. First, exemplary programs attend to the macro-, community-, and individual-level determinants of newcomers' health and use a population health approach that aims to make structural changes to economic, social, and physical environments; improve access to services; strengthen communities; and strengthen women and men in a gender-sensitive manner. Second, such interventions pay attention to the intersections between experiences of migration and other social identifiers that influence health such as gender, race, ethnicity, socio-economic status, and geographic location. Third, they embrace targeting and tailoring strategies to ensure acceptability and uptake. And, finally, promising practices use community-based participatory approaches in research and health promotion interventions conducted by, for, and with women and men on issues that are relevant to their communities while seeking positive social change and healthy behaviours.

Girls' Health Promotion: The Girls Action Foundation Approach

Nancy Poole and Tatiana Fraser

The Girls Action Foundation is a national umbrella organization and virtual network for girls' empowerment initiatives in Canada. As described on its website, the Girls Action Foundation leads and seeds girls' programs across Canada, builds girls' and young women's skills and confidence, and inspires collective action to change the world. Girls Action currently reaches over 60,000 girls and young women across Canada, in urban, remote, and northern communities, through a network of over 200 partnering organizations. Leadership skills, media literacy, sexual health, and violence prevention are fostered through all-girls spaces, resources, and encouragement for girls to be agents of change in their own social networks and communities.

Girls Action programs employ a unique multifaceted framework, each facet of which is drawn from critical social theory (see Chapter 3), with its focus on emancipatory knowledge (as described, for example, by Freire [2006] and hooks [1994]) and applied to the realm of girls (see http://www.girlsactionfoundation.ca/en/amplify-designing-spaces-and-programs-for-girls). The five facets or principles of the Girls Action framework, with short explicatory excerpts from the Girls Action website (www.girlsactionfoundation.ca/), are:

1. *Popular Education*
   "The Girls Action approach favours grassroots and critical educational approaches designed to recognize girls' knowledge and invites girls to be experts in their own lives."
2. *Interlocking Feminist Analysis*
   "An interlocking feminist analysis recognizes and takes into account the multiple and intersecting impacts of policies and practices on different groups of women because of their race, class, ability, sexuality, gender identity, religion, culture, refugee or immigrant status, or other status. Only by recognizing the differing locations and varying histories of individuals can we begin to build relationships and mobilize for social change together."
3. *Social Action and Change*
   "In working towards social justice, the Girls Action approach promotes transformative change directed towards altering existing social structures and frameworks. Social action and change are achieved through the sharing of similar and diverse experiences, demystifying issues through education, encouraging and supporting action-oriented living strategies and critical thinking skills."
4. *Critically Asset-Based*
   "Working from a positive-oriented lens that emphasizes the assets and capacities of girls' own realities and experiences, the Girls Action approach builds on girls' strengths and community resources. This asset-based approach embraces a social, political and

economical reflexivity and a critical perspective while acknowledging that girls face certain structural barriers not limited to institutionalized racism, poverty and homophobia, and other forms of structural and personal violence."

5. *Organic*

"The Girls Action approach is continuously shaped by young women's input and feedback. A fluid spiral of learning, reflecting, researching, doing and evaluating informs this work on both organizational and programming levels."

Health Promotion with Gender in Mind

While health promotion in general has not, to date, fully articulated how to integrate gender within its vision and practice (Pederson, Ponic, Greaves et al., 2010; Reid, Pederson & Dupéré, 2007), clearly this is health promotion with gender in mind. One can feel the energy of girls being enabled and empowered to increase control over their health, *and* the determinants of their health in these principles. The Girls Action approach fully recognizes the role of gender-specific spaces when enacting popular education methods—for example, when starting conversations on highly gendered experiences such as violence against girls in dating relationships, identifying patterns of violence, learning together about the dimensions of violence, and strategizing and acting for change:

> Creating an empowering and supportive space for girls and young women to get together and talk about their experiences of violence is important in breaking isolation. It allows issues of violence to be seen as a societal problem and not an individual problem. Such spaces empower girls to find ways to take action against the roots of violence, while coping with lived experiences of violence. We also know that there aren't enough of these spaces. (Girls Action Foundation, 2010)

Creating an environment in which girls feel physically and emotionally safe to express themselves has been identified as an important element of effective girls' groups (LeCroy & Daley, 2001) and structured support groups overall have shown positive results on a range of health-related issues for girls (Azzarto, 1997; Dollete, Steese, Hossfeld et al., 2004).

Girls Action embeds a gender-based analysis within an intersectional one, recognizing "that the girls in our programs are diverse in terms of their race, socio-economic status, ability, sexuality, gender identity, religion, culture, Aboriginal, refugee, immigrant or other status, and much more." Such an analysis recognizes how health and other inequities play out:

> Reena Virk could not "fit in" because she has nothing to "fit" into. She was brown in a predominately white society, she was supposedly overweight in a society that values slimness to the point of anorexia, and she was different in a society that values "sameness" and uniformity. And she was killed by those who considered her difference an affront to their sense of uniformity. (Jiwani, 2010)

In such ways, attention to the multiple interlocking locations of girls and women is effectively integrated. And yet even as inequities are named, there is a conscious commitment within the Girls Action framework to accentuate the positive and to build supportive networks and community among girls, taking into account diversity and complexity, in order to catalyze action to address inequities. This linking of feminist analysis with an asset-based approach that extends girls' strengths, resiliency, and leadership potential is particularly salient. Such approaches in helping girls to form close relationships, find a valued place in a constructive group, and use available support systems are evidenced in the wider literature on resiliency and empowerment (Watkins, 2002).

Cross-setting Work with an Empowerment Focus

The girls' groups affiliated with Girls Action are located in multiple settings in schools and communities. Some groups have a specific mandate to bring together girls with shared experiences such as the *gurlz Antidote club* for multiracial and Indigenous girls in Victoria (http://gurlz.antidotenetwork.info/), or Gashanti UNITY for Somali young women in Toronto (http://gashantiunity.ca/). Others are bringing together girls who live in the same region, such as Faro Girls Night Out in Faro, or the Tri-County Women's Centre in Yarmouth (http://tricountywomenscentre.org), while some have specific mandates, such as artistic endeavours like Rock Camp for Girls Montreal in Montreal (http://girlsrockmontreal.org), or sciences and technology like DiscoverE in Edmonton (http://discovere.ualberta.ca), or Les Scientifines in Montreal (http://scientifines.com).

The organic nature of Girls Action supports such local, contextualized work in multiple settings. A non-prescriptive, organic approach allows for attention to the issues relevant in different locations and settings, the localized determinants of health (Poland, Krupa & McCall, 2009), and widens the capacity for changing such settings. The Girls Action approach represents health promotion for a new generation in its focus on empowerment at individual, organizational, and community/political levels (Keleher, 2007). Girls are helped to develop communication skills, critical thinking, and leadership skills, and to take these forward into creating zines and campaigns for change. For example, Take Back the Tech! is a collaborative campaign that promotes creative and strategic use of technology in the fight to end violence against women.[3]

Conclusion

The linking of popular education methods with feminist analysis and social action across the Girls Action Foundation network is health promotion-oriented empowerment in a highly transformative manifestation.

Conclusions from Chapter: Bringing People Back in

Ann Pederson

The subtitle of this chapter, "Bringing People Back in," is an allusion to George Homans's presidential address to the American Sociological Association in 1964 entitled, "Bringing Men Back in" (Homans, 1964), in which he argued that structural functional theory, a school of sociological thought that dominated North American sociology in the early part of the twentieth century, described a society in which there were no actors, only social norms and roles. The challenge, Homans argued, was to bring "men" back in to social theory in order to explain social action and social change. This is one of the challenges of health promotion practice—to ensure that it is undertaken in ways that respect, understand, and engage appropriately with the particularities of a given population (or the population as a whole) while avoiding essentializing certain aspects of the population (such as their being female or from a particular cultural community) and attending to context. This is the crux of the structure-agency debate in health promotion practice (see Chapter 3)—recognizing the capacity of individuals and communities for active engagement with the factors and conditions that shape their health while recognizing the constraints imposed by social structure.

While we would no longer use the term "men" to describe an entire population, the purpose of this chapter was to consider what happens when health promotion practice starts with a group of people—a population—rather than with a setting or an issue. I think what we find when we talk about approaches to health promotion from a population lens are projects that emphasize particular, sometimes distinct, characteristics of people, which link to their access to resources (information, finances, time, services) and ability to control the determinants of their health—with two important caveats. The first caveat is that though the characteristics that identify people as a population may be aspects of themselves as individuals, a population approach is not necessarily an individualistic one. Second, the attributes that are important to health often have their effects because of context, be that a historical moment, particular society, set of social norms, or social setting (see Chapter 7). Thus, engaging with health promotion using a population lens does not necessarily mean restricting interventions to those directed at individuals or to individual aspects of people within the population. But it does mean seeing the people who are the population of interest in all their humanity and recognizing it within one's work. Interventions targeted at specific population groups are premised on the idea that one size does not fit all. This introduces the importance of targeting and tailoring health promotion practices and embracing an intersectional approach (see Chapter 4).

The promising practices illustrated in this chapter share all these dimensions as well as one more: These exemplary interventions address, in various ways, the determinants of health themselves, not just the downstream effects of those determinants on the health of a particular population. By addressing housing first, designing cities to be age-friendly, offering employment and training to immigrant women, and examining the context of girls' lives, these projects go far beyond health education and social marketing approaches to health promotion. Rather, they each illustrate a way of addressing root causes of marginalization, including poverty, racism, and gendered violence.

As the examples in this chapter illustrate, effective programs also avoid assuming that all girls, immigrants, older adults, or homeless people are alike. Rather, these examples illustrate that a focus on populations enables programmers, policy-makers, and researchers to explore the factors that contribute to this group being at greater risk than some others for certain experiences or health problems. But they do so with a complex and detailed understanding of the composition of the population of interest. In particular, as these examples illustrate, it is not simply a function of being a member of a particular population group that shapes health experiences but rather the social experiences that accompany that particular population group's experiences. Thus, these interventions are compelling because they focus on addressing social processes of marginalization that generate vulnerability or on those that foster self-efficacy and empower resistance. Thus, several of these interventions adopt engagement and empowerment approaches to enable individuals and communities to determine their own priorities and generate their own action plans. In sum, the examples in this chapter align with many of the principles of a "vulnerable populations" approach to health promotion—targeting both health risks and the determinants of those risks, linking to sectors beyond the formal health sector, and engaging with members of the population of interest (Frohlich & Potvin, 2008).

Finally, while we editors separated the entry points of issues, populations, and settings for individual examination, an intervention that is most likely to succeed will encompass all three aspects in its design and implementation to some degree. The value of exploring each entry point independently is that it allows us to reflect on a particular aspect of health promotion practice and its contribution to health promotion, reducing some of the complexity that confronts anyone trying to seriously understand how a given intervention works in a particular context with a particular group of people. Given the pressure on health promotion programs to demonstrate effectiveness, being able to establish guidelines for each aspect of an intervention will likely enhance our ability to have an impact through our programs.

Notes

1. See www.mentalhealthcommission.ca
2. See a video about this project at http://www.nouvelles.umontreal.ca/multimedia/forum-en-clips/mieux-comprendre-les-immigrants-diabetiques-pour-mieux-les-soigner.html
3. See http://www.kickaction.ca/

References

Alley, D., Liebig, P., Pynoos, J., Banerjee, T., Choi, I.H. (2007). Creating elder-friendly communities: Preparations for an aging society. *Journal of Gerontological Social Work, 49*, 1–18.

Awofeso, N. (2003). The healthy cities approach—Reflections on a framework for improving global health. *Bulletin of the World Health Organization, 81*, 3. http://www.celebrites.waw.pl/page-Healthy_city

Azzarto, J. (1997). A young women's support group: Prevention of a different kind. *Health & Social Work, 22*(4), 299–305.

Baradaran, H.R., Knill-Jones, R.P., Wallia, S. et al. (2006). A controlled trial of the effectiveness of a diabetes education programme in a multi-ethnic community in Glasgow. *BMC Public Health, 6*, 134.

Bashir, S. (2002). Home is where the harm is: Inadequate housing as a public health crisis. *American Journal of Public Health, 92*(5), 733–738.

Bird, C., Sullivan, G., Wenzel, S., Ridgely, M., Morton, S., Miu, A. (2002). Predictors of contact with public service sectors in homeless adults with and without alcohol and drug disorders. *Journal of Studies on Alcohol, 63*(6), 716–725.

Bradford Hill, A. (1965). The environment and disease: Association or causation? *Proceedings of the Royal Society of Medicine, 58,* 295–300.

Canadian Council on Social Development (CCSD). Retrieved from: www.ccsd.ca

Centre for Addiction and Mental Health (CAMH), Population and Life Course Studies Unit. (2005). Does student substance use vary by immigrant status? *eBulletin.6*(1). http://www. camh.net/Research/Areas_of_research/Population_Life_Course_Studies/eBulletins/ebv6n1_ ImmigrantStudents_2003OSDUS.pdf

Choudhury, S.M., Brophy, S., Fareedi, M.A. et al. (2009). Examining the effectiveness of a peer-led education programme for Type 2 diabetes and cardiovascular disease in a Bangladeshi population. *Diabetic Medicine, 26,* 40–44.

Chui, T, Maheux, H. & Tran, K. (2007). *Immigration in Canada: A portrait of the foreign-born population, 2006 census.* Cat. no. 97-557-XIE. Ottawa: Statistics Canada.

Commission on the Social Determinants of Health (CSDH). (2008). *Closing the gap in a generation: Health equity through action on the social determinants of health.* Geneva: World Health Organization.

Daykin, N. & Naidoo, J. (1995). Feminist critiques of health promotion. In B. Bunton, S. Nettleton & R. Burrows (Eds.), *The sociology of health promotion: Critical analyses of consumption, lifestyle, and risk* (pp. 60–69). New York: Routledge.

Dollete, M., Steese, S., Hossfeld, B., Russell, N., Taormina, G., Matthews, G. et al. (2004). *Executive summary: A national multi-setting study of changes in adolescent girls' sense of connection, self-image, and sense of competence during a girls' circle.* A study by Maya Dollete and Stephanie Steese of the Dominican University of California, San Rafael, in collaboration with Girls Circle Association, a project of the Tides Center.

Fawcett, S., Schultz, J., Watson-Thompson, J., Fox, M. & Bremby, R. (2010). Building multi-sectoral partnerships for population health and health equity. *Prevention and Chronic Diseases, 7*(6). Retrieved from: http://www.cdc.gov/pcd/issues/2010/nov/10_0079.htm

Federal, Provincial, and Territorial Committee of Officials (Seniors). (2006). *Healthy aging in Canada: A new vision, a vital investment. From evidence to action.* Background paper. Retrieved from: http://www. phac-aspc.gc.ca/seniors-aines/publications/public/healthy-sante/vision/vision-bref/index-eng.php

Federal, Provincial, Territorial Ministers Responsible for Seniors. (2007). *Age-friendly rural and remote communities: A guide.* Public Health Agency Canada. Retrieved from: http://www.phac-aspc.gc.ca/ seniors-aines/publications/public/healthy-sante/age_friendly_rural/index-eng.php

Frankish, C.J., Hwang, S. & Quantz, D. (2005). Synthesis paper: Lessons in prevention and treatment of homelessness in Canada. *Canadian Journal of Public Health, 96,* S23–S30.

Frankish, J., Quantz, D., Stevenson, S. & Clemmer, S. (2003). Development of a homelessness research agenda: Lessons from BC. *Journal of Urban Health, 79*(4), S153.

Freire, P. (2006). *Pedagogy of the oppressed* (30th anniversary ed.). New York: Continuum.

Frohlich, K.L. & Potvin, L. (2008). The inequality paradox: The population approach and vulnerable populations. *American Journal of Public Health, 98*(2), 216–221.

Georgiades, K., Boyle, M.H. & Duku, E. (2007). Contextual influences on children's mental health and school performance: The moderating effects of family immigrant status. *Child Development, 78*(5), 1572–1591.

Girls Action Foundation. (2010). *Why girls? Why violence prevention?* Montreal: Girls Action Foundation. Retrieved from: http://girlsactionfoundation.ca/files/WHY_GIRLS_VIOLENCE_ PREVENTION_eng-lowres.pdf

Green, L.W. & Kreuter, M.W. (2004). *Health program planning: An educational and ecological approach* (4th ed.). New York: McGraw-Hill.

Hancock, T. (1997). Healthy cities and communities: Past, present, and future. *National Civic Review, 86*(1), 11–21. doi: 10.1002/ncr.4100860104

Hill, A. (1965). The environment and disease: Association or causation? *Proceedings of the Royal Society of Medicine, 58*(1965), 295–300.

Homans, G.C. (1964). Bringing men back in. *American Sociological Review, 29*, 809–818.

hooks, b. (1994). *Teaching to transgress: Education as the practice of freedom.* New York: Routledge.

Hwang, S. (2001). Homelessness and health. *Canadian Medical Association Journal, 164*(2), 229–233.

Hwang, S., Tolomiczenko, G., Kouyoumdjian, F.G. & Garner, R.E. (2005). Interventions to improve the health of the homeless: A systematic review. *American Journal of Preventive Medicine, 29*(4), 311–321.

Hyman, I. (2007). *Immigration and health: Reviewing evidence of the healthy immigrant effect in Canada.* CERIS Working Paper no. 55. Toronto: Joint Centre of Excellence for Research in Immigration and Settlement. Retrieved from: http://ceris.metropolis.net/

Hyman, I. &Guruge, S. (2002). A review of theory and health promotion: Strategies for new immigrant women. *Canadian Journal of Public Health, 93*(3), 183–187.

Hyman, I. & Jackson, B. (2011). Patterns of migrants' health. In Health Canada, Migrant Health. *Health Policy Research Bulletin* (January). http://www.hc-sc.gc.ca/sr-sr/pubs/hpr-rpms/index-eng.php

Hyman, I., Zaidi, Q., Sivasamy, S., Yesmin, K., Zhou, Y. & Kljujic, D. (2010). *Migration and diabetes: Preliminary findings for the migration and diabetes study.* Report submitted to the Public Health Agency of Canada, Ottawa.

Jiwani, Y. (2010). Reena Virk: The erasure of race. Quoted in *Why Girls? Why Violence Prevention.* Montreal: Girls Action Foundation. Retrieved from: http://www.vancouver.sfu.ca/freda/articles/virk.htm

Keleher, H. (2007). Empowerment and health education. In H. Keleher, C. MacDougall & B. Murphy (Eds.), *Understanding health promotion.*216–233. Melbourne: Oxford University Press.

Keller, I.M. & Kalache, A. (1997). Promoting healthy aging in cities: The Healthy Cities project in Europe. *Journal of Cross-Cultural Gerontology, 12*, 287–298.

Koch, A & Tyrrell, C. (2007). An Evaluation of the Peer Outreach Worker Program at Access Alliance Multicultural Community Health Centre. Access Alliance Multicultural Community Health Centre. Toronto, Ontario: AAMCHC

Lawton, J., Ahmad, N., Hanna, L. et al. (2008). "We should change ourselves, but we can't": Accounts of food and eating practices amongst British Pakistanis and Indians with Type 2 diabetes. *Ethnicity & Health, 13*, 305–319.

Lawton, M.P. & Nahemow, L. (1973). Ecology and the aging process. In C. Eisdorfer & L. Nahemow (Eds.), *The psychology of adult development and aging* (pp. 464–488). Washington: American Psychology Association.

LeCroy, C.W. & Daley, J. (2001). *Empowering adolescent girls: Examining the present and building skills for the future with the Go Grrrls Program.* New York: W.W. Norton.

Lee, K. (2000). *Urban poverty in Canada: A statistical profile.* Ottawa: Canadian Council on Social Development.

Liard, G. (2007). *Shelter: Homelessness in a growth economy: Canada's 21st Century paradox.* Calgary: Sheldon Chumir Foundation for Ethics in Leadership.

McMurray, A. (2007). Building the evidence base: Research to practice. In A. McMurray (Ed.), *Community health and wellness: A socio-ecological approach* (pp. 347–375). Marickville, New South Wales: Mosby-Elsevier.

Mental Health Commission of Canada. *At Home/Chez Soi.* Retrieved from: www.mentalhealth-commission.ca

Newbold, K.B. (2005). Self-rated health within the Canadian immigrant population: Risk and the healthy immigrant effect. *Social Science and Medicine, 60*, 1359–1370.

Ng, E., Wilkins, R., Gendron, F. & Berthelot, J.M. (2005). Dynamics of immigrants' health in Canada: Evidence from the National Population Health Survey. In *Healthy today, healthy tomorrow? Findings from the National Population Health Survey.* Statistics Canada, Cat. no. 82-618. Ottawa: Statistics Canada.

Nutbeam, D. (1998). *Health promotion glossary* (rev. ed.). Retrieved from: http://www.who.int/hpr/NPH/docs/hp_glossary_en.pdf

Patterson, M., Somers, J.M., McIntosh, K., Shiell, A. & Frankish, C.J. (2008). *Housing and support for adults with severe addictions and/or mental illness in British Columbia.* Vancouver: Centre for Applied Research in Mental Health and Addiction.

Pederson, A., Ponic, P., Greaves, L., Mills, S., Christilaw, J., Frisby, J., Humphries, K., Jackson, B.E., Poole, N. & Young, L. (2010). Igniting an agenda for health promotion for women: Critical perspectives, evidence-based practice, and innovative knowledge translation. *Canadian Journal of Public Health, 101*(3), 259–261.

Picot, G., Hou, F. & Coulombe, S. (2008). Poverty dynamics among recent immigrants to Canada. *International Migration Review, 42*(2), 393–424.

Plouffe, L. & Kalache, A. (2010). Towards global age-friendly cities: Determining urban features that promote active aging. *Journal of Urban Health: Bulletin of the New York Academy of Medicine, 87,* 5.

Poland, B., Krupa, G. & McCall, D. (2009). Settings for health promotion: An analytic framework to guide intervention design and implementation. *Health Promotion Practice, 10,* 505–517.

Pottie, K., Ng, E., Spitzer, D., Mohammed, A. & Glazier, R. (2008). Language proficiency, gender, and self-reported health: An analysis of the first two waves of the Longitudinal Survey of Immigrants to Canada. *Canadian Journal of Public Health, 99*(6), 505–510.

Public Health Agency of Canada (PHAC). (2006). World Health Organization, Global Age-Friendly Cities project, brochure. Retrieved from: http://www.phac-aspc.gc.ca/seniors-aines/pubs/age_friendly/index.htm

Raphael, D., Anstice, S., Raine, K., McGannon, K., Rizvi, S.K. & Yu, V. (2003). The social determinants of the incidence and management of Type 2 diabetes mellitus: Are we prepared to rethink our questions and redirect our research activities? *International Journal of Health Care Quality Assurance, 16*(3), 10–20.

Reid, C., Pederson, A. & Dupéré, S. (2007). Addressing diversity in health promotion: Implications of women's health and the intersectional theory. In M. O'Neil, A. Pederson, S. Dupéré & I. Rootman (Eds.), *Health promotion in Canada: Critical perspectives* (2nd ed.) (pp. 75–90). Toronto: Canadian Scholars' Press Inc.

Spallek, J., Zeeb, H. & Razum, O. (2010). Prevention among immigrants: The example of Germany. *BioMed Central Public Health, 10*(92), 191–192.

Speller, V., Wimbush, E. & Morgan, A. (2005). Evidence-based health promotion practice: How to make it work. *Promotion and Education* (Suppl. 1), 15–20, 56–57.

Spitzer, D.L. (2005). Engendering health disparities. *Canadian Journal of Public Health, 96* (Suppl. 2), S78–S96.

Statistics Canada. 2008/2009. *Canadian Community Health Survey: Healthy aging, 2008/9.* Ottawa: Ministry of Industry.

Statistics Canada. (2010). *Population projections for Canada, provinces, and territories 2010 to 2036 and 2061.* Ottawa: Ministry of Industry.

Tsemberis, S., Gulcur, L. & Nakae, M. (2004). Housing first, consumer choice, and harm reduction for homeless individuals with a dual diagnosis. *American Journal of Public Health, 94*(4), 651–656.

Turcotte, M. & Schellenberg, G. (2007). *A portrait of seniors in Canada, 2006.* Ottawa: Minister of Industry. Retrieved from: http://www.statcan.ca/bsolc/english/bsolc?catno=89-519-XIE#formatdisp

United Nations Programme on Aging. (2010). Retrieved from: http://social.un.org/index/Ageing.aspx

Vissandjée, B., Desmeules, M., Cao, Z., Abdool, S. & Kazanjian, A. (2004). Integrating ethnicity and migration as determinants of Canadian women's health. *BioMed Central Women's Health* (Suppl. 32). http://www.biomedcentral.com/1472-6874/4/S1/S32

Vissandjée, B., Thurston, W., Apale, A. & Nahar, K. (2007). Women's health at the intersection of gender and the experience of international migration. In M. Morrow, O. Hankivsky & C. Varcoe (Eds.), *Women's health in Canada: Critical perspectives on theory and policy* (pp. 221–243). Toronto: University of Toronto Press.

Vissandjée, B., Yared, Z., Rabasa-Lhoret, R., Primeau, M.D., Villefranche, M. & Messier, V. (2010). *Migration and diabetes: Preliminary findings for the Migration and Diabetes Study.* Report submitted to the Public Health Agency of Canada, Ottawa.

Watkins, M. L. (2001). Listening to girls: A study in resilience In R. R. Greene (Ed.), *Resiliency: An Integrated Approach to Practice, Policy, and Research* (pp. 115-132). Washington, DC: NASW Press.

WHO. (1986). *Ottawa Charter for Health Promotion.* Geneva: WHO. Retrieved from: http://www.who.int/hpr/NPH/docs/ottawa_charter_hp.pdf

WHO. (2002). *Active ageing: A policy framework.* Geneva: WHO. Retrieved from: http://www.who.int/ageing/publications/active/en/index.html

WHO. (2006). *Global Age-Friendly Cities project.* Brochure published by the Public Health Agency of Canada. Retrieved from: http://www.phac-aspc.gc.ca/seniors-aines/pubs/age_friendly/index.htm

WHO. (2007a). *Global Age-Friendly Cities: A guide.* Geneva: WHO. Retrieved from: http://www.who.int/ageing/publications/Global_age_friendly_cities_Guide_English.pdf

WHO. (2007b). WHO Age-Friendly Cities project methodology. Vancouver protocol. Retrieved from: http://www.who.int/ageing/publications/Microsoft%20Word%20-%20AFC_Vancouver_protocol.pdf

Critical Thinking Questions

1. What are the strengths and limitations of approaching health promotion from a population perspective?
2. Is a population perspective necessarily an "at-risk" group approach? Why or why not?
3. When would a population approach to practice be useful? Not useful? Why?
4. What theoretical or methodological tools are discussed elsewhere in this book that could be resources for addressing health promotion interventions with populations?

Resources

Further Readings

Covington, S.S. (2004). *Voices: A program for self-discovery and empowerment for girls. Facilitator Guide.* Carson City: The Change Companies. Retrieved from: http://www.stephaniecovington.com/b_voices.php

> The *Voices* curriculum is based on the realities of girls' lives and the principles of gender responsivity; it is also grounded in theory, research, and clinical experience. The *Voices* curriculum advocates a strength-based approach and uses a variety of therapeutic approaches, including psycho-educational, cognitive-behavioural, and expressive arts. The program includes modules on self, connecting with others, healthy living, and the journey ahead. It is used in many settings (e.g., outpatient and residential substance abuse treatment, schools, juvenile justice, and private practice).

Girls Action Foundation. (2010). *Amplify toolkit.* Montreal: Girls Action Foundation. Retrieved from: http://www.girlsactionfoundation.ca/en/amplify-toolkit-1

> The *Amplify Toolkit* is a compilation of over 15 years of Girls Action's expertise in delivering and supporting girls' programs, as well as the endless knowledge and insights collected from their national

network members. The result is innovative best practices, tips, and activities for anyone wanting to start or strengthen a girls' program.

LeCroy, C.W. & Daley, J. (2001). *Empowering adolescent girls: Examining the present and building skills for the future with the Go Grrls program.* New York: W.W. Norton & Company. Retrieved from: http://www.public.asu.edu/~lecroy/gogrrrls/curriculum.htm

Empowering Adolescent Girls describes the developmental framework underlying the Go Grrls program. It describes the following developmental tasks critical for a healthy adolescent transition to adulthood: achieving a competent gender-role identification, establishing an acceptable body image, developing satisfactory peer relationships, establishing independence through responsible decision-making, understanding sexuality, learning how to obtain help and access resources, and planning for the future.

Relevant Websites

Active Aging: A Policy Framework

http://whqlibdoc.who.int/hq/2002/WHO_NMH_NPH_02.8.pdf

Developed by WHO's Aging and Life Course program as a contribution to the Second United Nations World Assembly on Aging, held in April 2002, the report discusses the rapid worldwide growth of the population over age 60; the concept and rationale for "active aging"; the factors that determine healthy active aging; and seven key challenges associated with an aging population. It provides a policy framework for active aging and concrete suggestions for key policy proposals.

Age-Friendly Communities: Tools for Building Stronger Communities

http://afc.uwaterloo.ca/index.html

This website, developed by a number of partners in the Kitchener/Waterloo region (Ontario), provides tools and resources to help local communities find solutions to becoming more age-friendly in a way that best suits their unique needs. It provides tips, tools, and instructional videos under the following headings: Getting Started, Principles, Community Sectors, Building Blocks, Community Stories, and Resources.

Age-Friendly Communities Initiative: Public Health Agency Canada

http://www.phac-aspc.gc.ca/sh-sa/ifa-fiv/2008/initiative-eng.php

This website provides an overview of the Age-Friendly initiatives launched by the WHO and in Canada with links to two useful guides, *Age-Friendly Rural and Remote Communities: A Guide* and *Global Age-Friendly Cities: A Guide*, information on which is included in this section.

Age-Friendly Manitoba

http://www.agefriendlymanitoba.ca/

This attractive website is a one-stop resource centre that provides age-friendly communities with information, discussions, resources, and identifies key people to assist communities in becoming more age-friendly. It describes the Age-Friendly Manitoba Initiative, whose goal is to make Manitoba the most age-friendly province in Canada.

Age-Friendly Rural and Remote Communities: A Guide

http://www.phac-aspc.gc.ca/seniors-aines/alt-formats/pdf/publications/public/healthy-sante/age_friendly_rural/AFRRC_en.pdf

This practical guide was developed to complement the WHO's *Global Age Friendly Cities Guide* to assist Canadian rural and remote communities to become more age-friendly. The report describes the findings obtained through focus groups with older adults (age 60+) in 10 rural and remote communities across Canada, and provides checklists of age-friendly features appropriate to these settings.

Canadian Best Practices Portal

http://cbpp-pcpe.phac-aspc.gc.ca/

The Canadian Best Practices Portal was launched in 2006 by the Centre for Chronic Disease Prevention within the Public Health Agency of Canada. The website for the Portal describes the site as "a compendium of community interventions related to chronic disease prevention and health promotion that have been evaluated, shown to be successful, and have the potential to be adapted and replicated by other health practitioners working in similar fields." Of the 339 "best practices" featured in the Canadian Best Practices Portal, 10 directly targeted immigrant or ethnic populations in Canada (at the time of writing).

Girls Action Foundation

www.girlsactionfoundation.ca

This website serves as an online national network for girls, young women, and partner organizations that work with and support girls and young women across the country. Members have access to groups, blogs, and e-newsletters that foster knowledge exchange and resource sharing, collaborations, and new initiatives. The site also features a public online resource centre with access to downloadable publications related to girls and young women, from research reports to zines to manuals on designing spaces and programs for diverse groups of girls and young women. Linked to the Girls Action's website is kickaction.ca, an online community space for girls and young women who are engaged in community action across Canada. The site provides a space for girls to connect, access resources, and profile their creative work.

Global Age-Friendly Cities: A Guide

http://www.who.int/ageing/publications/Global_age_friendly_cities_Guide_English.pdf

Beginning with the concept of an age-friendly city and its connection with active aging, the report describes the research process conducted with seniors, caregivers, and service providers in 33 cities worldwide, and presents the major issues and concerns in each of eight domains of urban living: (1) outdoor spaces and buildings; (2) transportation; (3) housing; (4) social participation; (5) respect and social inclusion; (6) civic participation and employment; (7) communication and information; and (8) community support and health services. A checklist of age-friendly features in each domain is provided.

Healthy Aging in Canada: A New Vision, a Vital Investment, from Evidence to Action

http://www.phac-aspc.gc.ca/seniors-aines/publications/public/healthy-sante/vision/vision-bref/index-eng.php

This discussion brief, published by the Federal, Provincial, Territorial Committee of Officials (Seniors), describes a new vision for healthy aging in Canada and makes the case for investing in healthy aging now. It summarizes what we know and don't know, and suggests the implications for policy and practice in five key areas of focus: (1) social connectedness, (2) physical activity, (3) healthy eating, (4) falls prevention, and (5) tobacco control. Lastly, it describes a framework for action and suggests some key opportunities for moving ahead.

It Gets Better Project

www.itgetsbetter.org

In September 2010, well-known columnist and author Dan Savage posted a video on the YouTube site that he had created with his partner, Terry. The video was intended to provide hope to young people facing harassment, particularly lesbian, gay, bisexual, transgender (LGBT) kids and teens, following several highly publicized suicides. In mere months, thousands of videos have been made and posted to the site. Through the reach of the Internet, this promising practice to promote the well-being of LGBT youth reaches young people worldwide. This project is a grassroots initiative that works with the power of contemporary social media to communicate a positive, life-affirming message; it has not yet been evaluated in a conventional sense, but it is breaking new ground as a health promoting strategy.

Mental Health Commission of Canada: At Home

http://www.mentalhealthcommission.ca/English/Pages/homelessness.aspx

This website outlines the details of the MHCC of Canada's At Home-Chez Soi research project, including what is happening in each of the five city sites: Moncton, Montreal, Toronto, Vancouver, and Winnipeg. The site offers links to the rest of the MHCC activities and resources, as well as the websites of research and organizations affiliated with the At Home-Chez Soi demonstration project.

Municipalités amies des aînés (MADA)

http://www.mfa.gouv.qc.ca/fr/aines/mada/Pages/mun-amies-aines.aspx

This site provides information on the implementation of age-friendly communities in Quebec (the MADA approach).

National Collaborating Centre for the Determinants of Health

http://www.nccdh.ca

A lack of information on successful interventions addressing migration status and ethnic affiliation has been identified as a serious knowledge gap by the National Collaborating Centre on the Determinants of Health. See: National Collaborating Centre for Determinants of Health. (2008). *Evidence review: The influence of socio-economic status and ethno-racial status on the health of young children and their families.* Antigonish: Author.

World Health Organization: Social Determinants of Health—Women and Gender Equity

http://www.who.int/social_determinants/themes/womenandgender/en/index.html

The WHO Commission on Social Determinants of Health sponsored several knowledge networks, which in turn generated reports to the Commission on specific social determinants. The Women and Gender Equity Knowledge Network report focused on the mechanisms and processes through which gender inequities contribute to the poor health of millions worldwide. Girls and women, as well as boys and men, are damaged as a result of gender inequality. "Because of the numbers of people involved and the magnitude of the problems, taking action to improve gender equity in health and to address women's rights to health is one of the most direct and potent ways to reduce health inequities and ensure effective use of health resources."

Youth Net/Réseau Ado

http://www.youthnet.on.ca/

Youth Net/Réseau Ado is a bilingual regional mental health promotion and intervention program run by youth, for youth in eastern Ontario. Their objective is to reach out and help youth develop and maintain good mental health, as well as healthy coping strategies for dealing with stress, while decreasing stigma around mental illness and its treatment. They do this through education and intervention.

CHAPTER 10

Promising Practices in Aboriginal Community Health Promotion Interventions

Charlotte Reading and Jeff Reading

The World Health Organization defines health promotion as "the process of enabling people to increase control over their health and its determinants, and thereby improve their health" (WHO, 2007, p. 10). Within an Aboriginal context, health promotion is most promising when it involves collective processes that address inequities in health determinants, such as education, self-determination, environmental stewardship, and economic security (Boyer, 2006; Chandler & Lalonde, 1998; Loppie Reading & Wien, 2009; NAHO, 2002). Aboriginal (First Nations, Inuit, and Métis) are all terms recognized in the *Constitution Act* of Canada (1982), Section 35(2), and are used in this chapter to describe the Indigenous peoples of Canada and their descendants. The unique historic, political, and economic complexities within which Aboriginal peoples pursue health promotion necessitate a collaborative approach that incorporates multiple constructions of health and distinct cultural values.

Among Aboriginal peoples living in Canada, a number of similar historical circumstances have shaped the health and well-being of populations. Most notably, all three Aboriginal groups have undergone a process of colonization, which included the dispossession of ancestral lands, the imposition of colonial institutions, and the disruption of traditional lifestyles. It is critical that health professionals and policy-makers gain a respectful appreciation of how these historical, political, and social inequities shape the health promotion needs of Aboriginal communities. Otherwise, health promotion programs can represent disrespectful practice and reflect another form of colonial oppression.

Aboriginal Constructions of Health

The most noteworthy preface to any discussion of Aboriginal health is that a universal Aboriginal paradigm (i.e., belief system) does not exist. Nevertheless, despite diversity in geography, language, and social structure, Aboriginal peoples do share certain values, which are philosophically distinct to Indigenous cultures. Similarly, before any attempt is made to understand Aboriginal constructions of health, it is essential that we appreciate language as a foundation for viewing the world. Through language, Indigenous philosophies construct the existential whole as interdependent and reciprocally related domains, which are typically portrayed as verbs rather than nouns. For instance, whereas in European lexicons, rain is constructed as a distinct element of nature (i.e., water), Indigenous languages may well describe "the process of water falling from the sky to meet the earth" (Leavitt, 1995; Young, 1984).

Indigenous metaphysics situate the human body where physical and spiritual realms overlap. Hence, we are individually and collectively shaped by activities in both realms that sometimes require healing that is liminal or "possessed of the ability to move between and among these states" (Kelm, 1998, p. 84). Complete health is achieved only through harmony with the Creator, family, community, and nature (Long & Fox, 1996). This harmony extends to our ancestors as well as to the children not yet born, thus symbolizing respect for ancient wisdom as well as connection and concern for the environment that must one day sustain our children's children's children. This paradigm, based on unity, interrelatedness, and balance, differs considerably from Western Cartesian-based notions of health, which often deconstruct the physical body in order to isolate and examine its individual parts (Long & Fox, 1996). [1]

Within many Indigenous cultures, a circle is used to represent the cyclical and dynamic nature of human life, which reflects many stages—birth, growth, death, and decay, as well as the mind, heart, body, and spirit (Leavitt, 1995). The circle also symbolizes an intimate connection among beliefs, knowledge, feelings, and actions, as well as among the individual, family, community, culture, and the cosmos. In recent years, some Aboriginal peoples in Canada have adopted the medicine wheel as a symbol of this holistic model. However, it is important to note that this symbol does not hold meaning for all Indigenous peoples.

Health Promotion and Aboriginal Peoples in Canada

When viewed together, the most promising community health promotion interventions among Aboriginal peoples in Canada share some commonalities that include the incorporation of Indigenous concepts, Indigenous contexts, and Indigenous processes.

Indigenous Concepts
Holism
Many Indigenous cultures embrace a gestalt paradigm, often reflected in value themes of holism, which emphasizes the complete person in the entirety of his or her life; personalism, which places value on individual autonomy and freedom; relationality, which acknowledges responsibility for the self, community, environment, and cosmos; as well as balance and harmony, which acknowledges the sacredness of all existence and unconditional respect for humans and non-humans alike (Gunn Allen, 1986; Klein & Ackerman, 1995; McMillan, 1995).

Indigenous knowledge systems are predicated on the belief that many truths exist and are manifest in subjective life experiences. The humility of Indigenous cultures is evidenced in belief systems that not only acknowledge all life as equal and related but that do not necessarily recognize humans as the most important beings in the cosmos (Oakes, Riewe, Koolage, Simpson & Schuster, 2000).

Reciprocity
In general, Indigenous cultures reflect a philosophical structure that positions the life of an individual within a network of family, community, and nation. In particular, the social norms

of many Indigenous cultures differ considerably from Euro-Canadian culture with respect to the concept of reciprocity, which tends to be conceptualized in more relative terms and considers each individual a vital thread in the social fabric of the community (Paul, 2000). Traditional norms emphasize collectivity and the fulfillment of social roles through action within social networks. Identity is thus embedded in the context of relationships, which are rooted in reciprocity and complementarity. Thus, separation from one's social network can be detrimental to identity and self-concept, which may ultimately be harmful to health and well-being (Barrios & Egan, 2002; Yellow Horse Brave Heart, 2001).

Plurality

Conceptualized by Elder Albert Marshall (Eskasoni Mi'kmaq First Nation, Cape Breton, NS), two-eyed seeing offers an alternative to the existing divisiveness between Indigenous and Western approaches to health promotion. Rather than viewing these culturally distinct approaches as incommensurate with one another, Elder Marshall advises that we view health from "one eye with the strengths of Indigenous knowledges and ways of knowing, and from the other eye with the strengths of Western (or Eurocentric, conventional, or mainstream) knowledges and ways of knowing ... and to using both these eyes together, for the benefit of all." In this way, two-eyed seeing health promotion strategies can draw from the perspectives of both Indigenous and Western thought, rather than the domination or assimilation of either.

Willie Ermine conceptualizes plurality as "the ethical space," which "is formed when two societies, with disparate worldviews, are poised to engage each other. It is the thought about diverse societies and the space in between them that contributes to the development of a framework for dialogue between human communities" (Ermine, 2007, p. 193).

Indigenous Contexts
Social Determinants of Aboriginal Health

The underlying principle of health promotion emphasizes the notion that health and/or illness occurs with specific contexts. According to the World Health Organization:

> ... the social determinants of health are the conditions in which people are born, grow, live, work and age, including the health system. These circumstances are shaped by the distribution of money, power and resources at global, national and local levels, which are themselves influenced by policy choices. The social determinants of health are mostly responsible for health inequities—the unfair and avoidable differences in health status seen within and between countries. (World Health Organization, 2011, para. 1)

The physical, emotional, mental, and spiritual health and well-being of Aboriginal peoples is influenced by a myriad of intersecting determinants in politically, historically, socially, and culturally distinct ways. In addition to experiencing deleterious living conditions that create additional health challenges as well as constrain choices about health behaviours, Aboriginal individuals and communities experience inequities that often restrict access to resources that might address those challenges (Loppie Reading & Wien, 2009).

Indigenous Processes
Community Control

To some degree, Aboriginal health promotion interventions continue to be undertaken by "outsiders" who do not consult with nor engage community members. This form of "helicopter health promotion" occurs when practitioners develop interventions, then fly into communities to implement and evaluate the extent to which the programs are "successful" using criteria that are not relevant to Aboriginal communities.

Evolving within the context of ethical conditions for health research, Aboriginal communities have affirmed the right to *control* the process of interventions undertaken about, with, and for them. In this case, control refers to "the aspirations and rights of First Nations [and other Aboriginal] Peoples to maintain and regain control of all aspects of their lives and institutions extending to research, information and data" (NAHO—First Nations Centre, 2005, p. 5).

Community Engagement

Aboriginal community engagement represents a process by which members take actions aimed at benefiting the entire community. Indigenous values of relationship, reciprocity, and collective vision underpin this process, whereby community members collaborate to move the community toward positive change. In the context of Aboriginal health promotion, community engagement reflects a critical component of self-determination, which represents a legitimate aspiration among all Indigenous peoples.

When political and professional stakeholders collaborate with Aboriginal communities in the development and implementation of health promotion interventions, true partnerships can emerge in an atmosphere of mutual trust. Collaborative partnerships enhance the degree to which Aboriginal communities share decision-making power, as well as help to ensure that health promotion interventions are undertaken in a respectful, relevant, reciprocal, and culturally appropriate manner, with benefits shared among all partners.

Cultural Responsiveness

When Aboriginal communities initiate, develop, and control the processes and products of health promotion interventions, the integration of culturally responsive practice is enhanced. However, the cultural diversity of Aboriginal peoples across Canada requires the engagement of local perspectives in order to adequately appreciate and address the diversity of distinct contexts in which health promotion interventions occur. In particular, the so-called "pan-Aboriginal" (Health Council of Canada, 2010) approach to health promotion might posit that all Aboriginal peoples view tobacco as culturally significant, and that promoting respect for the sacredness of tobacco might be a means of reducing its non-traditional or recreational consumption. While this approach seems logical and is convenient for a national-level campaign, it lacks the sensitivity to community-specific belief systems. Therefore, any "Aboriginal approach" must focus on the process of community engagement while not making assumptions about the specific cultural or spiritual protocols of exceedingly diverse Aboriginal communities.

Capacity-Building

Historically and, to a certain extent, currently, fewer health promotion interventions are developed and implemented in Aboriginal communities than in non-Aboriginal communities (McLennan & Khavarpour, 2004). As well, there are limited opportunities for the participation of Aboriginal peoples in the development and implementation of interventions within their own communities, and health promoters rarely provide opportunities to enhance capacity-building within community-based interventions. Aboriginal community capacity-building in research involves activities that enhance a community's ability to effect change (Reading & Nowgesic, 2002). Likewise, health promotion processes must include community-level capacity-building similar to the process of research engagement in which "Research that engages the community and that addresses concerns relevant to the people, that builds on traditional knowledge, and that enhances local capacity holds the greatest promise of contributing to that goal" (Brant-Castellano & Reading, 2010, p. 13). In the context of health promotion, opportunities for community members to acquire new and useful information, as well as to develop or enhance their skills, represent critical components of successful Aboriginal health promotion interventions.

Promising Practices

The following examples describe innovative, community-based, and collaborative actions addressing diabetes, food security, and service access for Aboriginal populations. The four promising practice profiles, selected from a background paper written for the Canadian Heart Health Strategy and Action Plan (Scott, 2007), are grounded in the distinct cultural concepts, contexts, and approaches of their respective Aboriginal communities.

1. The Kahnawake Schools Diabetes Prevention project is a multi-component school intervention that involves parents in collaboration with hospital physicians, dieticians, local universities, and school officials (Macaulay, Paradis, Potvin et al., 1997). For more information, see http://www.ksdpp.org (Also see Chapter 16.)
2. Initiated between 2000 and 2005, the Tui'kn Initiative in Cape Breton, Nova Scotia, represents a cross-jurisdictional collaboration between five First Nations communities, as well as local health authorities and Dalhousie University, to create an Indigenous model of primary health care. For more information, see http://www.tuikn.ca
3. Food security in Canada's North has been addressed through two northern initiatives: (1) the Food Mail program (Glacken & Hill, 2009), initiated in the 1960s, subsidizes the cost of shipping nutritious food to remote northern communities; and (2) the Community Freezer program, initiated in 2001, uses collaborative policy and interventions to reinforce a subsistence economy and traditional ethical codes. For more information, see http://nutritionnorthcanada.ca/index–eng.asp

4. Since 2003, the Heart and Stroke Foundation of Saskatchewan provides stroke-related outreach and services to health care providers in Aboriginal communities. For more information, see http://www.heartandstroke.sk.ca/site/c.inKMILNlEmG/b.3657349/k.1EC/First_Nations_Inuit__M233tis_Resources.htm

Kahnawake Schools Diabetes Prevention Project

In response to advice from community Elders to address the epidemic of diabetes within the Mohawk community of Kahnawake, in 1993, community members collaborated with physicians, dietitians, researchers, and school officials to develop the Kahnawake Schools Diabetes Prevention project (KSDPP). With active participation of a local advisory board, the KSDPP provides a holistic and culturally appropriate, classroom-based health education program on nutrition, fitness, diabetes, understanding the human body, and healthy lifestyles, as well as a home support program for parents and caregivers on nutrition, physical activity, and healthy lifestyles.

Although initially developed as a three-year pilot project to increase healthy eating and physical activity among elementary school students (grades 1–6), the KSDPP has since expanded to serve all community school children. The collaborations have also expanded to include mutually beneficial research partnerships with local universities, as well as capacity-building by providing training for service providers from other communities.

This community-controlled program embraces a pluralistic model of health promotion through the incorporation of Indigenous and Western theories, including social learning theory, the precede-proceed model, the *Ottawa Charter for Health Promotion*, and traditional Indigenous teachings. In addition to the physical health-related objectives, KSDPP strives to maximize community engagement through information-sharing, capacity-building, and collective decision-making.

Cape Breton Island, Nova Scotia

The Tui'kn Initiative represents collaboration between five First Nations communities in Cape Breton, Dalhousie University's medical school, and provincial health authorities, with the aim of increasing community members' access to physician and nurse practitioner services, improving local control of health information, and enhancing a more collaborative approach to health programming among communities. Through community engagement and management, as well as capacity-building, this initiative focuses on addressing the root causes of limited service access and considers the cultural context and relevance of health interventions.

Access to physician care was established through community-based and mobile primary care teams, including having doctors available for clinical hours and home visits, in-patient care, support for program development, and occasional after-hours service. Compliance with drug regimes increased in small, remote communities as a result of access to a mobile blood-collection service, including blood monitoring associated with drug treatments, especially for diabetes. With the support of Dalhousie University's Population Health Research Unit, capacity was developed within local Aboriginal health team members, who were trained to manage community health information and an electronic patient record system. The integration of regional and local health planning also provides support for decision-making related to program development and evolution.

Food Security in Canada's North

While the following examples of food security initiatives in Canada's North have not been systematically reviewed, they do reflect promising practice because of the creative and collaborative policy climate that supported them, as well as their reinforcement of subsistence economy and traditional ethical codes. Beginning in 2001, the Food Mail pilot project was collaboratively established by Indian and Northern Affairs Canada (INAC), Health Canada, the Government of Nunavut, Canada Post, and the Kugaaruk Hamlet Council. The aim of this initiative was to improve food security and promote healthy eating by reducing the postage rate for priority perishables from $0.80 per kilogram to $0.30 per kilogram.

The project, which is now available in approximately 145 communities in Canada, includes nutrition education, as well as retail training in proper food handling and storage. Nutritionally void foods, such as potato chips and candy, do not qualify. With an eye to future evaluation of the program, dietary recalls were completed by community members to determine the average diet. Baseline data were also collected on food-purchasing practices; opinions about the quality, variety, and cost of certain foods; and reasons for not buying more fresh fruit and vegetables. Finally, demographic and household food security information was gathered using a modified version of the United States Department of Agriculture Food Security Module. On May 21, 2010, the Government of Canada announced that a new program called Nutrition North Canada would replace the Food Mail program effective April 1, 2011 (Aboriginal Affairs and Northern Development Canada, 2011).

In 2001, the Community Freezer program established community freezers, which are accessible to all members to facilitate the storage of harvested foods. Successful hunters make donations to the community freezer and withdrawals are not monitored, so as to minimize the stigma of food insecurity.

Another creative example of community support for country foods are hunter-support programs that offer a financial subsidy (for gas and hunting equipment) to hunters who make communal contributions of harvested foods. For example, the Cree Income Security program funds hunters and trappers according to the time they spend out on the land. Similarly, the Northern Quebec Hunter Income Support program, administered by the Kativik regional government, purchases harvested food, which is distributed free of charge to those who cannot hunt.

The Inuit Hunting, Fishing, and Trapping Support program, which was designed by community members, invests in harvesting equipment (such as boats) that is available for communal use and endeavours to encourage Inuit hunting, fishing, and trapping activities, and to ensure that Inuit communities have access to the products of such activities. Similarly, the five-year Nunavut Hunter Support program (1993–1998), which was cost-shared by Nunavut Tungavik Incorporated and the Government of the Northwest Territories, provided capital funding in the form of a lump-sum payment (up to $15,000) to a limited number of full-time hunters to help cover costs related to equipment.

Although Canada appears to lead the world in developing effective Aboriginal hunter and trapper-support programs, best practices for unique situations are still emerging to address income support, incentive, and regulation. In order to reinforce and sustain traditional food practice, as well as to offer opportunities to benefit from participation in both subsistence and cash economies, flexible work schedules, subsistence leave, and job-sharing options must be available for those who harvest from the land and support communal food security.

Heart and Stroke Foundation of Saskatchewan

After a strategic planning exercise in 2002, the Heart and Stroke Foundation of Saskatchewan engaged in active outreach with Aboriginal communities through a series of workshops for community-based health service providers across the province. They have translated their stroke warning signs material into Cree and Dene and have encouraged Aboriginal representation on their Stroke Strategy Steering Committee. As a result of their proactive outreach efforts, requests from the community have increased dramatically, including those for training to deliver the foundation's Living with Stroke and Heart to Heart programs, thus building capacity at the local level and enhancing the foundation's relationship with Aboriginal communities.

Conclusion

Aboriginal peoples in Canada, including First Nations, Inuit, and Métis, are culturally diverse, geographically dispersed, and undergoing rapid social, cultural, and economic transitions. In the face of challenging obstacles, these four inspirational, community-based intervention projects demonstrate the urgent need to balance the development of community health promotion initiatives with broader socio-cultural public policy to create healthy environments for Aboriginal peoples.

The success of these interventions can be attributed, at least in part, to the appreciation and application of Indigenous concepts, contexts, and processes. Initially, incorporation of the distinct perspectives of Indigenous and Western paradigms reflects a more pluralistic alternative to the existing divisiveness between Indigenous and Western approaches to health promotion. Most notably, it is clear that, in developing and implementing these successful health promotion interventions within Aboriginal communities, policy-makers as well as program planners and practitioners considered the distinct contexts that influence all dimensions of health among Aboriginal peoples and communities.

Over the past three decades, social theorists and researchers have confirmed that control over one's life (i.e., self-determination), linked to addressing profound disparities, is key to improving health and well-being (Ermine & Hampton, 2007). Repressive colonial structures and systems have diminished opportunities for self-determination among Aboriginal peoples, thereby deleteriously influencing all other determinants of health. In the case of health promotion, self-determination involves Aboriginal community control over and active engagement in all decisions and activities related to health interventions.

Ultimately, successful Aboriginal community health promotion initiatives, such as those highlighted in this chapter, involve the entire community, which, in addition to ensuring that community needs are addressed, has the potential to increase uptake, provide a sense of ownership, engender community pride, and promote aspirations toward self-determination.

Note

1. See the works of René Descartes at http://plato.stanford.edu/entries/descartes-works/

References

Aboriginal Affairs and Northern Development Canada. *Nutrition North Canada*. Retrieved from: http://nutritionnorthcanada.ca/index-eng.asp

Adelson, N. (2005). The embodiment of inequity: Health disparities in Aboriginal Canada. *Canadian Journal of Public Health, 96*(Suppl. 2), S45.

Barrios, P. & Egan, M. (2002). Living in a bicultural world and finding the way home: Native women's stories. *Affilia, 17*, 206–228.

Boyer, Y. (2006). *Self-determination as a social determinant of health*. Discussion document for the Aboriginal Working Group of the Canadian Reference Group reporting to the WHO Commission on Social Determinants of Health. Vancouver: National Collaborating Centre for Aboriginal Health.

Brant Castellano, M. & Reading, J. (2010). Policy writing as dialogue: Drafting an Aboriginal chapter for Canada's tri-council policy statement: Ethical conduct for research involving humans. *The International Indigenous Policy Journal, 1*(2), 1–20.

Chandler, M. & Lalonde, C. (1998). Cultural continuity as a hedge against suicide in Canada's First Nations. *Transcultural Psychiatry, 352*, 191–219.

Ermine, W. (2007). The ethical space of engagement. *Indigenous Law Journal, 6*(1), 193–203.

Ermine, W. & Hampton, E. (2007). Miyo-mahcihowin: Self-determination, social determinants, and Indigenous health. In B. Campbell & G. Marchildon (Eds.), *Medicare: Facts, myths, problems, and promise* (pp. 342–348). Toronto: James Lorimer and Company.

Glacken, J. & Hill, F. (2009). *The Food Mail pilot projects—achievements and challenges*. Ottawa: Minister of Indian Affairs and Northern Development and Federal Interlocutor for Métis and Non-status Indians.

Gunn Allen, P. (1986). *The sacred hoop: Recovering the feminine in American Indian traditions*. Boston: Beacon Press.

Health Council of Canada. (2010). Health Council of Canada update: Improving the health and well-being of Aboriginal peoples in Canada. Toronto: Health Council of Canada.

Kelm, M. (1998). *Colonizing bodies: Aboriginal health and health in British Columbia*. Vancouver: UBC Press.

Klein, L. & Ackerman, L. (Eds.). (1995). *Women and power in Native North America*. London: University of Oklahoma Press.

Leavitt, R. (1995). *Malliseet and Micmac: First Nations of the Maritimes*. Fredericton: New Ireland Press.

Long, D. & Fox, T. (1996). Circles of healing: Illness, healing, and health among Aboriginal people in Canada. In D. Long & O. Dickason (Eds.), *Visions of the heart: Canadian Aboriginal issues*. 239–269. Toronto: Harcourt Brace.

Loppie Reading, C. & Wien, F. (2009). *Health inequalities, social determinants, and life course health issues among Aboriginal peoples in Canada*. Ottawa: Public Health Agency of Canada—National Collaborating Centre for Aboriginal Health.

Macaulay, A., Paradis, G., Potvin, L., Cross, E., Saad-Haddad, C., McComber, A., Desrosier, S., Kirby, R., Montour, L., Lamping, D., Leduc, N. & Rivard, M. (1997). The Kahnawake Schools Diabetes Prevention project: Intervention, evaluation, and baseline results of a diabetes primary prevention program with a Native community in Canada. *Preventive Medicine, 26*(6), 779–790.

Marshall, A. (2008). *Two-eyed seeing*. Retrieved from: http://www.brasdorcepi.ca/two-eyed-seeing

McLennan, V. & Khavarpour, F. (2004). Culturally appropriate health promotion: Its meaning and application in Aboriginal communities. *Health Promotion Journal of Australia, 15*(3), 237–239.

McMillan, A. (1995). *Native peoples and cultures of Canada: An anthropological overview* (2nd ed.). Vancouver: Douglas & McIntyre.

NAHO—First Nations Centre. (2005). *Ownership, control, access, and possession (OCAP) or self-determination applied to research: A critical analysis of contemporary First Nations research and some options for First Nations communities.* Ottawa: NAHO.

National Aboriginal Health Organization (NAHO). (2002). *Improving population health, health promotion, disease prevention, and health protection services and programs for Aboriginal people.* Ottawa: NAHO.

Oakes, J., Riewe, R., Koolage, S., Simpson, L. & Schuster, N. (Eds.). (2000). *Aboriginal health, identity, and resources.* Winnipeg: Departments of Native Studies and Zoology and Faculty of Graduate Studies, University of Manitoba.

Paul, D. (2000). *We were not the savages: A Mi'kmaq perspective on the collision between European and Native American civilizations.* Halifax: Fernwood.

Reading, J. & Nowgesic, E. (2002). Improving the health of future generations: The Canadian Institutes of Health Research, Institute of Aboriginal Peoples' Health. *American Journal of Public Health. 92*(9), 1396–1400.

Scott, K. (2007.) *Canadian heart health strategy and action plan* (pp. 8–12). Theme Working Group 4, Background Paper, Aboriginal Health. Unpublished manuscript, Public Health Agency of Canada.

World Health Organization (WHO). (2007). The Bangkok Charter for Health Promotion in a Globalized World. *Health Promotion International, 21*(S1), 10–14.

World Health Organization (WHO). (2009). *Milestones in health promotion statements from global conferences.* Geneva: WHO.

World Health Organization (WHO). (2011). Retrieved from: http://www.who.int/social_determinants/en/

Yellow Horse Brave Heart, M. (2001). Culturally and historically congruent clinical social work assessment with native clients. In R. Fong & S. Furuto (Eds.), *Culturally competent practice: Skills, interventions, and evaluations* (pp. 163–177). Boston: Allyn & Bacon.

Young, T. (1984). Indian health services in Canada: A socio-historical perspective. *Social Science and Medicine, 18,* 257–64.

Critical Thinking Questions

1. What are the fundamental elements of promising health promotion practice in Aboriginal communities? Why are these elements important to consider when developing and implementing Aboriginal health promotion?

2. In what ways might community engagement facilitate successful health promotion programs in Aboriginal communities? What are some examples of community engagement strategies with Aboriginal peoples?

3. What are the unique historical and cultural contexts within which social determinants influence the health of Aboriginal peoples in Canada? Why is it important to consider these contexts when developing and implementing health promotion interventions?

4. In what ways might integration of concepts such as two-eyed seeing and the ethical space facilitate successful health promotion interventions among Aboriginal peoples?

5. In what ways might the health promotion interventions described in this chapter also represent actions of self-determination?

Resources

Further Readings

Boyer, Y. (2006). *Self-determination as a social determinant of health.* Discussion document for the Aboriginal Working Group of the Canadian Reference Group reporting to the WHO Commission on Social

Determinants of Health. Hosted by the National Collaborating Centre for Aboriginal Health and funded by the First Nations and Inuit Health Branch of Health Canada, Vancouver

The author discusses the historical and political determinants of Aboriginal peoples' health as well as the important role self-determination (i.e., control over individual and collective events) plays in achieving health.

Loppie Reading, C. & Wien, F. (2009). *Health inequalities, social determinants, and life course health issues among Aboriginal peoples in Canada.* Ottawa: Public Health Agency of Canada—National Collaborating Centre for Aboriginal Health.

The authors describe a model for understanding the ways in which social determinants influence the health of Aboriginal peoples over the life course.

McLennan, V. & Khavarpour, F. (2004). Culturally appropriate health promotion: Its meaning and application in Aboriginal communities. *Health Promotion Journal of Australia, 15*(3), 237–239.

The authors explore the importance of spirituality, community cohesion, and identity to the promotion of health and well-being among Australia's Indigenous peoples.

National Aboriginal Health Organization (NAHO). (2002). *Improving population health, health promotion, disease prevention, and health protection services and programs for Aboriginal people.* Ottawa: NAHO.

The author identifies key issues for improving population health, health promotion, disease prevention, and health protection services and programs for Aboriginal peoples.

Related Websites

Health Canada: First Nations, Inuit, and Aboriginal Health

http://www.hc-sc.gc.ca/fniah-spnia/promotion/index-eng.php

Health Canada is dedicated to helping First Nations peoples and Inuit care for, improve, and maintain their health. They offer unique programs and services to reflect the cultures of First Nations and Inuit that respect their physical, mental, emotional, and spiritual needs, as well as family and community backgrounds.

Native Youth Sexual Health Network (NYSHN)

http://www.nativeyouthsexualhealth.com/

NYSHN is a North America–wide organization working on issues of healthy sexuality, cultural competency, youth empowerment, reproductive justice, and sex positivity by and for Native youth. NYSHN works with Indigenous communities across the United States and Canada to advocate for and build strong, comprehensive, and culturally competent sexuality and reproductive health education programs in their own communities. They are a peer-based network of individuals, families, communities, and Aboriginal society at large. Training, advocacy, program creation, and direct youth and community engagement are their core duties. NYSHN also works directly with service providers, organizations, agencies, adults, and Elders and allied communities.

CHAPTER 11

Promoting Health through the Settings Approach

Michel O'Neill, Paule Simard, Nathalie Sasseville, Jodi Mucha, Barbara Losier, Lorna McCue, Douglas McCall, Marthe Deschesnes, Daniel Laitsch, François Lagarde, Trevor Hancock, Marie-Claude Pelletier, Martin Shain, Alison Stirling, and Manon Niquette

The Settings Approach to Health Promotion

Michel O'Neill

As mentioned earlier, in order to analyze the practice of health promotion in Canada, the editors of this book have decided to look at these entry points: *issues, populations,* and *settings* as proposed by Frohlich and Poland (2007) in their chapter in the second edition and again in Chapter 7 of this book. In the second edition of the book, Ilona Kickbusch wrote:

> For me, the most important sentence in the *Ottawa Charter* remains the positioning of health within society: *Health is created in the context of everyday life—where people live, love, work and play.* Today one might add where we travel, shop and Google. This simple sentence in the *Ottawa Charter* is the expression of the de-territorialization of health out of the health care system into the social arena and the market. (2007, p. 365; italics in the original)

There is probably no better way to begin discussing the settings approach than with this quote. It suggests a variety of places in people's day-to-day lives where health and illness are produced. During the mid-1980s, the idea emerged that it is in such settings that the new health promotion movement, put forward by the World Health Organization (WHO, 1986), had to implement the actions suggested by the *Ottawa Charter.* The first setting where WHO got involved was in the city through the healthy cities movement, which was started in 1988. Soon after, it was through the school, the hospital, the prison, the university, and many other settings, including less expected ones like nightclubs (Bellis, Hughes & Lowey, 2002) or ecosystems (Parkes & Horowitz, 2009), that the approach was developed and put in place. For some (Poland, Green & Rootman, 2000; Dooris, 2005; Poland, Krupa & McCall, 2009), the settings approach is the preferred way through which health promotion theory and practice can be linked.

In this chapter, we will first look at how the approach has been used in Canada in five types of settings—four more classical (cities and towns; schools; hospitals and other health care settings; workplaces) and a less conventional but most important one (the virtual setting). Indeed, the virtual world ranges from visioconferencing to brain research, with obviously the Internet as a central channel for most of it, through which a vast and increasing number of people "live, love, work and play" for significant parts of their lives. For us, it is thus a real setting that health promoters need to understand and use much more than they have done so up to now (O'Neill, 2009; Catford, 2011).

In each type of setting, the general issues raised by how to promote health are first pointed out, followed by at least one practical example of a health promotion "promising practice" in that context. In the conclusion, building on these examples as well as on the international literature to which several Canadians have been prominent contributors, we will propose a few general characteristics of the settings approach, present a few of its main achievements, and discuss some challenges that it is currently facing.

Healthy Cities, Towns, and Communities in Canada: The Current Situation and Challenges

Paule Simard, Nathalie Sasseville, Jodi Mucha, Barbara Losier, and Lorna McCue

Emergence of the Concept

As an integral part of the international movement of health promotion, the healthy cities approach, for its original formulators, was based on a holistic and ecological vision of health (Hancock, 1993; Hancock & Duhl, 1988). For them, an expanded concept of health emphasized the importance of its multiple determinants and was preoccupied with reducing social inequalities in health. The originality of the approach was to highlight the role that local governments can play to address the factors that determine health (De Leeuw, 2009; Hancock, 2009; Deplancke, 2009; O'Neill & Simard, 2006; Simard, 2005).

Out of Duhl and Hancock's seminal ideas, first presented in Toronto in 1984 at a conference called "Beyond Health Care, Healthy Toronto 2000," the European Office of the WHO was seduced by the concept and launched its Healthy Cities program on that continent in 1986 (Hancock & Duhl, 1988). According to its initiators, "a healthy city is one that is engaged in a process of creating, expanding and improving those physical and social environments and community resources which enable people to mutually support each other in performing all the functions of life and developing to their maximum potential" (Hancock & Duhl, 1988, p. 41). This project later moved beyond WHO and became a vast international movement currently involving several thousands of cities and communities on all continents (Tsouros, 1992; De Leeuw, 2009).

The Movement in Canada

In Canada, the Healthy Cities initiative evolved in a specific way and was labelled the "Healthy Communities" movement in order to include municipal communities of all sizes as well as communities other than cities (linguistic, unorganized territory, schools, etc.). However, unlike many other countries with national networks, the Healthy Cities/Communities movement has been operating mostly as a set of provincial networks rather than as a unified Canadian one.

In 2010, four provincial networks of Healthy Cities/Towns/Communities existed in British Columbia, Ontario, Acadian New Brunswick, and Quebec. Alberta, Saskatchewan, Manitoba,

Nova Scotia, and Newfoundland were also involved in Healthy Communities or similar approaches, but did not have formal networks in place (Deplancke, 2009; Hancock, 2009).

With some variations, the actions of these four networks all rely on the principles promoted by the WHO for the movement (WHO, 1992; Deplanke, 2009): community participation, multi-/intersectoral partnerships, political commitment of local authorities, and implementation of healthy public policies. To those, Hancock (2009) recently proposed to add a fifth one: asset-based community development. However, the provincial networks do diverge in how their initiatives are deployed, due to the peculiarities and challenges of their own jurisdictions (Deplancke, 2009). A project involving them has helped to document their characteristics.[1] Here is a brief glimpse of what they look like (see the Resources list at the end of the chapter for their websites, which provide hundreds of concrete examples of the wide range of activities undertaken).

British Columbia Healthy Communities (BCHC) was created in 2005 through funding from the provincial Ministry of Health, a first network having been funded for a short period in the 1990s. BCHC builds on community capacity to create healthy communities and places emphasis on the youth leadership role within their communities. Currently, the network works on the basis of special projects and supports partners through informal "memberships" to promote individual and community health.

Created in 1992, the Ontario Healthy Communities Coalition works with communities to build strong, equitable, and sustainable communities through education, engagement, and collaboration. The coalition has over 400 members, including individuals, organizations, municipalities, networks, and provincial associations. The coalition offers services and publications in both French and English.

Since the launching of the province's first Healthy City (Rouyn-Noranda) in 1987, many large and small municipalities have joined the Quebec *Réseau québécois de villes et villages en santé* (RQVVS), a provincial network incorporated in 1990. In 2010, there were 201 RQVVS municipal members with hundreds of projects in a variety of areas ranging from environment and poverty to access to health services. The RQVVS works primarily with the municipalities or regional county municipalities that are its regular members. It also supports health and social service practitioners working in the province's public health facilities so they can in turn assist the municipalities. The Healthy Communities movement is one of the key strategies of the "community development" (*développement des communautés*) approach put forward by the province's Public Health National program (Ministère de la santé et des services sociaux du Québec, 2008).

The *Mouvement Acadien des communautés en santé du Nouveau-Brunswick* (MACS-NB) is a French-language provincial network that has operated since 2000. Inspired by the Quebec model with which it has very close ties, MACS-NB has developed an original approach by working with different types of communities (municipalities, non-municipal territories, schools, community organizations, etc.) on their collective well-being through action on the social determinants of health (like housing, education, etc.). With 56 members (communities, groups, and schools), MACS-NB is also active in the *Santé en français* movement aiming at insuring equity in health and access to health services in Canada for the francophone minorities.

A Promising Practice at the National Level

Despite some attempts in the 1990s, there is currently no Canada–wide Healthy Cities/ Communities network. Only since May 2009 have closer contacts between the provincial networks been developed through a joint initiative to demonstrate the usefulness of the approach for chronic disease prevention.[2] One of this project's goals is to explore the idea of formalizing a national Healthy Cities/Towns/Communities network. So far, this project has helped to highlight the common principles as well as the diverse strategies used in all four networks, which are summarized in Figure 11.1.

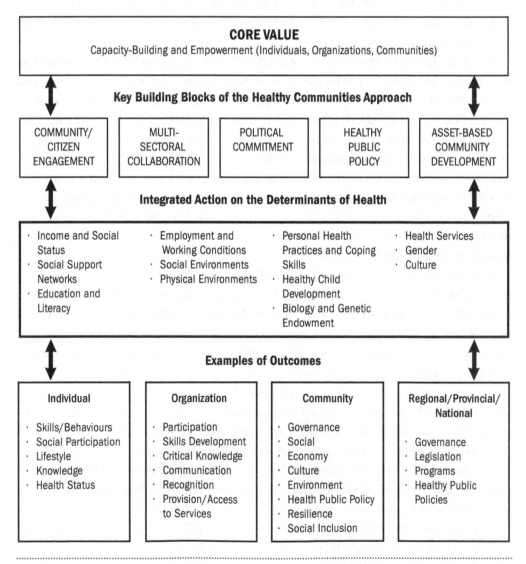

FIGURE 11.1: The Healthy Communities Approach: A Framework for Action

Source: Developed collaboratively by the Ontario Healthy Communities Coalition, BC Healthy Communities, Réseau Québécois de Villes et Villages en Santé, Mouvement Acadien des Communautés en Santé du Nouveau-Brunswick.

This joint venture is interesting in a number of respects such as: obtaining national and international recognition to ensure sustainable federal and provincial funding; sharing expertise among networks for the renewal of the approach; and disseminating the tools developed by different partners.

Despite Canada's leadership role in the origins of the global movement as well as the resilience of some of its provincial networks, several challenges remain for Healthy Communities in Canada. First is the sustainability of the joint effort undertaken by the four networks, particularly as some of them experience financial insecurity. Second, in order to establish a countrywide movement in a nation as large as Canada, it is necessary to go beyond the diverse approaches, languages, and strategies used by each network. A final challenge is to include similar initiatives in the other provinces or territories, even if they do not have a formal Healthy Communities network.

Addressing Complexity, Capacity, and Context to Support Educators: School Health Promotion in Canada

Douglas McCall, Marthe Deschesnes, and Daniel Laitsch

The Emergence of Comprehensive School Health Programs

Despite the diversity of geography, cultures, language, single-issue approaches, and multiple government/agency jurisdictions, school health promotion (SHP) in Canada has developed in similar ways across the country since the late 1980s. Canadian researchers, practitioners, and officials were part of the worldwide movement that defined comprehensive, coordinated, and "whole school" strategies in those first years, with Canadian wording being an important part of one of the first SHP publications issued by the World Health Organization (WHO, 1991). Two decades later, Canadians are again part of the global discussion, this time reflecting a shift from promoting evidence-based and building multi-intervention programs on selected health issues to sustaining those efforts through ecological systems-based approaches; such approaches recognize that schools are an inseparable part of a complex web of multiple relationships and interactions within their neighbourhoods, with other agencies and the families they serve, as well as with the front-line delivery points of bureaucratic, multi-level systems (BC Ministry of Education, n.d.; Canadian Association for School Health, 2007; Deschesnes et al., 2010a, 2010b; McCall & Doherty, 2004; Laitsch, Taylor & Rootman, 2006; McCall, 2006; Palluy et al., 2010; see also Chapter 5 of this book for a discussion of the ecological approach to health promotion).

These Canadian reflections are similar to others around the world (Keshavarz et al., 2010), where attention is being drawn to issues such as neighbourhood context, coordination, capacity-building, complexity, integration of health promotion within the core mandates of schools, systems change, sustainability, implementation processes, and organizational as well as professional development. These new ideas suggest that SHP is more than simply implementing a program or set of programs *in* the school setting. Instead, it is more about combining interventions at multiple levels across several systems to improve the health *of the entire setting* (Dooris et al., 2007).

The apparent chaos depicted in Figure 11.2, produced by the Canadian SHP research program (McCall & Doherty, 2004), illustrates the many people, places, and processes that relate to schools. Sorting out this complexity requires new thinking and new types of research. Based on this new approach to SHP, a few examples of Canadian promising practices are presented below.

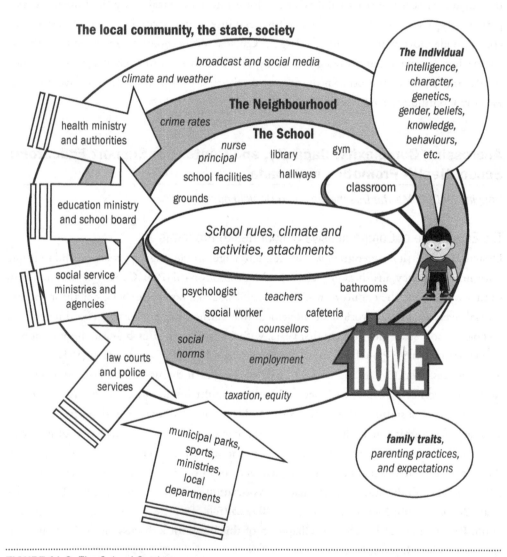

FIGURE 11.2: The School Setting

The complex ecology of the school setting is depicted in this simple version of a diagram developed by Canadian researchers. Health status and behaviours are largely determined by the interaction among individual, family, school, and community/societal factors.

Within the school, each day is different for each child and these experiences are derived from many physical environments within the school, by several adults and other students that accumulate differently for the many students attending each school.

The more complex version of this diagram can be found at http://www.schools-for-all.org/page/Ecological%2C+Systems-based+Appro aches+to+Schools+%28EE%29

Source: McCall, D. & Doherty, M. (2004). *Developing a research agenda in school health promotion.* Surrey: School Health Research Network. Retrieved from: www.docstoc.com/docs/document-preview.aspx?doc_id=43532100

Four Examples of Promising Practices

The goal of the New Approaches, New Solutions (NANS) strategy in Quebec (Janosz et al., 2010) is to reduce the impact of social inequalities on high school students' achievement. The capacity-building strategy helps local schools, supported by school boards, agencies, and ministries, to implement programs that match their local contexts. Health status, social behaviours, and related conditions are positioned as impediments to learning rather than as independent goals. The strategy is based on an "action model" that expects and welcomes changes to programs as they are implemented in complex, local situations. Between 2002 and 2008, most participating schools saw significant gains related to socialization of their students in more positive norms and beliefs about schooling and their life goals, but not enough to influence their dropout rates. Schools that clearly displayed the core characteristics of the strategy (e.g., mobilization of staff, shared vision, planning, use of research-based information) showed significant promise in promoting student success, though they needed to strengthen their operations as well as their context to succeed in the face of severe socio-economic challenges.

Multi-level modelling was used to determine the impact of a whole school approach to school nutrition in the Annapolis Valley of Nova Scotia (Veugelers & Fitzgerald, 2005), a project mentioned in Chapter 5 as a good illustration of the application of an ecological approach. Students in seven self-selected schools, which established a critical mass of multiple interventions, practised healthier eating, were more active, and had healthier body weights in comparison to other students in that province.

How to coordinate multiple programs is another key question raised by the new approach to SHP. The assignment of coordinators at all levels is one aspect of this coordination challenge. Card and Doyle (2008) assessed the role of school health coordinators facilitating co-operation between the school districts and health authorities in Newfoundland, and raised important questions about job descriptions, professional skills, and continuity.

An analysis of smoking programs in secondary schools in Prince Edward Island (Murnaghan et al., 2008) showed that school characteristics and student beliefs about policies may counteract comprehensive programming that included both policies and anti-smoking education. When younger students were housed in high schools with older students who smoked, the younger students were more apt to emulate those older students. When no-smoking policies were skirted by students who still smoked on school grounds without consequences, the students noticed and discounted those policies. The PEI study revealed that actions addressing the negative role modelling of senior students smoking, the age/grade at which students transfer from middle to high school, the influence of close friends, and the implementation of clear no-smoking rules are needed even within multi-intervention programs. This analysis of the interaction between local contextual influences, school grade levels/organization, and student characteristics could help to unravel some of the contradictory research about school-based smoking prevention programs.

Conclusion

Considerable progress has been made in the past two decades in understanding school health promotion. Individual interventions such as health education, school services, and agency/school policies can have limited but important benefits. We also know that coordinated, multiple-intervention programs are more effective. What we don't know is how to coordinate and sustain those programs within the ever-changing but nevertheless constant academically driven ecology of schools, and how to ensure that the necessary concomitant support for schools from health and other systems is also provided.

If policy-makers, officials, practitioners, and researchers do not shift their attention about school health to the more recent SHP approaches as suggested above, we run the risk of repeating mistakes from the past that we already know and could avoid. Like almost all comprehensive SHP programs, once the initial research funding and the ensuing support dry up, the interventions are at risk of waning and the ecology of the schools of reverting to their original state, much like a desert that will bloom temporarily when seasonal rains come, but will revert when the moisture disappears. Schools are and should be primarily focused on the academic achievement and safe custody of their students. So, health promotion programs will be seen as "add-ons" to these core mandates unless we show how student success and school effectiveness are increased by health and social development programs. Further, we need to better understand how schools truly function as complex, adaptive systems that can absorb incremental change while performing their primary duties. Unless we embed our SHP programs within the core operations of schools as well as within the core functions of health authorities, social service and other agencies, even the best and most effective programs are not likely to survive.

Health Promoting Hospitals and Health Care Services: The Case of the Montreal Network[3]

François Lagarde and Trevor Hancock

Origins of the Movement

Historically, hospitals and health services have evolved based on their ability to treat disease and maintain patient health. Yet paradoxically, hospitals and the health care system can and do cause harm to patients (Baker et al., 2004) and their families by, for example, transmitting types of disease through microorganisms like Methicillin-resistant Staphylococcus aureus (MSRA) or *C. difficile*; to staff[4] through occupational hazards that are specific to this setting (e.g., Ontario Nurses Association, 2010); and to the environment (Hancock, 2001) through, for example, unhealthy policies to wash hospital linen with environmentally unfriendly products.[5] At a minimum, these adverse effects must be prevented as the health care system has an ethical duty to "do no harm." More than that, hospitals and the health care system should be both healthy settings for their patients and staff, and influential organizations and partners in their communities—that is, they should be health-promoting organizations that improve the quality of their communities and the environment (Hancock, 1999, p. 327).

In 1993, the World Health Organization (WHO) initiated the International Network of Health Promoting Hospitals and Health Services (HPH) to reorient health care institutions by integrating health promotion and education, disease prevention, and rehabilitation services in curative care (WHO, 2010). The International Network now has more than 740 member institutions that strive to integrate health promotion concepts, values, and strategies within their organizational structure and culture. Specific evidence of the effectiveness of the HPH approach is limited primarily due to the lack of systematic research on the HPH framework or publication of findings (McHugh, Robinson & Chesters, 2010). However, it has been argued that the HPH philosophy is "based on strong evidence and methods to incorporate health promotion as a core principle in the organization" (Groene, 2005).

The Montreal Network of Health Promoting Hospitals and CSSSs

In 2005, the *Agence de la santé et des services sociaux de Montréal* (Montreal regional agency of health and social services) was recognized as the first HPH regional network outside the European continent. As of 2010, some 20 *Centres de santé et des services sociaux* (CSSSs—local health and social services centres) and hospitals are members of the Montreal Network of Health Promoting Hospitals and CSSSs. These institutions work most notably with users and their families, staff, and the community to: decrease the incidence of chronic disease, better meet the needs of an aging population, create and maintain a healthy workplace for staff, promote respectful actions toward the environment, and build healthy communities. Member institutions commit to the five WHO HPH standards: (1) management policy, (2) patient assessment, (3) patient information and intervention, (4) promotion of a healthy workplace, and (5) continuity and co-operation (Groene, 2006).

To help member institutions implement HPH standards, the Montreal Network has published a number of resources, including a guide to develop a written management policy for health promotion (Lagarde, 2009). Although the name and content of policy sections may vary from institution to institution, member organizations are encouraged to use the checklist shown in Box 11.1.

BOX 11.1:

A Checklist to Implement the Health in Hospitals Approach

- link with the quality management program
- link with the public health plan
- link with the sustainable development program
- adoption by the board of directors
- responsibility of the executive director
- health promotion included in the mission, vision, and organizational plans
- reminder that health promotion is everyone's responsibility
- regular item on the agenda of board meetings
- inclusion of health promotion measures and activities intended for human resources
- health promotion included in operational and clinical procedures, budgets, and communication activities
- staff and coordination mechanisms for health promotion
- assessment of the health promotion policy and related activities

---

Source: Lagarde, F. (2009). *Guide to develop a health promotion policy and compendium of policies.* Montreal: Agence de la santé et des services sociaux de Montréal.

The recommended consultation process leading to the adoption of the policy should involve a range of constituents: a users' committee; a council of physicians, dentists, and pharmacists; a council of nurses; a multidisciplinary council; a board of directors; the executive director and managers; community partners; and unions. The following are some key lessons learned and recommendations from institutions' experience in developing a health promotion policy in such settings (Lagarde, 2009):

- Establish a formal link between the quality management program and accreditation processes to cement the commitment from senior management. For example, the CSSS de la Montagne's policy states that the quality management department "monitors the consistency of health promotion guidelines with the CSSS continuous improvement objectives and with the quality standards of the accreditation process. The department also ensures that this component of the CSSS mission is represented in the planning conducted for different programs (clinical projects). Furthermore, it provides support for the assessment of outcomes resulting from health promotion activities, particularly through management accords" (Lagarde, 2009, p. 57).
- Take an inventory of existing health promotion measures to demonstrate the policy's relevance and rally opinion leaders.
- Define tasks to show how the policy will affect various departments and employees.
- Address requirements for expertise, training, and resources.
- Stay open to discussing health promotion issues and problems that directly affect the institution, such as workplace stress levels, as well as any lack of resources or dedicated budgets.
- Publish information regularly about the policy process, adoption, and impact. Testimonials from patients, families, staff members, physicians, and partners should also be published to demonstrate the relevance of adhering to health promotion.

The way in which the principles of the HPH international movement have been implemented in the Montreal area shows that it is quite feasible for hospitals and other types of health care facilities to become health promoting settings, provided they are well supported in the process. In this respect, the fact that they are included in a network is surely a positive factor and we can expect that not only will several more facilities join the Montreal network in the years to come but that it will also be the case for other networks in the rest of Canada and worldwide.

Promoting Health in the Workplace: GP²S and the Healthy Enterprise Standard[6]

Marie-Claude Pelletier and Martin Shain

Healthy Workplaces and the Development of Standards

During the last 25 years the field of workplace health promotion has evolved considerably from a time in the mid–1980s, when it meant little more than a collection of disconnected health programs, to the present when the concept of comprehensive workplace health promotion has become far more dominant. In addition, the focus has shifted over this period from an almost exclusive preoccupation with offering individual employees assistance in addressing their own identified health needs to a broader attention to the healthfulness of the environments, notably the psychosocial ones, in which people work. Accordingly, the scope of workplace health promotion (and also the scope of health *protection* in this setting) extends now to *mental* as well as to physical well-being (Shain & Suurvali, 2001; Santé Canada, 2004a, 2004b; Shain, 2009).

With the considerable increase over the past 10 years in human and monetary costs for organizations that are "non-healthy," either psychologically or physically, it is becoming increasingly necessary to integrate disease prevention and health promotion strategies as pillars of organizational performance. With nearly 17 percent of companies' payrolls devoted to the effects of disease and underperformance because of the "non-health" status of its workforce (Watson Wyatt Worldwide, 2001), the impact justifies the means, especially when in the Canadian context, we can expect a return of $1.50 to $3.43 per dollar invested (Renaud et al., 2008; PHAC, 2010) in structured interventions for prevention and health promotion. It is also necessary that these interventions be based on the best available practices. Having standards developed in a consensual manner is a good way to implement these best practices.

The development of standards for a healthy workplace also has important implications for public health policy. By raising the net health of the workforce through the implementation of standards, the net health of the population at large is also raised. We do not yet know how much it is raised because such measurements are complex. However, it is only logical to assert that there is a transfer of health or harm from the workplace to society, and that this results in gains or losses to the economy. The calculus for this transfer involves costs to our institutional systems of health care, social services, and even corrections. It also involves impacts upon domestic life and even the democratic functioning of communities. In addition, as legal pressures to create a psychologically safe and healthy workplace increase, the development of standards serves as a resource to employers who may otherwise be at a loss to understand the nature and extent of their duties.

The "Healthy Enterprise" Standard of (GP²S)

GP²S (from the French *Groupe de Promotion et de Prévention en Santé,* The Group for Promotion of Prevention Strategies in Health), a non-profit organization established in 2004 by the Quebec business community, is an information hub dedicated to the mobilization and support of employers around a comprehensive approach to workplace health promotion (GP²S, 2010a). GP²S seeks to improve health conditions in the workplace and the productivity of organizations through the integration of structured initiatives to promote health and influence management practices by promoting a workplace environment conducive to health.

In order to do so, GP²S recruited a group of key stakeholders and experts from all relevant sectors to develop a standard (GP²S, 2010b). The standard *Healthy Enterprise Prevention, Promotion, and Organizational Practices Contributing to Health in the Workplace* was launched as a world première in February 2008 and has been operational since March 2009. The purpose of this standard is: (1) to provide a guide that identifies best practices to improve health and productivity in the workplace and (2) to officially recognize companies that successfully implement the standard with a certification awarded by the BNQ (*Bureau de normalisation du Québec*).[7]

The standard covers four fields of activity known to have a significant impact on health: (1) lifestyle, (2) the balance between work and private life, (3) the work environment, and (4) management practices. These four fields deal with responsibility and behavioural changes concerning health at the *personal* level, but also—mainly with the creation of a physical and social environment—at the whole organizational level through mobilization and empowerment. While this process involves senior management and supervisors as prime movers, the whole workforce is engaged in the identification and resolution of issues.

With this in mind, the five steps for implementation of the standard are:

1. Obtaining the commitment of senior management.
2. Creating a health and wellness committee.
3. Collecting data (individual and organizational).
4. Implementing the program.
5. Evaluating the program.

The minimal time frame required to apply for certification is 12–18 months, the time necessary to implement the steps and processes. Two levels of certification are possible: Healthy Enterprise (40 requirements) and Healthy Enterprise-Elite with 20 additional requirements.

Through its consciousness-raising and mobilization activities with partners qualified to support employers in their initiatives, GP²S has seen a growing number of players who have acquired the expertise and developed a service offer to support employers. Various programs are currently being developed as well. This mobilization has created a fertile breeding ground for employers wishing to encourage a healthy and productivity culture within their companies, as shown in Figure 11.3.

Employers who have used the Healthy Enterprise guide have been quick to observe significant results (GP²S, 2010c, pp. 13–15). Among others, they observed changes in their employees' level of commitment, degree of satisfaction, and health behaviour, as well as an evolution of the culture within the workplace. There were also significant reductions in costs related to illness, production, and absences, as well as occupational health and safety program fees. Be they tangible or intangible benefits, the positive and significant results obtained by employers who have implemented a structured approach to health promotion allow us to conclude, once again, that it really pays to take care of employees' health.

Promoting Health in Virtual Settings

Alison Stirling and Manon Niquette

Encompassed mainly by the Internet and the newer interactive Web 2.0 platforms (such as wikis, blogs, social-networking sites, video-sharing, and mobile e-technologies), the virtual setting is changing health promotion practice as well as the public's expectations and capabilities. Virtual opportunities are plentiful for health promotion (HP) to communicate and

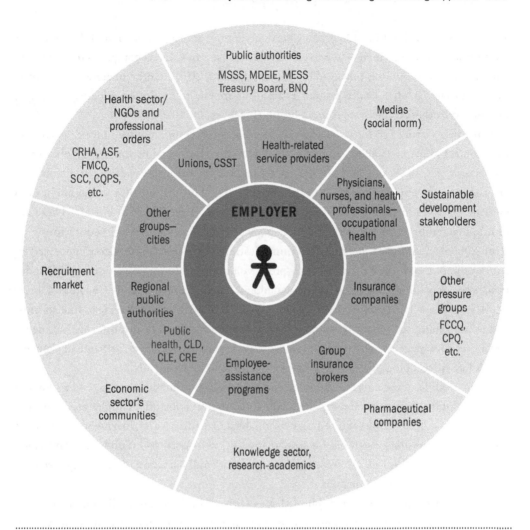

FIGURE 11.3: A Framework to Create a Facilitating Environment for the Employer to Promote Cohesive and Convergent Actions in Workplace Health Promotion

engage with wide audiences through multiple strategies and channels. More than 83 percent of Canadians regularly use the Internet, and 70 percent of them search online for health information (Statistics Canada, 2010; Underhill & McKeown, 2008). Ninety-five percent of youth are online every day (Flicker et al., 2008), and "78% of the Quebec internauts (Quebecers 18 years old or more who use the Internet at least once a week) have used at least one social networking site" (CEFRIO, 2010; free translation). A scan of Canadian HP organizations' websites finds that most are using the Internet to promote health and provide expert-selected quality resources to the public, members, and other health professionals rather than as a place to interact with people. A smaller number, particularly youth-serving groups, health foundations, and social marketing enterprises, are using interactive Web 2.0 platforms and social media to pull in content and public participation. In July 2010, Canada had the world's greatest number of Facebook users in proportion to its population; the United Kingdom was in second place and the US in third (CEFRIO, 2010). Canadians are not as heavy users of mobile devices for sending and receiving email—16 percent of Internet users in Canada compared to 34 percent among the seven countries surveyed (Fleishman-Hillard, 2010). Unfortunately, there is little evidence that Canadian health promoters are using mobile technologies to educate, engage, or empower others to further promote health (Lefebvre, 2009).

Canadian virtual HP initiatives can be viewed as being on a continuum of "participatory control" between expert-directed HP and lay-directed social media sites (Robinson & Robertson, 2010). At one end are the government and institution websites and web portals that provide expert-vetted health information (e.g., HealthLink BC) to the public, and evidence sources for health professionals (e.g., Canadian Best Practices Portal). There are online behaviour-change interventions (e.g., Stupid.ca), healthy lifestyle education (e.g., Kino-Québec), and social marketing communications (ParticipACTION.com) provided by a mix of public and private sectors. Non-profit voluntary health organizations' and foundations' sites are adding interactive forums and blogs. Three examples are the Canadian Cancer Society and its virtual community Smokers Helpline, which offers phone, online forums, and texting supports; the Heart and Stroke Foundation's tailored health information, news, and a Facebook page where stroke survivors connect; and, finally, PasseportSanté in Quebec, which has videos, blogs, fact sheets, and experts for healthy living advice.

In the middle of the continuum, there is a convergence of media formats, and a blurring between public, voluntary, and private sector interests. A couple of examples are: Abilities. ca, a magazine, foundation, and resource for disabled Canadians, and SharingStrength.ca for breast cancer survivors. Both offer a combination of web-based and mobile text and video resources and links, as well as opportunities to network and chat, and both are supported by foundations and private companies.

At the other end are the lay public-led sites with multiple social media applications for content sharing, networking, mobile access, and exchange. Peer-support groups, such as the francophone Groupe Maman (*Mouvement pour l'autonomie dans la maternité et pour l'accouchement naturel*), the Facebook initiative "Allaitement," as well as GayFathers-toronto.com and Rezo (http://www.rezosante.org)—community health organizations for gay and bisexual men—are interesting examples of this type around two types of issues.

The virtual world has empowering potential for individuals to find health information that is contextually relevant, to identify friends, to locate supports and online communities, and to engage in actions for change, all with little expert direction from health promoters (Eysenbach, 2008; Korp, 2006; Robinson & Robertson, 2010). The challenges for Canadian HP in the virtual setting are to balance targeted communications with diverse populations' interests and quality control of content with collaborative filtering of links toward high-quality information.

Promising Practices in Virtual Health Promotion

TeenNet/Youth Voice Research Group, based at the University of Toronto, uses a variety of social media to create "accessible, responsive, and health promoting systems for youth and young adults on health issues."[8]

La gang allumée, a Quebec-based youth coalition against smoking, offers a dynamic website, videos, and online communities for youth 11–17 years.[9]

These HP interventions possess, at one degree or the other, the five elements reflecting good practices (Kreps & Neuhauser, 2010; Flicker et al., 2008) in communications approaches and health promotion principles as described in Box 11.2.

BOX 11.2:

Five Principles to Develop Appropriate Online Health Promotion Interventions

- interactive and responsive, valuing active audience participation in process and content
- interoperable in multiple settings and strategies to meet diverse needs and social contexts
- engaging and dynamic, having the target audience as part of the intervention, content, or project
- contextually tailored for large groups and individuals alike, and customized to their interests and needs
- inclusive, accessible, participatory, and empowering

Source: Kreps, G.L. & Neuhauser, L. (2010). New directions in eHealth communication: Opportunities and challenges. *Patient Education and Counseling, 78*, 329-336.; Flicker, S., Maley, O., Ridgley, A. et al. (2008). Using technology and participatory action research to engage youth in health promotion. *Action Research, 6*, 285-303.

A key challenge for promoting health in the virtual setting is thus to involve people as collaborators and participants, and to offer empowering social health resources and networks. With this in mind, there is absolutely no doubt that the virtual world is rapidly becoming one of the key settings where "people live, love, work and play" in Canada and elsewhere, and health promoters should be not only aware of it but learn how to be active participants in it.

Conclusion

Michel O'Neill

In the sections above, five types of settings have been discussed as well as how interventions in each can promote health. What can be derived from these discussions is that settings are "places," not just in the physical or geographical sense, but also in the sense that people are interacting in them. And each setting is a place that functions in a given context, but is also unique and different from other settings with which it may share similarities.

The settings approach is described in Box 11.3.

Given these characteristics, the settings approach is thus seen by some of its proponents as one of the key ways in which health promotion practice can be organized (Poland, Krupa & McCall, 2009), despite the difficulty of proving its effectiveness (Dooris, 2005). It is inspired by some of the most acknowledged theoretical models in the field (ecological theory, systems theory, complexity theory), provides an organized framework usable in a variety of health promoters' real-life work situations, and is quite sensitive to context without denying the usefulness of the evidence-based approach to program development, which is currently very popular in public

---

BOX 11.3:

Key Features of the Healthy Settings Approach

- Takes place in the real lives of people, where their day-to-day activities occur (i.e., where they live, work, love, play, etc.)
- Allows people to contextualize the intervention to the reality of each setting
- Proposes comprehensive approaches based on an ecological and open systems vision
- Proposes interventions that aim to change individuals and organizations as well as the environments in which the setting is based
- Proposes to do so by involving as many stakeholders of the setting and its environment as possible

---

Source: Adapted from Poland, B., Green, W.L. & Rootman, I. (2000). *Settings for health promotion: Linking theory and practice.* Thousand Oaks: Sage; Dooris, M. (2005). Healthy settings: Challenges to generating evidence of effectiveness. *Health Promotion International, 26*(1), 55–65; Dooris, M., Poland, B., Kolbe, L. et al. (2007). Healthy settings: Building the evidence for whole system health promotion—Challenges and future directions. In D. McQueen & C.M. Jones (Eds.), *Global perspectives on health promotion effectiveness.* New York: Springer; Poland, B., Krupa, D. & McCall, G.S. (2009). Settings for health promotion: An analytic framework to guide intervention design and implementation. *Health Promotion Practice, 10*(4), 505–516.

health and health promotion (Poland, Krupa & McCall, 2009). Consequently, as it proposes a structured way to intervene in individuals' lives and in the environments in which they live, it is surely one of the powerful ways to organize the practice of health promotion on a day-to-day basis notably because for most of the settings, as seen above, there are strong national and international networks involving practitioners and researchers that may be joined by whoever is interested.

Notes

1. Healthy Communities, Healthy Nation: An Inter-provincial Healthy Communities Approach to Chronic Disease Prevention, a project funded by the Coalitions Linking Action and Science for Prevention (CLASP) of the Canadian Partnership against Cancer.
2. Ibid.
3. The authors wish to thank Louis Côté (chair of the Governance Board of the International Network of Health Promoting Hospitals and Health Services) and Françoise Alarie (assistant coordinator of the Montreal Network) for their valuable input.
4. In 2006, just over 1 million people in Canada worked directly in health occupations; this represented 6 percent of the total Canadian workforce (Canadian Institute for Health Information, 2007).
5. With respect to reducing harm to the environment, the Canadian Coalition for Green Health Care has been quite successful in Ontario in helping hospitals to become environmentally responsible corporate citizens and is now expanding nationally.
6. The authors wish to thank Dr. Mario Messier (scientific director for GP²S) for his valuable input.
7. The *Bureau de normalisation du Québec* (BNQ) develops consensual standards, implements certification programs, and registers management systems. Retrieved from: www.bnq.qc.ca
8. Retrieved from: http://www.teennetproject.org
9. Retrieved from: http://lagangallumee.com

References

Baker, G.R., Norton, P.G., Flintoft, V. et al. (2004), The Canadian Adverse Events Study: The incidence of adverse events among hospital patients in Canada. *CMAJ, 170*(11), 1678–1686.

BC Ministry of Education. (n.d.). *Healthy schools network overview.* Retrieved from: http://www.healthy-schoolsnetwork.org/

Bellis, M.A., Hughes, K. & Lowey, H. (2002). Healthy nightclubs and recreational substance use: From a harm minimization to a healthy settings approach. *Addictive Behaviors, 27*(6), 1025–1035.

Canadian Association for School Health. (2007). *Comprehensive school health: A Canadian consensus statement* (2nd ed.). Surrey: Canadian Association for School Health.

Canadian Institute for Health Information. (2007), *Canada's health care providers.* Ottawa: CIHI.

Card, A. & Doyle, E. (2008). School health coordinators as change agents. *Health & Learning 3*(1), 3–8.

Catford, J. (2011). The new social learning: Connect better for better health. *Health Promotion International, 26*(2): 133–135.

CEFRIO. (2010). L explosion des médias sociaux au Québec. *Netendances 2010, 1,* 4. Retrieved from: http://www.cefrio.qc.ca/fileadmin/documents/Publication/NETendances-Vol1-1.pdf

De Leeuw, E. (2009). Evidence for healthy cities: Reflection on practice, method, and theory. *Health Promotion International, 24*(Suppl. 1), i19–i36.

Deplancke, E. (2009). *Healthy communities report: A report on Healthy Community initiatives in Canada and around the world and how to apply these strategies in Haldimand and Norfolk Counties.* Ontario, Canada: Haldimand-Norfolk Health Unit.

Deschesnes, M., Trudeau, F. & Kebe, M. (2010a). Factors influencing the adoption of a Health Promoting School approach in the province of Quebec, Canada. *Health Education Research, 25*(3), 438–450.

Deschesnes, M., Couturier, Y., Laberge, S. et al. (2010b). How divergent conceptions among health and education stakeholders influence the dissemination of healthy schools in Quebec. *Health Promotion International 25*(4), 435–443.

Dooris, M. (2005). Healthy settings: Challenges to generating evidence of effectiveness. *Health Promotion International, 26*(1), 55–65.

Dooris, M., Poland, B., Kolbe, L. et al. (2007). Healthy settings: Building the evidence for whole system health promotion—Challenges and future directions. In D. McQueen & C.M. Jones (Eds.), *Global perspectives on health promotion effectiveness.* 327–353. New York: Springer.

Eysenbach, G. (2008), Medicine 2.0: Social networking, collaboration, participation, apomediation, and openness. *Journal of Medical Internet Research, 10*(22). Retrieved from: www.jmir.org/2008/3/e22

Fleishman-Hillard (2010). *Understanding the role of the Internet in the lives of consumers: Digital Influence Index Study.* Fleishman-Hillard/Harris Interactive, July 2010. Retrieved from http: //digitalinfluence.fleishmanhillard.com/

Flicker, S., Maley, O., Ridgley, A. et al. (2008). Using technology and participatory action research to engage youth in health promotion. *Action Research, 6,* 285–303.

Florence, M.D., Asbridge, M. & Veugelers, P.J. (2008). Diet quality and academic performance. *Journal of School Health, 78,* 209–215.

Frohlich, K. & Poland, B. (2007). Points of intervention in health promotion practice. In M. O'Neill, A. Pederson, S. Dupéré & I. Rootman (Eds.), *Health promotion in Canada: Critical perspectives* (2nd ed.) (pp. 46–60). Toronto: Canadian Scholars' Press Inc.

GP²S. (2010a). Retrieved from: www.gp2s.net

GP²S. (2010b). Retrieved from: http://www.gp2s.net/documents/documentation/brochure_corporative.pdf

GP²S. (2010c). *La santé au travail, une avenue rentable pour tous. Mémoire présenté au ministre des finances du Québec.* Retrieved from: http://www.gp2s.net/index.php?option=com_content&task=blogcateg ory&id=40&Itemid=88

Groene, O. (2005). Health promotion in hospitals—From principles to implementation. In O. Groene & M. Garcia-Barbero (Eds.), *Health promotion in hospitals: Evidence and quality management* (pp. 3–20). Geneva: World Health Organization.

Groene, O. (2006). *Implementing health promotion in hospitals: Manual and self-assessment forms.* World Health Organization. Retrieved from: www.euro.who.int/__data/assets/pdf_file/0009/99819/ E88584.pdf

Hancock, T. (1993). The Healthy City: Concept to application. Implications for research. In J.K. Davies & M.P. Kelly (Eds.), *Healthy cities. Research and practice.* 148-162.London/New York: Routledge.

Hancock, T. (1999). Healthy and health-promoting hospitals. *Leadership in Health Services/International Journal of Health Care Quality Assurance, 12*(2), viii–xix.

Hancock, T. (2001). *Doing less harm: Assessing and reducing the environmental and health impact of Canada's health care system.* Toronto: Canadian Coalition for Green Health Care. Retrieved from: www. greenhealthcare.ca

Hancock, T. (2009). *Act locally: Community-based population health promotion.* Report for the Canadian Senate Sub-committee on Population Health. Ottawa, Canadian Senate Sub-committee on Population Health.

Hancock, T. & Duhl, L. (1988). *Healthy cities: Promoting health in the urban context.* WHO Healthy Cities Paper 1. Copenhagen: FDAL.

Janosz, M., Belanger, J., Dagenais, C., Bowen, F., Abrami, P.C., Cartier, S.C., Choinard, R., Fallu, J.-S., Desbiens, N., Lysenko, L. & Turcotte, L. (2010). Evaluation of the new approaches, new solutions intervention strategy: Summary of the final report. Montreal: Groupe de recherche sur les environments scolaires, Université de Montréal.

Keshavarz, K., Nutbeam, D., Rowling, L. et al. (2010). Schools as social complex adaptive systems: A new way to understand the challenges of introducing the health promoting schools concept. *Social Science & Medicine, 70*(10), 1467–1474.

Kickbusch, I. (2007). Health promotion: Not a tree but a rhizome. In M. O'Neill, A. Pederson, S. Dupéré & I. Rootman (Eds.), *Health promotion in Canada: Critical perspectives* (2nd ed.) (pp. 363–366*)*. Toronto: Canadian Scholars' Press Inc.

Korp, P. (2006). Health on the Internet: Implications for health promotion. *Health Education Research, 21*, 78–86.

Kreps, G.L. & Neuhauser, L. (2010). New directions in eHealth communication: Opportunities and challenges. *Patient Education and Counseling, 78*, 329–336.

Lagarde, F. (2009). *Guide to develop a health promotion policy and compendium of policies.* Montreal: Agence de la santé et des services sociaux de Montréal.

Laitsch, D., Taylor, M. & Rootman, I. (2006). Systems thinking, capacities, and change. Keynote panel presentation at the 2006 National Invitational Conference and Seminars of the Joint Consortium for School Health, May 25, Vancouver.

Lefebvre, C. (2009). Integrating cell phones and mobile technologies into public health practice: A social marketing perspective. *Health Promotion Practice, 10*, 490–493.

Memoire to the Minister of Finance, Mr. Raymond Bachand. Retrieved from: www.gp2s.net/documents/memoires/memoire_gp2s.pdf, pp. 13 and 14.

Ministère de la santé et des services sociaux du Québec. (2008). *Programme national de santé publique 2003–2012 (mise à jour 2008).* Quebec: Ministère de la santé et des services sociaux du Québec.

McCall, D. (2006). An ecological and systems approach to school health promotion. Surrey: School Health Research Network, Canadian Council on Learning.

McCall, D. & Doherty, M. (2004). *Developing a research agenda in school health promotion.* Surrey: School Health Research Network. Retrieved from: www.docstoc.com/docs/document-preview.aspx?doc_id=43532100

McHugh, C., Robinson, A. & Chesters, J. (2010). Health promoting health services: A review of the evidence. *Health Promotion International, 25*(2), 230–237.

Murnaghan, D., Leatherdale, S., Sihvonen, M. et al. (2008). A multi-level analysis examining the association between school-based smoking policies, prevention programs, and youth smoking behavior: Evaluating a provincial tobacco control strategy. *Health Education Research, 23*, 1016–1028.

O'Donnell, M.P. (2002). *Health promotion in the workplace* (3rd ed). Toronto: Delmar, a division of Thomson Learning.

O'Neill, M. (2009). L'internet comme lieu d'intervention en santé publique: Pourquoi? Pour qui? Par qui? *Santé Publique, 21*(Supp. 2), 3–4.

O'Neill, M. & Simard, P. (2006). Choosing indicators to evaluate healthy cities projects: A political task? *Health Promotion International, 21*(2), 146–152.

Ontario Nurses Association. (2010). *Submission to the Expert Advisory Panel to review Ontario's occupational health and safety system.* Toronto: ONA. Retrieved from: www.ona.org/documents/File/politicalaction/ONASubmission_ExpertAdvisoryPanelToReviewOntarioOccupationalHealthAndSafetySystem_201006.pdf

Palluy, J., Arcand, L., Choinière, C. et al. (2010). Réussite éducative, santé et bien-être: Agir efficacement en contexte scolaire. Synthèse de recommandations. Montreal: Institutnational de santé publique du Québec. Retrieved from: www.inspq.qc.ca/pdf/publications/1065_ReussiteEducativeSanteBienEtre.pdf

Parkes, M.W. & Horowitz, P. (2009). Water, ecology, and health: Ecosystems as settings for promoting health and sustainability. *Health Promotion International, 24*(1), 94–102.

Poland, B., Green, W.L. & Rootman, I. (2000). *Settings for health promotion: Linking theory and practice.* Thousand Oaks: Sage.

Poland, B., Krupa, G. & McCall, D.S. (2009) Settings for health promotion: An analytic framework to guide intervention design and implementation. *Health Promotion Practice, 10*(4), 505–516.

Public Health Agency of Canada (PHAC). (2010). *Active living at work.* Retrieved from: http://www.phac-aspc.gc.ca/alw-vat/studies-etudes/develop-eng.php

Renaud, L., Kishchuk, N., Juneau, M., Nigam, A., Tétreault, K. & Leblanc, M.-C. (2008). Implementation and outcomes of a comprehensive worksite health promotion program. *Canadian Journal of Public Health, 99*(1), 73–77.

Robinson, M. & Robertson, S. (2010). Young men's health promotion and new information communication technologies: Illuminating the issues and research agendas. *Health Promotion International, 25*, 363–370.

Rowling, L. & Jeffreys, V. (2006). Capturing complexity: Integrating health and education research to inform health-promoting schools policy and practice. *Health Education Research, 21*(5), 705–718.

Shain, M. (2009). The psychologically safe workplace: Emergence of a corporate and social agenda in Canada. *International Journal of Mental Health Promotion, 11*(3), 324–327.

Shain, M. & Suurvali, H. (2001). *Investing in comprehensive workplace health promotion: A resource.* Ottawa: Health Canada.

Simard, P. (2005). *Perspective pour une évaluation participative des villes et villages en santé.* Quebec: Institut national de santé publique du Québec.

Santé Canada. (2004a). *Guide d'élaboration et de réalisation du système de promotion de la santé en milieu de travail pour les moyennes et les grandes entreprises.* Retrieved from: http://www.hc-sc.gc.ca/ewh-semt/pubs/occup-travail/model-guide-modele/index-eng.php

Santé Canada. (2004b). *Modèle de promotion de la santé dans les petites entreprises: Guide d'élaboration et de réalisation du système de promotion de la santé en milieu de travail pour les petites entreprises.* Retrieved from: http://www.hc-sc.gc.ca/ewh-semt/pubs/occup-travail/small-guide-petite/index-eng.php

Statistics Canada. (2010). *Canadian Internet Use Survey.* Retrieved from: http://www.statcan.gc.ca/daily-quotidien/100510/dq100510a-eng.htm

Tsouros, A. (Ed.). (1992). *World Health Organization Healthy Cities project: A project becomes a movement. Review of progress, 1987 to 1990.* Copenhagen: FADL Publishers for World Health Organization, Healthy Cities Project Office.

Underhill, C. & McKeown, L. (2008). Getting a second opinion: Health information and the Internet. *Health Reports, 19*, 23-25.Cat. no. 82-003. Ottawa: Statistics Canada.

Veugelers, P.J. & Fitzgerald, A.L. (2005). Effectiveness of school programs in preventing childhood obesity: A multilevel comparison. *American Journal of Public Health, 95*(3), 432–435.

Watson Wyatt Worldwide. (2001), *Staying at work 2000/2001—The dollars and sense of effective disability management*. Cat. no. W-337. Vancouver: Watson Wyatt Worldwide.

WHO. (1986). *Ottawa Charter for Health Promotion*. Geneva: World Health Organization.

WHO. (1991). Comprehensive school health education: Suggested guidelines for action. *Hygie, 11*(3), 8–16.

WHO. (1992). Reflections on progress: A framework for the Healthy Cities Project Review. Copenhagen: WHO Europe.

WHO. (2010). *Purpose and goals of the HPH Network*. Retrieved from: www.who-cc.dk/goals-and-purpose-of-the-hph-network

Critical Thinking Questions

1. What are the main characteristics of the settings approach to health promotion?
2. Some authors propose that the settings approach could be the best way to link to theory and practice in health promotion. Do you agree? Why?
3. Pick one of the five settings covered in the chapter. What do you think of the degree of advancement of what we know about how to intervene in such a setting?
4. Do you think the virtual setting is comparable to the other settings? Why or why not?
5. Pick a setting different from the five covered in the chapter. How could it be used to promote health?

Resources

Further Readings

The Settings Approach in General

Poland, B., Krupa, G., & McCall, D.S. (2009) Settings for health promotion: An analytic framework to guide intervention design and implementation. *Health Promotion Practice, 10*(4), 505–516.

In this award-winning paper, Poland, Krupa, and McCall propose a template to look at settings for research, especially for intervention purposes.

Healthy Schools

Rowling, L. & Jeffreys, V. (2006). Capturing complexity: Integrating health and education research to inform health-promoting schools policy and practice. *Health Education Research, 21*(5), 705–718.

This article is helpful in understanding the new approach to school health promotion.

Healthy Workplaces

O'Donnell, M.P. (2002). *Health promotion in the workplace* (3rd ed.). Toronto: Delmar, a division of Thomson Learning.

The third edition of the book *Health promotion in the workplace* is an excellent introduction to the subject. It offers to students and practitioners alike a framework for studying workplace health promotion, while at the same time reviewing some significant conclusions that have been reached in the field.

Virtual

Robinson, M. & Robertson, S. (2010). Young men's health promotion and new information communication technologies: Illuminating the issues and research agendas. *Health Promotion International, 25*, 363–370.

Robinson and Robertson (2010) consider the structural potential of new forms of Web 2.0 applications to engage young men in health promotion, and to include health literacy skills and reach marginalized people.

Relevant Websites

The Settings Approach in General

Healthy Settings Development Unit, University of Central Lancashire

http://www.uclan.ac.uk/schools/school_of_health/research_projects/eph/healthy_settings.php;

The Healthy Settings Development Unit aims to support and facilitate the holistic and integrated development of healthy settings.

Healthy Communities

Healthy Communities Provincial Networks

For British Columbia: http://www.bchealthycommunities.ca/content/home.asp
For New Brunswick: http://www.macsnb.ca/
For Ontario: http://www.ohcc-ccso.ca/
For Quebec: http://www.rqvvs.qc.ca/

The above are websites for the current provincial networks for healthy communities.

Healthy Hospitals

Canadian Coalition for Green Health Care

www.greenhealthcare.ca

This is the website for the Canadian Coalition for Green Health Care which is committed to adopting environmentally friendly and sustainable health care delivery.

Healthy Schools

World School Health Encyclopedia and Knowledge Exchange Program

www.schools-for-all.org

A shared workspace, wiki-based encyclopedia and multi-partner exchange program promoting health, learning, social development, equity, safety and sustainability through schools.

Healthy Workplaces

Planning Wellness

Part 1: http://www.welcoa.org/freeresources/pdf/aa_v5.4.pdf
Part 2: http://welcoa.org/freeresources/pdf/aa_v5.6.pdf

Planning wellness, parts 1 and 2 are two special reports produced by L.S. Chapman and Welcoa (Wellness

Council of America). They offer the reader a comprehensive resource with practical insights related to planning health promotion programs in the workplace. The administrative and legal context is for the US, but most of the information is relevant to health promotion programs in Canada.

Virtual

Canadian Breast Cancer Foundation

http://www.cbcf.org

The Canadian Breast Cancer Foundation uses multi-channel strategies—including their Finding Hope blog, videos on YouTube, and Twitter—to seek support and spread news, and online communities in Facebook for sharing stories and hope among breast cancer survivors.

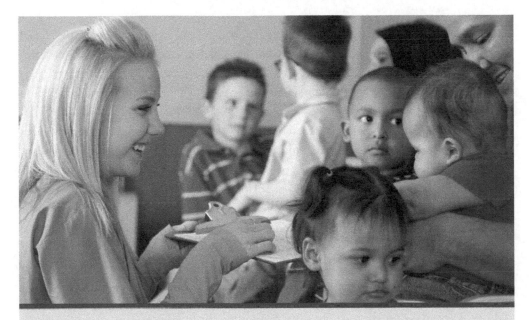

PART III

Additional Topics to Consider in Reflecting on Health Promotion Practice

In Part III, other topics of central importance to the practice of health promotion are addressed. We will discuss issues such as reflexivity, evaluation, and ethics, which are key dimensions for practice. We will also discuss the question of professionalization as health promotion is a relatively young field of practice. In addition, we will discuss practice areas and give concrete examples of HP practice. A chapter dedicated to health promotion practice addresses health inequalities, and another offers reflections on health promotion from the perspectives of a few key professions.

In Chapter 12, Boutilier and Mason offer key advice on why and how health promotion practitioners, whether their job is in intervention, research, policy-making, or even teaching contexts, would benefit immensely from being reflexive about it.

In Chapter 13, Hyndman and O'Neill address an issue that has gained a lot of attention internationally since 2007 with the Galway Consensus on health promotion competencies, as well as nationally in Canada: Should health promotion become a profession and, if so, what would be the consequences? This has major implications for the practice in the field and should of great interest to current as well as future practitioners in the country.

In Chapter 14, Raphael looks at the implications of health inequities for the practice of health promotion. Since 2007, the issue of health inequities has received a lot of attention in Canada and abroad, notably because of the report of WHO's Commission on the Social Determinants of Health in which several Canadians played a central role. The impact of Canada's political climate on health inequities since the second edition a few years ago is also addressed, providing food for thought about the importance and feasibility of developing health promotion practices with this issue in mind.

Chapter 15 addresses a topic that is too often forgotten in health promotion practice—its ethical dimension. Massé and Williams-Jones strongly remind the reader that health promotion is in some respects a moralizing practice, grounded in values and beliefs about what is "good" for the health of an individual or a population and imposing upon them information or behaviours that might have significant unexpected negative effects. Reflecting on the ethical dilemmas of health promotion practice is thus an important and neglected element, and the authors provide useful suggestions for how to go about it.

In Chapter 16, Potvin and Goldberg invite the practitioner to consider evaluation in a very different light than how it is often presented. Giving precise examples, they argue for a reflexive approach that takes into account the context of the intervention as well as how evaluation can be a transformative force to innovate and improve one's practice.

Finally, Chapter 17, edited by Sophie Dupéré, brings together reflections on health promotion from the perspectives of a few key professions and practice areas. The authors discuss the place and challenges of health promotion in their respective fields and provide some promising practices.

Robert Perrault first looks at the challenges of increasing clinical prevention in medical practice and describes an innovative intervention. Then Hills and Dallaire discuss the long and intimate relationship between nursing and health promotion, a link that is emphasized by Burgess, who suggests that nurse practitioners are well positioned to engage in and advance health promotion actions and interventions. Following that, Kadija Perrault and Anderson explore the potential of health promotion for the various professions working in rehabilitation, providing two examples of promising practices in their domain. Whereas these four first sections address health promotion practice among current health professions, the four subsequent ones look at other, sometimes overlooked types of practitioners.

In the first, Ponic and Frisby discuss community development as a foundational strategy for health promotion because of its potential for individual, organizational, and social change; they provide an example illustrating that it is often a long-term endeavour requiring time, resources, and a willingness to embrace complexity. In the second, St-Pierre and Mendell look at the need for health promoters to develop new knowledge and skills in policy-making and propose health impact assessments as a promising practice to do so. Villedieu then reflects on how journalism has evolved to address health issues, followed by Hershfield and Renaud, who discuss how the professionals in health communication can promote health; the three latter sections address the ways in which the provision of information to individuals and populations through various means is a critical part of health promotion practice. The chapter concludes with a section on what is very frequently advocated for in health promotion—interprofessional practice—in which Morin and Dumont raise the potential but also the challenges of this way of practising.

At the end of this third part, the reader will have reflected on several key dimensions important for the practice of health promotion and, hopefully, will have seen, in a reflexive way, how this can have an impact on his or her own current or future practice. The descriptions of "promising practices" from different practice areas should also provide the reader with a more global picture of health promotion practice in Canada and ideas to develop or modify specific interventions to reduce health inequalities.

CHAPTER 12

The Reflexive Practitioner in Health Promotion:
From Reflection to Reflexivity

Marie Boutilier and Robin Mason[1]

Introduction

When we were invited to write this chapter on reflective practice in health promotion, we expected to draw heavily upon our previous experience and writings to distill lessons and guidelines for others. Now, as we finish, we are reminded of how risky it is to act on assumptions at a project's beginnings. Upon reflection, we have found that we brought different disciplines, questions, and writing styles to this project, and this has led us to examine reflexivity in health promotion as both a solitary and collaborative process, practised within different modes and mediums. In this chapter we review some understandings of and foci for reflection, and focus on the "how to" of reflective practice in health promotion in different modes—verbal and visual—and the ways in which our own reflections might shed light on the reflective process for others.

Cycles and Spirals: Reflection and Reflective Practice

Historically, reflection was initially defined as the "active persistent and careful consideration or any belief or supposed form of knowledge in the light of the grounds which support it" (Dewey, 1933, p. 118), emerging from a state of doubt and involving "the kind of thinking that consists in turning a subject over in the mind and giving it serious thought" (Moon, 1999, p. 12). In this model, reflection is a cycle that concludes with the testing or evaluation of a determined action and then begins again—the inspiration for Lewin's (1946) spiral of action research. Later, Schön (1983) recognized that in the action of real-life problem-solving, professionals must "reflect *in* action" when faced with complex problems. Thoughtful experimentation becomes part of the process of problem-solving—a form of "research"—occurring in an iterative and cyclical process.

The act of questioning and experimenting with strategies occurs in an ongoing cyclical process until the question is reframed (often in collaboration with others) and change occurs. Not only does reflection expand the professional's tacit knowledge tool kit for problem-solving, it can contribute to theory development, self-development, decision-making, empowerment, and other outcomes that are unexpected as new ideas or images are applied in practice (Moon, 1999). In addition, it serves as a preventive process in being drawn into repetitive and routine thinking and solutions, missed opportunities, and boredom or burnout (Schön, 1983).

There is the risk that reflexivity may become too inward-looking, self-absorbed, and over-individualized in "hermeneutic narcissism" (Maton, 2003), losing its intent of transformative knowledge development. It can "become a disembodied process because it involves turning ourselves into objects of study" (Cunliffe & Easterby-Smith, 2003, p. 34). Or, "the often lofty theoretical justifications for greater reflexivity can manifest themselves as a license to write about our most beloved topic—ourselves ... shad[ing] into personal therapy" (Haggerty, 2003, p. 159). In plain language, the risk is that our reflexive undertakings will focus on our personal emotions and psyches rather than being accompanied by critical analysis of our practice and its context. Haggerty points out that the assumption of self-awareness requisite to reflexivity sidesteps the truism (following Freud) that we cannot be fully aware of our assumptions and, in reflexivity, we may unwittingly "rationaliz[e] unconscious motivations and prejudices" (2003, p. 159). For this reason, we offer the caveat that reflexivity is meant to focus largely on professional practice, with some boundaries drawn by the individual between personal and professional issues. This is integral to "professionalism" for most people and becomes more or less intuitive, but is a point that bears articulation.

For health promoters, the challenges for reflection are found in the combination of collaboration, multidisciplinary strategies, and values (including a professional ethic of service to communities), all practised within the context of the employing organization. When health promotion entails evaluation research, it draws on professional training, but can also be grist for reflection and creativity.

Foci for Reflection in Health Promotion: Power and Collaboration

Health promotion practice often requires the "messiness" of collaboration. Collaboration is seldom defined, but involves working across differences of discipline, culture, community, and practice. Challenges to collaboration include power, expertise, and control (Gondolf, Yllo & Campbell, 1997; Rovegno & Bandhauer, 1998; Boutilier, Cleverly & Labonté, 2000); different work cultures, language of practice, time constraints, and outcome expectations (Buckeridge et al., 2002); and discipline and institutional expectations (Mason & Boutilier, 1996). The current acceptance of "professional-community collaboration" has led to "new roles" in community health (e.g., community trainers), with complex relationships negotiated around differences in power, skills, and understanding, and requiring increasingly critical reflection on the "messiness" of collaborative work (Dugdill et al., 2009). Regular individual and collective engagement in the process of reflection can help bring problematic or contentious issues to light, while honest commitment to the process also supports the development of trust in the individuals and organizations participating in the collaboration.

While reflective practice is usually an individual activity, the collaborative and inter-professional practices common in health promotion also lend themselves to reflection as a collaborative activity (O'Neill & Dupéré, 2006). Collaborative reflection involves collective consideration of issues, actions, and questions, including those that affect group interactions (Barr, 2005). Collaborative reflection offers the possibility of creating effective, successful working relationships, but requires investments of time, energy, and trust. As some caution, "rigourous [sic] reflection, especially when done in a process of social interaction with others, can be both exhilarating and painful. The question is, 'can collaborations succeed without it?'" (Bray, Lee, Smith & Yorks, 2000, p. 11).

When individuals engage in reflective practice, they deliberately examine their situations, behaviour, practices, and effectiveness within specific situations *after the fact*, so they become wiser at working within the complex and dynamic world of practice. Experienced professionals also engage in reflection *during action*, forming judgments, acting and reacting in the moment on the basis of past experience and learning—Schön's reflection-in-action (1983). When decisions are made on the basis of experience and the aims, means, and context are considered against the actual situation and probable outcomes, however, reflection may be considered to have begun *before the action* (Clarke, James & Kelly, 1996). This kind of reflection also builds on learnings from previous projects, merging with reflection-on-action. Not to be taken lightly are the resources needed for both kinds of reflective practice: the time and space to ask questions and speculate upon the answers.

BOX 12.1:

"What If?" Questions for Individual and Collaborative Reflection

The most important question that professionals ask might be "What if?" (Schön, 1983, p. 145). The question opens the door to creativity, artistic strategies, tacit knowledge, and "the swampy lowlands." Consider what questions could be asked in your reflections that highlight issues of values, discipline-based knowledge, tacit knowledge, resources, power, and collaborations in health promotion. These questions can be asked individually or collaboratively.

Examples of "what if" questions about collaborations include:

- What if different partners had collaborated? Who else should be here?
- What if you, for example, lived in this neighbourhood, had a child at this school, or worked in this hospital? How would the issue change for you?
- What if all the collaborators were employed by the same organization? Shared visible characteristics (e.g., race, gender, ability)? Had the same medical health issue? Lived in your neighbourhood? How do these differences shape our perspectives?
- What if all of your collaborators were at the same professional level, or paid the same amount as you are? Would it change the power dynamics?
- What if the collaborators don't share the same language? What if they are uncomfortable with writing? What images would capture the project vision? The process? How do partners' visions differ and what is shared? Why?
- What if you had been guided by a different theory or a different discipline-based training? What would you have done differently? Would the process and outcome be different? What have you read or heard about that is similar?
- What if you were to be engaged in this project for years to come? How would you feel? How would that change your strategies?
- What if you met in a different place? On different "turf"? How does place and space affect your collaboration?

- What if you had a different form of reporting about your project? For example, what would you emphasize in a documentary film on your project? In a play or short story? What is the narrative?
- What if you were working on a very short-term contract? What if you worked from home? What if you had a permanent job? How does career ambition and/or tenure colour some of your and your collaborators' perspectives?
- What and who are your most helpful resources? What are the biggest challenges?
- What if you were asked to do this again? Would you do it differently?

Moving beyond Projects:
Becoming a Reflective Health Promotion Practitioner

In this section we will explore some of the tools that can assist in becoming a reflexive practitioner. The literature offers some examples of how to begin, including: role-playing, video or audiotaping practice sessions, utilizing client feedback, and working with peer or mentor supervision (Evans, 1997; Kottkamp, 1990). There are also resources in participatory research evaluations that will also often apply to health promotion, such as group reflections and storytelling (Labonte & Feather, 1996; Ellis, Reid & Barnsley, 1990).

The most frequently used and easily accessible tool for health promoters is writing (Health Promotion Resource System, 2010). Writing is a powerful tool for learning from and reflecting upon experience. First, the act of writing itself engages both hand and brain integrating the right and left hemispheres in the action. Second, the physical act of converting thoughts into words upon a page demands the slowing down of thought; it allows for moving back into the past and invites musing about the future. While writing, we can pause the action, go back and revisit a thought, consider options and reformulate a sentence; in this way writing is itself often a reflective process (Kottkamp 1990).

There is also an increasing interest in the relationship between art and health, reflecting understandings both of different modes of learning and knowing, and of the mind–body relationship as seen, for example, in the online *International Journal of the Creative Arts in Interdisciplinary Practice* (http://www.ijcaip.com). Recent commentaries on Schön's work on reflective practice highlight the new strategies and professional roles in health, which endeavour to reflect and collaborate with communities (Dugdill et al., 2009), and construct new narratives drawing on arts-based knowledge (Bold & Chambers, 2009). Thus, apart from written journals, "new conversations" are emerging in different modes of professional reflection (Overby, 2009). These include photography (Bhosekar, 2009; Lemon, 2007), drawing-based journals (Tokolahi, 2010; Deaver & McAuliffe, 2009), other visual documentations (Jaruszewica, 2006), spatial poetics and imagery (McIntosh, 2008), weblogs (Hagerman, 2010, Sharma, 2010), and can be individual or collaborative (O'Neill & Dupéré, 2006). Visual modes of reflection are also appropriate where community members need to reflect but are reluctant to write (Ghaye, Melander-Wikman, Kisare et al., 2008), or in cultural contexts where visual images better articulate reflections, or where access to and use of pens and papers are problematic (Williams, 2009).

Writing, Writing, Writing ...

There are different forms that writing can take, including diaries, case records, or journals. While a diary is a list of daily activities with little space set aside for review of those activities, a case record contains detailed description of specific situations or projects. Kottkamp (1990) describes a case record as based on a problematic situation that includes responses to basic questions about the nature of the situation, the action taken, the alternatives considered, and the hoped for outcomes. Another useful layout involves a factual description of an event in one column and later reflections in a second column (Moon, 1999), akin to reflection on action. Journal writing shares features with case records, but expands the scope of reflection beyond problematic situations.

A journal contains the ongoing consideration of the individual in relation to others, the emotions evoked, the values in harmony or collision, and the skills possessed or wanting, in addition to questions about specific situations, the actions taken, the alternatives considered, and the hoped for outcomes. A journal may contain conversations, poetry, drawings, or songs that assist in making thoughts or feelings clear.

In addition to the descriptive documentation of situations and events, alternatives considered, and possible outcomes had these been followed, the journal includes a critical analysis of the political context in which actions unfold, one's knowledge, skills, expertise, values, and assumptions. It becomes the means by which observing, questioning, critiquing, synthesizing, and acting are integrated into daily practice, or reflection-in-action. From reflecting on the specifics of a project or problematic situation and in the midst of making choices in daily practice, one shifts into reflection as a way of encountering the world.

BOX 12.2:

Aids to Written Reflection

- Questioning what, why, and how one does things
- Asking what, why, and how others do things
- Seeking alternatives
- Keeping an open mind
- Comparing and contrasting
- Seeking the framework theoretical basis or underlying rationale
- Viewing from varying perspectives
- Asking for others' ideas and viewpoints
- Using prescriptive models only when adapted to the situation
- Considering consequences
- Hypothesizing
- Synthesizing and testing
- Seeking, identifying, and resolving problems

Source: Roth, R. (1989). Preparing the reflective practitioner: Transforming the apprentice through the dialectic. *Journal of Teacher Education, 40*(2), 31–35.

To begin journalling, one should set aside a block of time. Many find it works best to begin the entry with the date, place, and a summary of a specific situation, activity, or focus of reflection. Consider issues and questions such as the "What if" ones noted above. Emotional reactions are important considerations in that reality. If reflecting on a specific event or situation, consider the emotions related to entry, during the situation and now, upon reflection.

Reflections Past and Present: Journals and Diagrams

In writing this chapter we have inevitably reflected on our own reflective processes. One of us (RM) is a fairly consistent journal writer while the other (MB) uses journals more selectively and more often engages in diagrams that map out relationships, ideas, leading to decisions and strategies. We offer below examples drawn from our own reflections.

Journal Reflections (RM)

My career path has taken me to work in community social service settings, research centres, and a hospital. I have worked collaboratively on projects to address local hunger, youth unemployment, newcomer settlement issues, an organizational policy on intimate partner violence (IPV), and curriculum development. I have frequently found journalling a useful way of organizing my thoughts and experiences. In the excerpts below, written during a collaborative initiative focused on integrating education on IPV into a hospital setting, I consider the "place" and "ownership" of education in the larger hospital environment. At the time, I was the facilitator of an ad hoc group of front-line practitioners who decided to design and disseminate across the hospital a curriculum on IPV to improve care for patients who had experienced abuse. However, within the larger institutional structure, our group—and thus the project—were vulnerable; there was no funding for the group or the education program we had developed, no clear lines for reporting or accountability, and our group did not appear on any organizational chart. While I was a salaried employee and represented the group at meetings, neither my job title nor role profile included this group or the educational initiative; nor did any of the other members have "educator" listed in their role profiles or job responsibilities. However, there was an organizational policy that stated that responding to disclosures of IPV was everyone's responsibility, and that the institution was required to provide the education to support staff. So our group operated in a grey area both within and outside the traditional professional hierarchies and institutional structures. The policy said that staff members were to be educated about the issue, but no one had said that it was our group that should be fulfilling that mandate.

In order to preserve the anonymity of those to whom I refer in the journal, names and other identifiers have been removed. The original entries are marked by the border.

In rereading these two excerpts I am aware now of the responsibility I felt for ensuring our group's collaborative way of working was upheld in the face of a sometimes overwhelming bureaucracy and hierarchy. I believed an enormous trust had been placed in me to represent and speak out for the group; it was as their representative that I found my power and courage to speak out in meetings with senior administrators. Representing the group also meant

BOX 12.3:

Case Study: Reflections on a Practical Situation

May 30, 2001
Our group won an award for medical education. What a boost this was to group morale. And [it was] a lot of fun to get to go out to the award dinner. A number of people [named] stopped to congratulate the group. This should make it somewhat harder for them (the senior hospital administrators) to ignore us or take the program from us to Organizational Development as has been suggested via the rumour mill. Dr. A.A. said we should know there was tremendous support behind us. I don't know if this means behind the award or for the program itself.

June 12, 2001
The politics could kill you or, kill the project. Last week (June 7) at a formal meeting of [managers], Dr. B.B. quickly presented a series of overheads on women's health indicators for the hospital—one of which was based on the policy our group had developed—the indicator was a projected 75 percent of staff as attending one of our trainings. She turned to me and asked if I had anything to say. There had been no consultation or invitation to comment on the plan before the meeting and I was taken by surprise. Certainly in the wake of the earlier meeting it helped explain why they want to roll it out through the Organizational Development office. Our group doesn't have the support or resources to achieve 75 percent attendance. After the meeting I wrote her a note explaining how process, content, and values drive our project and the difficulties inherent in making it a mandatory program. Have to wait and see if there's a response. Then yesterday, C.C. came to see me from [a community organization] and told me that our formalizing education and trying to expand the training to organizations outside the hospital would create animosity and divisiveness among other hospitals and organizations.... Frustrating ... we wanted to share it with others, but it's just too competitive around funding and resources. I need to stay focused on the issue—helping and providing services to women. I think I better pull back from the community a bit and stay focused on the internal dissemination.

becoming highly attuned to (and even preoccupied by) the organizational politics and power dynamics. As an insider/outsider (a status achieved by default because the lines of reporting were unclear) I was afforded more power than other group members—for example, I did attend the same meetings as those who made key decisions for the organization—yet I had no access to the resources or infrastructure to help our group achieve its goals.

I also remember how conflicts with community partners added to my general frustration. As the first line of the second excerpt shows, I was exasperated by the politicking, which seemed to govern every aspect of my daily work life. In rereading this excerpt now, I recognize how reconciled I have become to the politics surrounding practice. The issue itself (IPV) is a politically sensitive one and those who work on it, particularly in hospital environments, are not usually accorded the support or recognition afforded those who specialize in other health issues. On the community side, the tension between comparatively well-resourced hospitals and poorly resourced community partners continues, although in my community we have developed ways of collaborating and supporting each other's work. I believe too that these collaborations have resulted in better understanding on each side of the demands and constraints of working in these very different sectors.

Visual Reflection (MB)

There are many modes of visual reflection, but diagramming with simple pen and paper, similar to journal-writing, is accessible to most health promoters. Reflections need not follow a prescribed format, but it may be helpful to observe how diagrams change and evolve over time within a project. My own diagrams often take on a "layering" effect over time, with expanded relationships and understandings eventually consistent with the spiral metaphor.

Rather than the traditional path of doctorate to academic post, my career has focused solely on research in different capacities and in a range of organizations and working arrangements. My written professional reflections have been somewhat sporadic and I have moved in and out of practice reflections, depending on the projects I worked on, stages of the projects, whether I am employed or working in a volunteer capacity, and the urgency of other dimensions of my life. My reflections have thus incorporated the logistics and "political economy of research," i.e., how the structures of the university mesh with research funding models and the division of labour in research (McQueen, 1994). This contingent nature of formal written reflections may hold for many people— the need for written reflection subsides when work is more or less routine, but a crisis or a decision point will stimulate the reflective process. The irony of this is that it is at these moments of possible crises that the time needed for reflection is in short supply.

As seen in Figure 12.1, my reflections often take the form of charting ideas and building models that first lay out and then link different dimensions of projects and issues. This reflective process goes through stages, with early diagrams having arrows flying in all directions as issues, collaborators, and readings are all brought together. Stepping back to look at the initial collage of ideas, organizations, interests, and so on leads to second or third diagrams that are cleaner and more legible. At this point it is often helpful to share the diagram with a colleague and work on it iteratively until we reach some conclusion or decision. Bringing in "fresh eyes" then helps us to understand where interests and perspectives intersect and diverge, and where possible future action lies, possibly building models or narratives to assess and guide the project.

The diagram included here was intended to capture relationships in a participatory research project and requires contextualization. It was an early diagram, drawn late in the project, trying to distill "lessons learned" for a conference presentation (Boutilier, Mason, Rootman et al., 1995). I was a research associate with a health promotion research unit, North York Community Health Promotion Research Unit (NYCHPRU), itself a partnership of the local public health unit and the University of Toronto. The project included a group of unemployed young people from Toronto's Jane-Finch neighbourhood who worked on federally funded literacy projects with Frontier College. NYCHPRU's Community Action Research Group (CARG) included two academics, named on the diagram: Irv (Rootman) and Ann (Robertson), nursing managers, two public health nurses, and Robin (Mason). The arrows indicate relationships and directions of influence and power.

Looking back, first, I remember how complex and exhilarating the project was, partly due to the non-academic emotional elements the young people brought—noted on the diagram as "anger, hope, and play." While Robin and I initially came to meetings ready to "work," we soon learned they needed time to joke around and "play" before talking about the research,

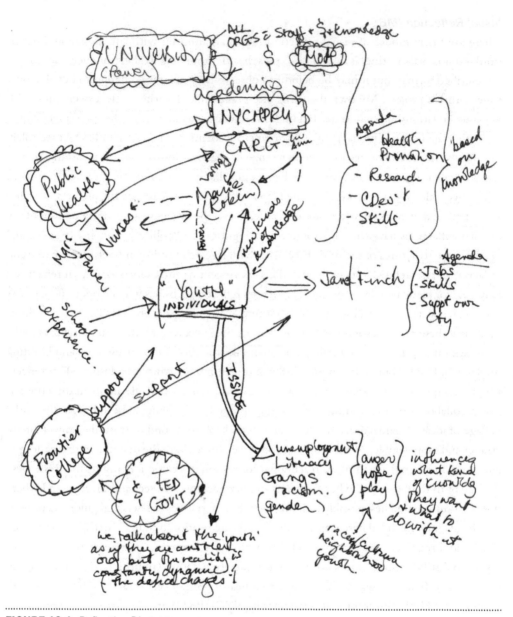

FIGURE 12.1: Reflective Diagram

which included expressions of anger and hope for change. Second, I notice the arrows from Frontier College are labelled "support" rather than "power" and now wish I had explored the dynamic of that distinction more at the time. Finally, Robin's name was in brackets because her involvement lasted several months on a student contract basis. In my mind it partially exempted her from some of the power dynamics and gave her a more neutral perspective. I now reflect that since then, I have been on contracts so I may be "bracketed" on research teams and power relationships, leading me to ask how that generates unique contributions to other projects. Thinking further about how this influenced my health promotion "practice," this project directly led to my observation that there are four "arenas" of health promotion practice: health and social services; community activism; policy (Boutilier, Cleverly & Labonté, 2000); the fourth being research itself, especially when it is participatory (Boutilier, 1996). The question remains for research as health promotion practice: How is "insider/outsider" status conferred in different spheres, e.g., am I an intellectual "insider" but an "outsider" to organizational politics, and how are specific interests (health-related, political, intellectual, social) integrated in each project?

Conclusions

We have examined health promotion reflection, how to reflect, and considered how the process of reflection can illuminate relationships, power, hierarchies, and improve practice. Reflection is integral to the repertoire of knowledge and understanding of what it means to promote health in a context of multiple interests. It becomes a key resource for health promoters as they develop expertise over time, becoming a part of one's professional identity and way of being a reflexive practitioner.

On reflection, the writing of this chapter itself has shaped our representation of reflexivity. While emphasizing the principles and values outlined in the *Ottawa Charter*, we are mindful of the practice of health promotion as lived experience for professionals committed to the health of the communities they serve. Reflection requires resources and facilitators, not the least of which is time.

We have focused on health promoters, but the processes of reflective practice described here apply to professional work in general. In health promotion, the importance of collaboration begs the question of whether processes and foci of reflection and reflexivity may differ across disciplines and professions, as influenced by their respective assumptions and values. While we see collaborative reflection as part of the health promotion reflective process, each individual and health promotion initiative will be unique according to the diversity of individuals, interests, organizations, values, personalities, and goals involved.

Afterword: Further Reflections

Prior to beginning work on this chapter, it had been several years since our last professional collaboration. In the interim we had each worked on other projects and in new collaborative relationships. In starting to work together again we found we could not immediately take up where we last left off. We found that we were challenged to re-examine our assumptions about our professional identities and ways of working together. We learned that we had benefited in different ways from our diverse experiences and now came together with new tacit knowledge that needed articulation for this new endeavour. Predictably, we required time and had to create a space in which to reflect, individually and together, in order to collaborate on this chapter. We recognize that the time and space to creatively explore and articulate ideas are critical in facilitating reflexivity.

Note

1. Authorship is alphabetical.

References

Barr, C. (2005). *Effective interprofessional education: Arguments, assumptions, and evidence.* Oxford: Blackwell.

Bhosekar, K. (2009). Using photographs as a medium to create spaces for reflective learning. *Reflective Practice, 10*(1), 91–100.

Bold, C. & Chambers, P. (2009). Reflecting meaningfully, reflecting differently. *Reflective Practice, 10*(1), 13–26.

Boutilier, M. (1996). *The effectiveness of community action in health promotion: A research perspective.* International Symposium on the Effectiveness of Health Promotion, Centre for Health Promotion, University of Toronto, Toronto.

Boutilier, M., Cleverly, S. & Labonté, R. (2000). Community as a setting for health promotion. In B. Poland, I. Rootman & L. Green (Eds.), *Settings for health promotion* (pp. 250–279). Thousand Oaks: Sage Publications.

Boutilier, M. & Mason, R. (1994) Paper presented at Health and Behaviour 1994, Queen's University, Kingston, March 1994.

Boutilier, M., Mason, R., Rootman, I., Robertson, A., Bresolin, L., Panhuysen, N., Tao, M., Sage, L. & Marz, C. (1995). Can the 2-step become a square dance? Participatory action research with community residents, agencies, public health, and the university. Annual Meeting of the Ontario Public Health Association.

Bray, J., Lee, J., Smith, L. & Yorks, L. (2000). *Collaborative inquiry in practice: Action, reflection, and meaning making.* Thousand Oaks: Sage Publications.

Buckeridge, D., Mason, R., Robertson, A., Frank, J., Glazier, R., Purdon, L. et al. (2002). Making health data maps: A case study of a community/university research collaboration. *Social Science & Medicine, 55*(7), 1189–1206.

Clarke, B., James, C. & Kelly, J. (1996). Reflective practice: Reviewing the issues and refocusing the debate. *International Journal of Nursing Studies, 33*(2), 171–180.

Cunliffe, A. & Easterby-Smith, M. (2003). From reflection to practical reflexivity: Experiential learning as lived experience. In M. Reynolds & R. Vince (Eds.), *Organizing reflection* (pp. 30–46). Burlington: Ashgate Publishing Co.

Deaver, S. & McAuliffe, G. (2009). Reflective visual journaling during art therapy and counselling internships: A qualitative study. *Reflective Practice, 10*(5), 615–632.

Dewey, J. (1933). *How we think.* Boston: Heath & Co.

Dugdill, L., Coffey, M., Coufopoulos, A., Byrne, K. & Porcellato, L. (2009). Developing new community health roles: Can reflective learning drive professional practice? *Reflective Practice, 10*(1), 121–130.

Ellis, D., Reid, G. & Barnsley, J. (1990). *Keeping on track: An evaluation guide for community groups.* Vancouver: The Women's Research Centre.

Evans, D. (1997). *Reflective learning through practice-based assignments.* Paper presented at the British Educational Research Association Annual Conference, September 11–14. Retrieved from: www. leeds.ac.uk/educol/documents/000000468.htm

Ghaye, T., Melander-Wikman, A., Kisare, M., Chambers, P., Bergmark, U., Kostenius, C. & Lillyman, S. (2008). Participatory and appreciative action and reflection (PAAR)—democratizing reflective practices. *Reflective Practice, 9*(4), 361–397.

Gondolf, E.W., Yllo, K. & Campbell, J. (1997). Collaboration between researchers and advocates. In G.K. Kantor & J.L. Jasinski (Eds.), *Out of the darkness: Contemporary perspectives on family violence* (pp. 255–267). Thousand Oaks: Sage.

Hagerman, K. (2010). *At the very root of it.* Retrieved from: http://attheveryrootofit.wordpress.com/

Haggerty, K. (2003) Ruminations on reflexivity. *Current Sociology, 51*(2), 153–162.

Health Promotion Resource System. (2010). *HP-101, Health promotion online course.* Retrieved from: http://www.ohprs.ca/hp101/main.htm

International Journal of the Creative Arts in Interdisciplinary Practice. Retrieved from: http://www.ijcaip.com

Jaruszewica, C. (2006). Opening windows on teaching and learning: Transformative and emancipatory learning precipitated by experimenting with visual documentation of student learning. *Educational Action Research, 14*(3), 357–375. Retrieved from: http://www.informaworld.com/smpp/title~db=all~content=t716100708~tab=issueslist~branches=14 - v14

Kottkamp, R.B. (1990). Means for facilitating reflection. *Education and Urban Society, 22*(2), 182–203.

Labonté, R. & Feather, J. (1996). *Handbook on using stories in health promotion practice.* Cat. no. H39-378/1996E. Ottawa: Minister of Supply and Services.

Lemon, N. (2007). Take a photograph: Teacher reflection through narrative. *Reflective Practice, 8*(2) 177–191.

Lewin, K. (1946). Action research and minority problems. *Journal of Social Issues, 2,* 34–46.

Mason, R. & Boutilier, M. (1996). The challenge of genuine power sharing in participatory research: The gap between theory and practice. *The Canadian Journal of Community Mental Health, 15*(2), 145–152.

Maton, K. (2003). Reflexivity, relationism & research: Pierre Bourdieu and the epistemic conditions of social scientific knowledge. *Space & Culture, 6*(1), 52–65.

McIntosh, P. (2008). Poetics and space: Developing a reflective landscape through imagery and human geography. *Reflective Practice, 9*(1), 69–78.

McQueen, D. (1994, June 16). *Visions of health promotion research.* Keynote address, Third Conference on Health Promotion Research, Calgary.

Moon, J. (1999). *Reflection in learning and professional development.* London: Kogan Page.

O'Neill, M. & Dupéré, S. (2006). Du carré à la spirale: Réflexions sur quelques années de participation du comité avec du collectif pour un Québec sans pauvreté. *The Canadian Journal of Program Evaluation, 21*(3), 227–234.

Overby, A. (2009). The new conversation: Using weblogs for reflective practice in the studio art Classroom. *Art Education, 62*(4), 18–24.

Reynolds, M. & Vince, R. (2004). *Organizing reflection.* Burlington: Ashgate Publishing Co.

Roth, R. (1989). Preparing the reflective practitioner: Transforming the apprentice through the dialectic. *Journal of Teacher Education, 40*(2), 31–35.

Rovegno, I. & Bandhauer, D. (1998). A study of the collaborative research process: Shared privilege and shared empowerment. *Journal of Teaching in Physical Education, 17,* 357–375.

Schön, D. (1983). *The reflective practitioner: How professionals think in action.* Boston: Basic Books.

Sharma, P. (2010). Enhancing student reflection using weblogs: Lessons learned from two implementation studies. *Reflective Practice, 11*(2), 127–141.

Tokolahi, E. (2010). Case study: Development of a drawing-based journal to facilitate reflective inquiry. *Reflective Practice, 11*(2), 157–170.

Williams, C. (2009). *A critical and participatory approach to gender equity among youth in Kibera, Kenya.* Thesis submitted to College of Nursing, University of Saskatchewan, Saskatoon.

Critical Thinking Questions

1. What are the underlying disciplines that form the bases of the knowledge and theoretical frameworks with which you frame questions and issues in health promotion?

2. What is the difference between reflecting on an issue and becoming a reflexive professional?

3. If you were to organize a collaborative reflection process, who would you involve? How would it happen? What questions would you start with?

4. What values are important to you in your work/professional life? Can you imagine a situation in which these are challenged in your work? What would be your first steps in working through it?

5. If you were designing a Type 2 diabetes educational initiative for an urban hospital setting, which stakeholders representing which interests would you consider as you developed your program? Who would be the target audience for the program? If you were designing a similar program for a low-income housing complex, which stakeholders representing which interests would you need to consider? In what ways would the program change depending upon where it was being delivered?

Resources

Further Readings

Gould, J. & Nelson, J. (2005). Researchers reflect from the cancer precipice. *Reflective Practice, 6*(2), 277–284.

Two researchers at a cancer research unit reflect together about the difficult emotional issues involved in working with cancer patients, power relations, and privilege, as well as facets of identity—race, class, gender, cultural capital, and personal biography.

McIntosh, P. (2010). *Action research and reflective practice: Creative and visual methods to facilitate reflection and learning.* London: Routledge.

Part one provides a historical overview of evidence-based medicine, and argues that evidence-based practice and research in health and social services must evolve to incorporate reflection; part two offers philosophical and practical guidance.

Reynolds, M. & Vince, R. (Eds.). (2004). *Organizing reflection.* Aldershot: Ashgate Publishing Ltd.

This collection examines reflection as important in organizational development. It applies reflection to communities of practice, collective reflection, critical reflection, and reflexivity; it also includes discussions of power relations, experience, and emotions.

Schön, D. (1983). *The reflective practitioner: How professionals think in action.* Boston: Basic Books.

This seminal work in the literature on reflective practice provides a "sociology of knowledge" approach to expertise and expert power. It rests on meticulous case studies of how professionals learn; its historical perspective maintains it as a paradigm-shaping work and a continuing resource for professionals, their teachers, and managers.

Relevant Websites

ItsLife

www.itslifejimbutnotasweknowit.org.uk/RefPractice.htm

UK teacher education site; extensive bibliography on reflective practice.

Learning and Teaching Unit, Manchester Metropolitan University Adult Education Web Site

www.ltu.mmu.ac.uk/ltia/issue11/index.shtml

Aims at widening participation in higher education through "activities and interventions aimed at creating a system that includes all who can benefit from it—people who might not otherwise view learning as an option, or who may be discouraged by social, cultural, economic, or institutional barriers."

CHAPTER 13

The Professionalization of Health Promotion in Canada:
Potential Risks and Rewards

Brian Hyndman and Michel O'Neill

Introduction

An early proponent of public health defined the discipline as "the science and art of preventing disease, prolonging life and promoting health through the organized efforts and informed choices of society, organizations, public and private, communities and individuals" (Winslow, 1920, p. 23). During the first half of the twentieth century, however, public health practice was focused primarily on dealing with preventing and responding to outbreaks of communicable disease. The period between the 1974 publication *A New Perspective on the Health of Canadians* (aka the Lalonde Report) and the 1986 release of the *Ottawa Charter for Health Promotion* fostered the expansion of health promotion, both as distinct field of practice within the broader public health sector and as a viable career option. New bureaucratic structures supporting the application of health promotion strategies and comprehensive approaches to addressing key risk factors for chronic disease, such as tobacco, alcohol, unhealthy dietary choices, and a sedentary lifestyle, were introduced at both the federal and provincial levels of government; graduate-level degree programs in Canada were launched; attempts to establish national- and provincial-level associations of health promoters were made (with varying degrees of success); and public health and social service organizations throughout Canada created positions with the term "health promotion" in the job title. In short, the nascent field of health promotion began to take on the attributes of a health profession.

The means by which a group achieves the status of a recognized profession has been a topic of study by sociologists for decades (e.g. Vollmer & Mills, 1966). Special attention has been given to the evolution of health professions, given their diversity and the dominance of medical professions in relation to others (Coburn, 1988; Freidson, 1977; Hoogland & Jochemsen, 2000; Jacob, 1999). These authors note that a health profession is usually defined by a set of common features, which are described in Box 13.1.

The extent to which these features have shaped the field of health promotion practice in Canada is the focus of this chapter. It provides an overview of both historical and current developments that have given rise to an occupational group loosely known as "health promoters," beginning with an introduction to educational opportunities in the field, followed by a discussion of professional associations, health promotion competencies, accreditation mechanisms, and concluding with discussion of the likelihood of health promotion becoming a regulated profession. It discusses the advantages and limitations associated with the ascription of key professional attributes to the field of health promotion in Canada. As will be seen,

---

BOX 13.1

Main Characteristics of a Profession

- The development of a specific body of knowledge that delineates the scope of the profession
- The profession is practised as a full-time occupation
- The establishment of university degree programs focused on teaching the profession
- The formation of local, regional, or national associations to promote the interests of the profession; ensure quality control (most often by means of an accreditation mechanism); establish a code of ethics; and protect the public from dangerous practices
- If concerns about public safety and the broader "public good" are paramount, then legislation is enacted to formally regulate the profession

---

Sources: Coburn, D. (1988). The development of Canadian nursing: Professionalization and proletarianization. *International Journal of Health Services, 18*(3), 437–456; Friedson, E. (1977). *Professional dominance: The social structure of medical care.* Chicago: Aldine Publishing Company; Hoogland, J. & Jochemsen, H. (2000). Professional autonomy and the normative structure of modern medicine. *Theoretical Medicine, 21*(5), 457–475; Jacob, J.M. (1999). *Doctors and rules: A sociology of professional values.* New Brunswick & London: Transaction Publishers.

potential advantages include greater recognition of health promotion as a distinct field of prac-tice and more developed infrastructure for building the knowledge base of health promotion, whereas potential drawbacks include barriers that could potentially exclude individuals with the potential to make important contributions to recognized health promotion strategies (e.g., community mobilization), as well as the risk of establishing attributes of professionalization that run counter to health promotion's key values of inclusion and equity.

As a potential way forward, we conclude by offering suggestions regarding possible approaches to solve the dilemmas associated with the view of health promotion becoming a distinct profession. Specifically, we propose that the recently developed Canadian (Ghassemi, 2009) and international (Barry et al., 2009) health promotion competencies could be used as a basis for engaging Canadian health promoters in a participatory dialogue aimed at striking a balance between the professional characteristics that are desirable and positive, while avoiding the negative attributes of professionalism that have the potential to seriously undermine the core values and concepts of health promotion practice.

Post-secondary Degree Programs in Health Promotion

The emergence of health promotion as a distinct field of practice within the Canadian public health sector led to the introduction of graduate-level degree programs for people interested in pursing health promotion as a career. Traditionally, public health education in Canada was highly constrained and limited to a small number of programs centred on schools of public health in Toronto and Montreal (Gaucher, 1979). In 1979, the first Canadian graduate program in health promotion, offered as an area of focus for a Master of Health Sciences degree, was established at the University of Toronto (Allison et al., 1995). By the beginning of the current century, several other universities across Canada had introduced graduate-level training in health promotion. These include for instance: a Master's in community health degree with an area of concentration in health promotion at Université Laval (established in 1989); a Master of Science degree program in health promotion studies with a distance learning option at the University of Alberta (established in 1996); and the transformation of a Master of Arts degree in health education to an MA in health promotion in 2006 at Dalhousie University (Wilson et al., 2000; Rootman, Jackson & Hills, 2007).

In addition to the development of specific degree programs, health promotion has emerged as an area of focus in undergraduate curricula offered through both health sciences faculties, as well as nursing and medical schools throughout Canada. A review conducted by Hills, Carroll, and Vollman (2007) found that the term "health promotion" appeared in the programs and course descriptions of 14 of the 16 medical curricula across Canada. In this context, health promotion was most often linked with disease prevention and epidemiology, and was usually subsumed under the broader labels of "population health" or "community health." Health promotion was thus framed as a "function" area of population/community health, with a related set of technical/intervention strategies (Hills, Carroll & Vollman, 2007).

While the incorporation of health promotion concepts and values into medical and health education curricula is encouraging, there is a risk that more specific training in health promotion may be marginalized by current developments affecting the nature and scope of educational opportunities for aspiring health promoters. This trend is somewhat offset, however, by the fact that support for strengthening the capacity of Canada's public health system was a recurrent theme of reports commissioned in the wake of the 2003 severe acute respiratory syndrome (SARS) outbreak (Naylor, 2003; Walker, 2004; Campbell, 2006). This concern for greater public health capacity in turn contributed to a number of academic institutions planning or implementing graduate-level training programs in public health using a "generalist" Master of Public Health (MPH) degree model. At the time of writing, during the fall of 2010, 11 Canadian universities had established, or were in the process of implementing, MPH degree programs (Public Health Agency of Canada, 2010).

This increased training capacity for public health professionals in Canada, while welcome, may come at the cost of further expansion of specialized degree opportunities for health promotion practitioners. In response to the upsurge of interest in MPH programs within Canadian universities, the federal Public Health Human Resources Task Group established a Working Group to develop guidelines for MPH programs in Canada. Their report follows the model of subsuming health promotion, along with disease prevention and epidemiology, and mentions health promotion only once as one of the "core content areas and competencies basic to public health" (MPH Guidelines Working Group, 2006, p. 8). Specific health promotion capacity areas, such as health communication, community mobilization, and policy development, are noticeably absent from the guidelines, which cite the draft (2006) version of the Canadian Public Health Workforce competencies (Public Health Agency of Canada, 2007) as the recommended template for guiding the development of MPH curricula.

As mentioned above, the establishment of post-secondary degree programs is a key attribute of an emerging profession; with respect to health promotion's development as a profession, we are of the opinion that conditions for this are currently not optimal at this time, given the insertion of health promotion into broader public health degrees rather than development of specific health promotion degrees. In the following three sections, we will assess the current status of other attributes of professionalism among trained practitioners who are actively engaged in health promotion. These include the establishment of professional associations, the development of discipline-specific competencies, and the extent to which these competencies could serve as the basis for possible accreditation mechanisms that may ultimately lead to health promotion becoming a regulated profession.

Professional Associations for Health Promoters

A professional association has been defined as a non-profit organization seeking to further a particular profession by advocating for the interests of individuals engaged in that profession while guarding the broader public interest (Harvey & Mason, 1995). Such bodies often strive to achieve a balance between these two seemingly conflicting priorities. As was noted previously, the existence of professional associations is one of the key features of a health profession. In the case of Canadian health promotion practice, the development and sustainability of professional associations has proven to be a constant and unresolved challenge.

Sporadic attempts have been made to establish a Canada-wide health promotion association since the release of the *Ottawa Charter* in 1986. In the late 1980s, efforts were made to expand the scope of the Canadian Health Education Society into a health promotion association, with interested members who were primarily graduates of Ontario and Atlantic university programs in health promotion. However, CHES proved to be unsustainable and was dissolved by 1991 (Ontario Prevention Clearinghouse, 2006).

More recently, the release of the proposed Canadian health promotion competencies (see below) has sparked interest in the development of a pan-Canadian health promotion network. Health promoters in Ontario, Manitoba, and Nova Scotia have engaged in informal discussions about the establishment of such a network since 2008. It was envisioned that the network would initially serve as a national advisory body overseeing the completion and adoption of a pan-Canadian set of health promotion competencies. However, the Public Health Agency of Canada's elimination of financial support for profession-specific competency development has slowed the development of the network, although discussions are still ongoing (Bursey, 2010).

There has been a similar lack of progress in the development of health promotion associations at the provincial and territorial levels. The lack of progress may be a function of the limited number of health promotion practitioners within the broader public health sector (especially in smaller Canadian provinces), as well as the role played by provincial public health associations in hosting and supporting networking opportunities for health promoters. A notable exception exists in the province of Ontario, where Health Promotion Ontario (HPO) has served as the primary association of health promoters since 1987.

The mission of Health Promotion Ontario, which evolved from a group of health promotion specialists within Ontario's public health units and a formal division within the Ontario

Public Health Association, is "to support the development of public health activities based on health promotion philosophy, practice and research" (HPO, 2010). HPO, among many things, maintains a members-only listserv, holds an annual conference, and conducts ongoing advocacy for the development of health promotion capacity in Ontario. One unique feature of HPO is that its membership is not restricted to individuals occupying designated health promotion positions; since 2005, membership in HPO has been open to any holder of a university degree (or equivalent training and experience) employed in an occupation that uses health promotion strategies and applies a variety of health promotion skills.

Health Promotion Competencies

Competencies guide the development of professional standards and systems of quality assurance. Since the 1970s, competency models have been increasingly used to clarify specific practice requirements for public health disciplines, including the practice of health promotion. An international review of health promotion competency frameworks by Battel-Kirk et al. (2009) found evidence of health promotion competencies and/or ongoing developmental work in Europe, Australia, New Zealand, the United States, and Canada. The study revealed that a number of countries have made significant advances in delineating competencies for health promotion practice, including, in some instances, the development of competency-based professional standards and quality assurance systems. However, overall progress has been uneven, with many countries lacking the necessary health promotion resources and infrastructure to engage in these developments.

Debates about the risks and benefits of specifying health promotion competencies have occurred within the Canadian health promotion community since the 1980s. It's important to note that these discussions were often framed within—or perhaps escalated to—the broader notion of "professionalizing" health promotion through the adoption of an accreditation system rather than the development of competencies per se (Ontario Prevention Clearinghouse, 2006). This illustrates the challenge of separating skills-based competencies defining health promotion practice from broader possible ramifications associated with professionalization (i.e., accreditation and potential regulation of the profession). In 2000, the Canadian Association of Teachers in Community Health, in conjunction with the Canadian Consortium of Health Promotion research, explored the issue of health promotion competencies at their fall symposium (Hills & O'Neill, 2003). While participants at this session concluded that health promotion competencies could be useful as broadly defined guidelines, there was concern that the rigid interpretation of competencies as professional standards of practice could prove detrimental to a field that was still evolving because it might curtail innovations in practice and knowledge development, as well as alienate other professions already involved in health promotion practice.

However, subsequent developments sparked an increased interest in a "made in Canada" solution to the question of health promotion competencies. Chief among these was the aforementioned renewal of public health in the wake of the SARS outbreak, which, among other things, resulted in the creation of the Public Health Agency of Canada (PHAC). In 2004, PHAC launched a competency-based approach to human resource planning (for public health) that culminated in the creation of core competencies for the public health workforce in Canada and provided grants to support the development of competencies for key public health areas, including health promotion (Public Health Agency of Canada, 2007). This opportunity was gladly seized upon because there was growing concern that health promoters working in the field of public health risked increased marginalization in the field of public health if they failed to take advantage of the opportunity to develop a set of competencies that expressed clearly the key concepts, values, and principles underlying health promotion practice (Hyndman, 2009).

In the spring of 2006, Health Promotion Ontario was thus funded by PHAC to develop a proposed set of pan-Canadian health promotion competencies. This work was guided by a review of competencies developed for health promoters in Australia (Shilton, Howat & James, 2003) and New Zealand (McCracken & Rance, 2000), as well as of an academic set of competencies developed for the (now defunct) MHSc degree program in health promotion at the University of Toronto. In addition, over 60 Canadian job descriptions for health promotion positions were reviewed to identify common requirements (Hyndman, 2009).

The information garnered from this review guided the development of a draft set of health promotion competencies that was initially released by HPO at its annual conference in May 2007. They were subsequently shared with an international audience at the nineteenth annual International Union for Health Promotion and Education (IUHPE) conference in Vancouver in June 2007. Participants at both events provided feedback that was used to further refine the competencies. Additional feedback was captured through an online survey completed by over 200 health promoters across Canada in the summer of 2007.

A revised version of the competencies was finally released by HPO in 2009 (Ghassemi, 2009). These competencies are listed in Box 13.2.

The revised pan-Canadian health promotion competencies coincided with the release of the international Galway Consensus Conference Statement on core competencies for health promotion and health education in 2009 (Barry et al., 2009). Jointly organized by the International Union for Health Promotion and Education (IUHPE), the Society for Public Health Education (SOPHE) and the US Centers for Disease Control, the purpose of the Galway Consensus Conference was to identify the core competency domains in health promotion practice.

A comparison of the pan-Canadian and Galway Consensus competencies by Hyndman (2009) reveals a number of commonalities as well as some notable differences. Both sets of competencies embrace the definition of health promotion embedded in the *Ottawa Charter* as the conceptual basis for, and the desired outcome of, health promotion practice. In addition, both competency statements acknowledge that health promotion is guided by a core set of values and principles that include a holistic socio-ecological approach to addressing health issues encompassing the social, economic, and cultural determinants of health.

The Galway Consensus Conference Statement identifies several audiences, including prac-titioners, researchers, academics, as well as policy- and decision-makers who have a stake in

BOX 13.2:

Proposed Pan-Canadian Health Promotion Competencies

All health promoters should be able to:

1. *Demonstrate knowledge necessary for conducting health promotion* that includes:
1.1. Applying a determinants of health framework to the analysis of health issues
1.2. Applying theory to health promotion planning and implementation
1.3. Applying health promotion principles in the context of the roles and responsibilities of public health organizations
1.4. Describing the range of interventions available to address public health issues
2. *Conduct a community needs/situational assessment for a specific issue* that includes:
2.1. Identifying behavioural, social, environmental, and organizational factors that promote or compromise health
2.2. Identifying relevant and appropriate data and information sources
2.3. Identifying community assets and resources
2.4. Partner with communities to validate collected quantitative and qualitative data
2.5. Integrating information from available sources to identify priorities for action
3. *Plan appropriate health promotion programs* that includes:
3.1. Identifying, retrieving, and critically appraising the relevant literature
3.2. Conducting an environmental scan of best practices
3.3. Developing a component plan to implement programs including goals, objectives, and implementation steps
3.4. Developing a program budget
3.5. Monitoring and evaluating implementation of interventions
4. *Contribute to policy development* that includes:
4.1. Describing the health, economic, administrative, legal, social, and political implications of policy options
4.2. Providing strategic policy advice on health promotion issues
4.3. Writing clear and concise policy statements for complex issues
5. *Facilitate community mobilization and build community capacity around shared health priorities* that includes:
5.1. Engaging in a dialogue with communities based on trust and mutual respect
5.2. Identifying and strengthening local community capacities to take action on health issues
5.3. Advocating for and with individuals and communities that will improve their health and well-being
6. *Engage in partnership and collaboration* that includes:
6.1. Establishing and maintaining linkages with community leaders and other key health promotion stakeholders (e.g., schools, businesses, churches, community associations, labour unions, etc.)
6.2. Utilizing leadership, team building, negotiation, and conflict resolution skills to build community partnerships
6.3. Building coalitions and stimulating intersectoral collaboration on health issues

7. *Communicate effectively with community members and other professionals* that includes:

7.1. Providing health status, demographic, statistical, programmatic, and scientific information tailored to professional and lay audiences

7.2. Applying social marketing and other communication principles to the development, implementation, and evaluation of health communication campaigns

7.3. Using the media, advanced technologies, and community networks to receive and communicate information

7.4. Interacting with, and adapting policies and programming that responds to the diversity in population characteristics

8. *Organize, implement, and manage health promotion interventions* that includes:

8.1. Training and coordinating program volunteers

8.2. Describing scope of work in the context of organization's mission and functions

8.3. Contribute to team and organizational learning

Source: Ghassemi, M. (2009). *Development of pan-Canadian discipline-specific competencies for health promoters: Summary report. Consultation.* Toronto: Health Promotion Ontario. Retrieved from: http://hpo.squarespace.com/storage/HP%20Competencies%20 Consultation%20Summary%20Report%20March%202009.pdf

promoting the health of the public. The proposed Canadian competencies, by contrast, were developed primarily for practitioners working in organizations with a health-promoting mandate, such as public health departments, community health centres, and regional health authorities. As such, they were intended to assist in developing competency-based job descriptions; in structuring the content of training and continuing education opportunities; and in increasing understanding of the skill set required for the planning, implementation, and assessment of health promotion interventions.

Features of health promotion practice in Canada influenced the positioning of key health promotion skills within broader domains of practice. While the Galway Consensus Conference Statement identifies advocacy as a primary domain of health promotion practice, the proposed Canadian competencies cite advocacy as a key competency area within the broader practice domain of community mobilization and capacity-building. This placement reflects a commitment to building capacity by advocating "with" communities as well as acknowledging a working reality that limits the extent to which health promoters can engage in direct advocacy within their organizations. Another distinction concerns the importance of evaluation and monitoring skills as a prerequisite for health promotion practice: While the Galway Consensus Conference Statement cites evaluation as a primary domain area, the proposed Canadian competencies positions evaluation as a subset of the practice domain related to planning. This was done to reinforce the importance of the "continuous quality improvement" cycle linking the effective planning of health promotion initiatives to evidence-informed practice.

To date, application of the pan-Canadian health promotion competencies has been limited. In 2008, for reasons that are not clear to the authors, PHAC failed to renew funding for the profession-specific competency work, and (at time of writing in fall 2010) has yet to reinstate its support. The resulting lack of resources has made it impossible to undertake the consultations needed to transform a "proposed" set of competencies into a final product, with pan-Canadian endorsement. There is nevertheless anecdotal evidence that the competencies are being used by several public health units in Ontario, primarily to develop job descriptions and to inform performance reviews (Burscy, 2010).

Health Promotion as a Regulated Profession: Are Competencies a Gateway to Credentialism and Colleges?

The development of health promotion competencies invariably gives rise to debate about the merits of taking further steps toward the professionalization of health promotion. These include the introduction of quality assurance mechanisms, such as a formal accreditation process by a recognized body, and the designation of health promotion as a regulated profession governed by a college established through legislation, which, in the Canadian context, would be at the provincial level.

One key area of debate, both in Canada and elsewhere, concerns the extent to which quality assurance mechanisms are needed to protect the "public good" by assessing proficiency in the domains of core health promotion competencies. The Galway Consensus Conference Statement recommends that each country or region develop or adopt quality assurance measures in accordance with prevailing political, economic, or cultural contexts (Barry et al., 2009).

To date, the health promotion field in Canada has taken a cautious stance on this issue. A 2006 discussion document prepared by the Ontario Prevention Clearinghouse (now known as Health Nexus) concluded that the development of formal accreditation mechanisms for health promotion would be rigorous, time-consuming, and potentially divisive due to concerns that had surfaced among health promotion practitioners whenever the issue was broached (Ontario Prevention Clearinghouse, 2006). In acknowledgement of this viewpoint, the proposed Canadian competencies are not intended to serve as an intermediary step toward mandatory accreditation processes to control the access into the health promotion field; rather, they are meant to inform and stimulate dialogue toward agreement on a requisite skill set for health promotion practice in Canada (Hyndman, 2009) that could be used to design academic programs or develop job descriptions.

The ultimate step along a gradient of professionalization is the designation of health promotion as a regulated profession. In Canada, regulated professions are those regulated under provincial or territorial *Health Professions Acts*, legislation established to protect the public's right to safe, effective, and ethical health care. Professional colleges are the regulating bodies established to ensure the accountability, performance, quality, and transparency of regulated health professionals. Most, but not all, regulations include controlled acts that, if performed by a non-regulated individual, could engender harm to a patient (Ontario Prevention Clearinghouse, 2006) and thus could become the object of a lawsuit for unlawful exercise of the profession.

It is the opinion of the authors of this chapter that the prospect of health promotion becoming a regulated profession in any Canadian jurisdiction is highly unlikely because such a process could elicit competing demands for similar status by public health practitioners in other areas of the field (e.g., epidemiologists, public health inspectors) or for the recognition of a generic public health profession. Moreover, the regulation of health promotion practice would probably fail to engender the support of a large segment of the health promotion field, which would view such a move as antithetical to health promotion's core values of participation, empowerment, and intersectoral collaboration. It could also alienate other already existing professions (e.g., nursing, nutrition, medicine, or social work), which are currently providing health promotion services, potentially generating energy-draining turf wars. The disadvantages of becoming a regulated profession thus seem more considerable than the potential benefits. A more likely, and probably more desirable, scenario is the emergence of a voluntary accreditation program. Kinesiology and evaluation are two examples of unregulated professions with voluntary accreditation programs currently existing in Canada that might serve as models for health promotion.

The Ontario Kinesiology Association is a voluntary association whose members must be graduates of a four-year Bachelor's program in kinesiology or human kinetics. The association requires member participation in its continuing standards program as a mandatory require-ment, and imposes upon members a code of standards and ethics designed to protect the public and the profession (Ontario Kinesiology Association, 2010). This approach ensures that all members are kept informed about emerging developments in the profession while simultan-eously ensuring consensus on standards to protect the interests of their clients.

By contrast, the Canadian Evaluation Society launched its credentialed evaluator (CE) designation in 2010. This designation program was created to define, recognize, and promote the practice of ethical, high-quality, and competent evaluation in Canada. Successful appli-cants for the designation are required to demonstrate evidence of a graduate-level degree or certificate, two years (full-time equivalent) of evaluation-related work experience over the past decade, and education and/or experience related to 70 percent of each of the five domains of competencies for Canadian Evaluation Practice (Canadian Evaluation Society, 2010).

There are potential advantages and drawbacks to the adoption of a voluntary accreditation program by Canadian health promoters of the same type as the certified health education specialist (NCHEC, 2010) in the US or similar ones elsewhere. The chief advantage is that it would provide practitioners with an opportunity to exercise greater control over defining the scope of health promotion practice, as opposed to having it defined for them by external funders whose interests may not be compatible with core health promotion values. It would also provide employers and academic programs with clear criteria for training and recruiting health promotion practitioners. Finally, this approach would help to reach a consensus on what health promotion is for Canada because by its very nature, it is not as neatly defined as more narrowly focused disciplines; indeed, the ambiguity of health promotion discourse has been identified as a perennial barrier to its development (O'Neill & Stirling, 2007).

A barrier to accreditation is that it is associated with considerable costs, including appli-cation fees, which may deter lower-income practitioners. This is an important considera-tion for a field that has long embraced equity and social justice as core values. Lastly, the degree of emphasis an accreditation mechanism would place on different dimensions of health promotion practice (e.g., policy development vs. community mobilization) could also be a concern. Would equal weight be given to all domains of health promotion practice? Would it offer sufficient flexibility to allow for subspecialization within a recognized competency area? These are but a few of the issues warranting careful consideration before any decisions about the adoption of an accreditation system are made, but it nevertheless seems to us the direction to move toward at this point.

Conclusion

The view of health promotion as a profession has long been a source of contention. Over two decades ago, the World Health Organization stated that health promotion is best performed by individuals with a wide variety of training and backgrounds, and suggested that it would be detrimental for health promotion initiatives to be delivered by one professional group at the exclusion of others (WHO, 1986). During health promotion's growth spurt in the wake of the *Ottawa Charter*, some early champions of health promotion viewed indicators of growing professionalism with a suspicion bordering on hostility. In a presentation to health workers in Adelaide, Australia, one pioneer of the Canadian health promotion movement (who subsequently recanted his words) decried "the proliferation of senior government departments; of journals and academic chairs; of new credentialing associations and research institutes; and bureaucracy's iron law of oligarchy, which transforms health promotion practitioners into health promotion managers, often at their own status-driven requests" (Labonté, 1994, p. 72).

Yet these concerns did not impede the field of health promotion from assuming some of the key attributes of a profession: more health promotion jobs were created; additional degree programs were launched; provincial departments and ministries of health promotion were created and restructured; and, more recently, proposed competencies outlining the scope of health promotion practice in Canada were developed. Given that key aspects of professionalism have long been a working reality within the field, there is a need to shift the discourse toward sustaining the desirable professional attributes that have the potential to advance it (e.g., greater recognition of health promotion within the broader health care system and recognized mechanisms promoting the common interests of the field), as well as the benefits of the populations receiving services from health promoters, while avoiding the negative attributes of professionalism (e.g., potential elitism and a rigidity that could stifle innovation) that have the potential to undermine health promotion's core values and concepts.

This conclusion is not new: It has been emphasized in previous literature examining health promotion as a distinct profession (McGhee, 1995; Ottoson et al., 2000). But it is an important message to convey to the Canadian health promotion community at a time when their scope of practice is being defined by both national and international sets of competencies, about which the consensus seems increasingly clear, which could serve as the basis for the development of more formal accreditation mechanisms.

One suggested way forward is to advocate for resources that would support the establishment and sustainability of the proposed pan-Canadian network of health promoters. This group could assume responsibility for coordinating a national dialogue among health promoters to reach consensus on a defined set of health promotion competencies, incorporating the best elements of the Canadian (Ghassemi, 2009) and international (Barry et al., 2009) versions. Decisions could then be made about the most effective means of using these competencies, including knowledge exchange events, training and professional development opportunities, and the establishment of provincial and territorial associations to advance the field of health promotion practice within their respective jurisdictions. In addition, the network could serve as a forum for reaching consensus on the feasibility of accreditation mechanisms.

This may seem like an overly ambitious agenda for an under-resourced field operating in a large and diverse country, in two official languages. However, inaction comes with considerable risks. In particular, PHAC's abandonment of discipline-specific competencies in favour of the more generic Public Health Workforce competencies, and the trend toward more generalist MPH degree programs at Canadian universities (although counter-examples exist, such as the specialization in health promotion of the Master's in community health, begun in September 2010 at Université Laval) have the potential to marginalize health promotion practice within the broader field of public health.

Almost a quarter century has passed since a dedicated group of individuals had the foresight to outline the key tenets of health promotion practice over the course of a five-day meeting in Ottawa. The resulting document, the *Ottawa Charter for Health Promotion*, sparked the development of an innovative new discipline that—for better or for worse—assumed some of the key characteristics of a health profession. It is time for Canadian health promoters to play a more proactive role in shaping the development of their chosen field of work. This will help to ensure that the core values that set health promotion apart from other health-related disciplines are not lost, and that its unique expertise is properly taught and employed.

References

Allison, K.R., McNally, D., DePape, D. & Kellner, M. (1995). The career paths of MHSc graduates in health promotion. *Canadian Journal of Public Health, 86*(1), 77–79.

Barry, M.M., Allegrante, J.P., Lamarre, M.C., Auld, M.E. & Taub, A. (2009). The Galway Consensus Conference: International collaboration on the development of core competencies for health promotion and health education. *Global Health Promotion, 16*(2), 5–11.

Battel-Kirk, B., Barry, M.M., Taub, A. & Lysoby, L. (2009). A review of the international literature on health promotion competencies: Identifying frameworks and core competencies. *Global Health Promotion, 16*(2), 12–20.

Bursey, G., past president, Health Promotion Ontario. (2010). Personal communication, August 5.

Campbell, A. (2006). *Spring of fear: The SARS Commission final report.* Toronto: Queen's Printer for Ontario.

Canadian Evaluation Society. (2010). *Professional designations program.* Retrieved from: http://www.evaluationcanada.ca/site.cgi?en:5:6

Coburn, D. (1988). The development of Canadian nursing: Professionalization and proletarianization. *International Journal of Health Services, 18*(3), 437–456.

Freidson, E. (1977). *Professional dominance: The social structure of medical care.* Chicago: Aldine Publishing Company.

Gaucher, D. (1979). La formation des hygiénistes à l Université de Montréal. 1910–1975: de la santé publique à la médecine preventive. *Recherches Sociographiques, 21*(1), 59–86.

Ghassemi, M. (2009). *Development of pan-Canadian discipline-specific competencies for health promoters: Summary report. Consultation.* Toronto: Health Promotion Ontario. Retrieved from: http://hpo. squarespace.com/storage/HP%20Competencies%20Consultation%20Summary%20Report%20 March%202009.pdf

Harvey, L. & Mason, S. (1995). *The role of professional bodies in higher education quality monitoring.* Birmingham: QHE.

Health Promotion Ontario (HPO). (2010). *Mission statement and summary of activities.* Retrieved from: http://hpo.squarespace.com/

Hills, M., Carroll, S. & Vollman, A. (2007). Health promotion and health professions in Canada: Toward a shared vision. In M. O'Neill, A. Pederson, S. Dupéré & I. Rootman (Eds.), *Health promotion in Canada: Critical perspectives* (2nd ed.) (pp. 330–346). Toronto: Canadian Scholars' Press Inc.

Hills, M. & O'Neill, M. (2003). Final report on the symposium for teachers of health promotion and community health, held on October 22, 2002. Retrieved from: http://www.utoronto.ca/chp/ CCHPR/workingpapers.htm

Hoogland, J. & Jochemsen, H. (2000). Professional autonomy and the normative structure of modern medicine. *Theoretical Medicine, 21*(5), 457–475.

Hyndman, B. (2009). Towards the development of skills-based health promotion competencies: The Canadian experience. *Global Health Promotion, 9*(2), 51–55.

Jacob, J.M. (1999). *Doctors and rules: A sociology of professional values.* New Brunswick & London: Transaction Publishers.

Labonté, R. (1994). Death of program, birth of metaphor: The development of health promotion in Canada. In A. Pederson, M. O'Neill & I. Rootman (Eds.), *Health promotion in Canada* (pp. 72–90). Toronto: W.B. Saunders.

McCracken, H. & Rance, H. (2000). Developing competencies for health promotion training in Aotearoa-New Zealand. *Promotion and Education, 7*(1), 40–43.

McGhee, G. (1995). Professionalization and the health promotion officer. *Health Education, 95*(5), 26–32.

MPH Guidelines Working Group. (2006). *Guidelines for MPH programs in Canada.* Ottawa: CIHR Institute of Population and Public Health-Public Health Agency of Canada, Office of Public Health Practice.

National Commission for Health Education Credentialing (NCHEC). (2010). *National Commission for Health Education Credentialing.* Retrieved from: http://www.nchec.org/

Naylor, D. (2003). *Learning from SARS: Renewal of public health in Canada.* Ottawa: National Advisory Committee on SARS and Public Health.

O'Neill, M. & Stirling, A. (2007). The promotion of health or health promotion? In M. O'Neill, A. Pederson, S. Dupéré & I. Rootman (Eds.), *Health promotion in Canada: Critical perspectives* (2nd ed.) (pp. 32–45). Toronto: Canadian Scholars' Press Inc.

Ontario Kinesiology Association. (2010). *Membership categories.* Retrieved from: https://www.oka. on.ca/index.php?page=becoming-a-member

Ontario Prevention Clearinghouse. (2006). *Ontario health promoters: Gains of organizing/risks of professionalizing. Commentary from the Ontario Prevention Clearinghouse.* Toronto: OPC.

Ottoson, J.M., Pommier, J., Macdonald, G., Frankish, J. & Dorion, L. (2000). The landscape in health education and health promotion training. *Promotion & Education, 7*(1), 27–32.

Public Health Agency of Canada. (2007). *Core competencies for public health in Canada.* Ottawa: PHAC.

Public Health Agency of Canada. (2010). *List of graduate programs in public health.* Retrieved from: http:// www.phac-aspc.gc.ca/php-psp/master_of_php-eng.php

Rootman, I., Jackson, S. & Hills, M. (2007). Developing knowledge for health promotion. In M. O'Neill, A. Pederson, S. Dupéré & I. Rootman (Eds.), *Health promotion in Canada: Critical perspectives* (2nd ed.) (pp. 123–138). Toronto: Canadian Scholars' Press Inc.

Shilton, T., Howat, P. & James, R. (2003). Review of competencies for Australian health promotion. *Australian Health Promotion Update* (October–November), 5.

Vollmer, H.M. & Mills, D.L. (1966). *Professionalization.* Englewood Cliffs: Prentice-Hall.

Walker, D. (2004). *For the public's health: A plan of action.* Final report of the Expert Panel on SARS and Infectious Disease Control. Toronto: Queen's Printer for Ontario.

Wilson, D., Glassford, R.G., Krupa, E., Masuda, J., Wild, C., Plotnikoff, R., Raine-Travers, K. & Stewart, M. (2000). Health promotion practice, research, and policy: Building capacity through the development of an interdisciplinary study centre and graduate program in Alberta, Canada. *Promotion & Education,* 7(1), 44–48.

Winslow, C.E.A. (1920). The untilled fields of public health. *Science, 51,* 23.

World Health Organization (WHO). (1986). A discussion document on the concepts and principles of health promotion. *Health Promotion International, 1,* 75.

Critical Thinking Questions

1. Name two attributes of a profession and discuss if health promotion has them or not.
2. In your view, should health promotion become a regulated profession in Canada? Why or why not?
3. What are the pros and cons to developing a voluntary accreditation program for health promoters in Canada?
4. If you look at the competencies proposed internationally for health promotion by the Galway Consensus (Barry et al., 2009) and the ones proposed for Canada (see Box 13.1), do you find that they are rather similar or rather different? Why?
5. Do you think all people claiming to practise health promotion in Canada should complete a Master's degree in this domain? Why or why not?

Resources

Further Readings

Barry, M.M., Allegrante, J.P., Lamarre, M.C., Auld, M.E. & Taub, A. (2009). The Galway Consensus Conference: International collaboration on the development of core competencies for health promotion and health education. *Global Health Promotion, 16*(2), 5–11.

The Galway Consensus is the current state of the international thinking about health promotion competencies.

Relevent Websites

Australian Health Promotion Association

www.healthpromotion.org.au

Australia is one of the few countries in the world where health promotion is a regulated profession. This website of the Australian Health Promotion Association provides a wealth of information about the association history, status, activities, and publications.

Health Promotion Ontario

http://hpo.squarespace.com/

Health Promotion Ontario is currently the only provincial association of health promoters in Canada. This website provides details on activities, publications, as well as links to other relevant health promotion sites and organizations.

National Commission for Health Education Credentialing

http://www.nchec.org/

This website provides a very interesting example of a voluntary accreditation process (the certified health education specialist—CHES) in a related field as applied in the US that could eventually serve as a model for similar processes in Canada.

CHAPTER 14

Implications of Inequities in Health for Health Promotion Practice

Dennis Raphael

Introduction

Health promotion has the goal of improving the health of a population. It is becoming increasingly clear that in wealthy developed nations such as Canada, the primary component of this effort involves reducing health inequities. One way to think about this is that the average health of the top 10 percent of Canadians represents the best that can be reasonably expected of the entire population. The primary health promotion task is to "level up" the health of the remaining 90 percent of the population, which falls below this 10 percent benchmark (Dahlgren & Whitehead, 2006; Whitehead & Dahlgren, 2006). While there is disagreement regarding how this levelling up may be accomplished, it is generally agreed these differences or inequalities in health are unjust and unfair.[1] They are considered health inequities (Braveman & Gruskin, 2003).

Health promoters should not forget about improving the health of the top 10 percent, but must recognize that their health issues are rather minor in the overall health situation. Actually, levelling up the health of the lower 90 percent may improve the health of the top 10 percent by improving the overall quality of societal functioning. That is, as measures are taken to reduce the health gap between the rich and everybody else, the increases in social cohesion and solidarity and reductions in class-related conflicts will promote the health of all (Wilkinson & Pickett, 2009).

How can the health of this 90 percent be levelled up? This question exposes a range of contentious issues concerning the nature of health promotion, means of intervention, and barriers to action. I argue that the most effective health promotion approach for reducing health inequities is contained in the *Ottawa Charter for Health Promotion* (World Health Organization, 1986) and reiterated by the Commission on the Social Determinants of Health (CSDH, 2008): *Create public policy that strengthens the prerequisites or social determinants of health.*

Status of Health Inequities in Canada

Health inequities in Canada are widespread and manifest in indicators of health status and injuries at every stage of the life course. The primary category for identifying health inequities is family or individual income: those of differing incomes experience differing health outcomes (Raphael et al., 2004). Two main methodological approaches identify health inequities related to income (Raphael et al., 2006). One approach identifies the average income received within a specific geographic area—such as a census tract, neighbourhood, or health care service area—and then details the health situations of those residing in these areas. These geographic areas are placed into equal population-sized groups from the wealthiest to the poorest such as quartiles (four groups), quintiles (five groups), or deciles (10 groups), and the health situation among groups is then compared.

The other approach categorizes individuals and families as a function of their income (e.g., high, upper-middle, middle, lower-middle, poor) and then examines their health outcomes. Overviews of the extent of income-related health equalities in Canada are available (Canadian Population Health Initiative, 2004a, 2008). A few examples are presented below to illustrate their extent in Canada.

Inequities in Death Rates or Mortality among Canadians

Figure 14.1 shows that how long Canadians live is strongly related to the average income of their neighbourhood (Wilkins, 2007). Men living in the poorest 20 percent of urban neighbourhoods live almost four and a half years less than those in the wealthiest 20 percent. The corresponding figure for women is almost two years.

Similar findings are seen for infant mortality rates, an especially sensitive indicator of overall societal health. Rates in the poorest 20 percent of urban neighbourhoods (7.1/1,000) are 40 percent higher than in the wealthiest 20 percent (5.0/1,000) (Wilkins, 2007).

The next findings illustrate one situation where health and extent of health inequities are improving and one in which they are decaying. Figure 14.2 shows declining death rates and income-related inequities for cardiovascular disease among urban Canadian men (Wilkins, 2007).

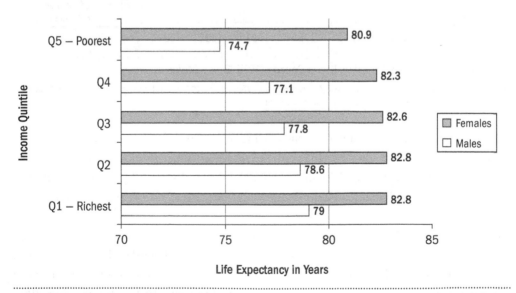

FIGURE 14.1: Life Expectancy of Males and Females by Income Quintile of Neighbourhood, Urban Canada, 2001

Source: Wilkins, R. (2007). *Mortality by neighbourhood income in urban Canada from 1971 to 2001.* Statistics Canada, Health Analysis and Measurement Group (HAMG). HAMG Seminar, and special compilations.

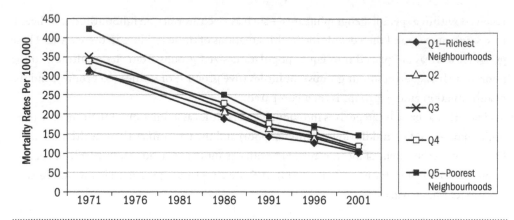

FIGURE 14.2: Ischemic Heart Disease Mortality, Urban Canada, 1971–2001, Males

Source: Wilkins, R. (2007). *Mortality by neighbourhood income in urban Canada from 1971 to 2001.* Statistics Canada, Health Analysis and Measurement Group (HAMG). HAMG Seminar, and Special Compilations.

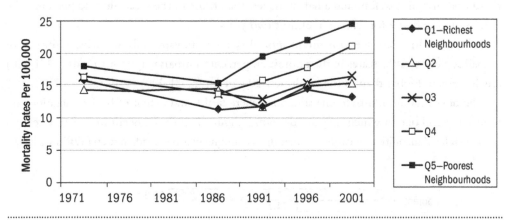

FIGURE 14.3: Diabetes Mortality, Urban Canada, 1971–2001, Males

Source: Wilkins, R. (2007). *Mortality by neighbourhood income in urban Canada from 1971 to 2001.* Statistics Canada, Health Analysis and Measurement Group (HAMG). HAMG Seminar, and Special Compilations.

Much of this is related to the improvement in living conditions from the immediate post–World War II period through to the 1980s. In Figure 14.3, however, both overall death rates and inequities for diabetes are increasing (Wilkins, 2007). Dying from diabetes may be more sensitive to changes in living conditions than heart disease whose effects may take decades to manifest.

Inequities in Illness and Injuries or Morbidity

Incidence of low birth weight differs as a function of average neighbourhood income (Wilkins, Houle, Berthelot & Ross, 2000). Rates are 40 percent higher in the poorest 20 percent of neighbourhoods (7.0/100) as compared to what occurs in the wealthiest 20 percent (4.9/100).

Figure 14.4 shows that children in the poorest Ontario neighbourhoods show injury rates 67 percent higher than children in the wealthiest neighbourhoods (Faelker, Pickett & Brison, 2000). These differences are apparent for minor, moderate, and extreme injuries.

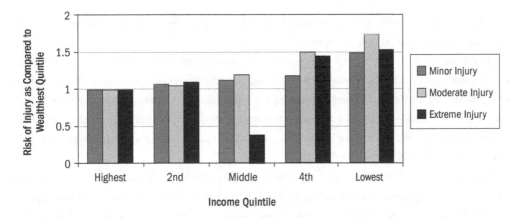

FIGURE 14.4: Association between Socioeconomic Status and Childhood Injury, by Severity of Injury, Ontario 1996

Source: Data adapted from Faelker, T., Pickett, W. & Brison, R.J. (2000). Socioeconomic differences in childhood injury: A population based epidemiologic study in Ontario, Canada. Injury Prevention, 6, 203–208, Table 4, p. 206.

Sources of Health Inequities

Health inequities are primarily a result of exposures to varying quality living conditions, which have come to be known as the social determinants of health (see Box 14.1) (Raphael, 2009a). Wealthy, high-income Canadians enjoy the best health because their living conditions are better than those experienced by other Canadians. These conditions affect health through pathways associated with material deprivation, psychosocial stress and lack of control, and adoption of maladaptive coping behaviours. These differences in living conditions and their manifestation as health inequities occur all the way from the top to the bottom of the Canadian socio-economic ladder.

Many Canadian health promoters' programs of practice say little, if anything, about living conditions and the importance of attempting to influence the public policies that create them (Raphael, 2008b). They work to improve health care systems' capacity to deal with

---

BOX 14.1:

Social Determinants of Health with Particular Relevance to Health Inequities in Canada

- Aboriginal status
- disability status
- early life
- education
- employment and working conditions
- food security
- gender

- health care services
- housing
- income and its distribution
- race
- social safety net
- social exclusion
- unemployment and employment security

Source: Mikkonen, J. & Raphael, D. (2010). *Social determinants of health: The Canadian facts.* Retrieved from: www.thecanadianfacts.org/

health inequities or believe they can prevent health inequities by promoting "healthy lifestyle choices," "social capital," or "resiliency."

The belief is that reducing risk behaviours (i.e., adopting healthy lifestyle choices), building connections and networks among individuals and communities (i.e., building social capital), and enhancing individual coping strategies (i.e., promoting resiliency) can improve health and reduce inequities without addressing the upstream determinants of both these mediating processes and their resultant health inequities. Critiques of these approaches are available (Muntaner, Lynch & Davey Smith, 2000).

It may be more useful to adopt a structural analysis of how health inequities come about. Here, health inequities—as well as the mediating outcomes of lifestyle choices, social capital, and resiliency—are due to the workings of the economic system, a governmental apparatus that maintains or reinforces these inequalities, and a public discourse that justifies them (Grabb, 2007). It can be reasoned, then, that health inequities can be reduced by changing or modifying the economic system, adjusting how governments operate, and shifting how these issues are understood by policy-makers and the public.

Health Inequities and Health Promotion Practice

Health inequities result primarily from differences in Canadians' living conditions. There are at least seven different ways in which "health promoters"—broadly defined—can take on the task of reducing health inequities. Table 14.1 outlines these different approaches.

Approach 1: Health Inequities and Access to and Quality of Health Care and Social Services

In this approach health inequities result from health care and social service issues. Particular individuals have less access to necessary services, or these services may be of less than optimal quality. Health promoters strive to reduce barriers to care and improve the quality of these services. "Health promoting" hospitals is part of this approach.

Some examples are addressing the health needs of homeless individuals, managing chronic diseases among vulnerable communities, and providing primary health care to immigrant groups, among others. Public health agencies provide preventive health services, and social service agencies support at-risk individuals and communities.

These activities are important, but do rather little to reduce health inequities. Moreover, limiting research and activity to these issues neglects the sources of health inequities. It can reinforce already dominant care emphases, obscuring the role that living conditions play in creating health inequities.

Approach 2: Health Inequities and Modifiable Medical and Behavioural Risk Factors

Modifying individual risk factors has been a primary concern of health promoters. Although, as noted in Chapter 1, the 1974 Lalonde Report identified risk behaviours as only one of four health fields, the healthy lifestyles approach came to dominate health promotion activity in Canada (Legowski & McKay, 2000).

TABLE 14.1: Health Promotion Approaches Directed toward Reducing Health Inequities

Health Inequities Interpretation	Key Health Promotion Concept	Health Promotion Practice Approach	Practical Implications of the Approach
1. Health inequities result from differences in access and quality of health and social services.	Health inequities can be reduced by strengthening health care and social services.	Create "health promoting" hospitals, clinics, and social service agencies.	Focus is limited to promoting the health of those already experiencing health inequities.
2. Health inequities result from differences in important modifiable medical and behavioural risk factors.	Health inequities can be reduced by enabling people to make "healthy choices" and adopt "healthy lifestyles."	Develop and evaluate healthy living and behaviour modification programs and protocols.	Healthy lifestyle programming may ignore the material basis of health inequities and widen existing health inequities.
3. Health inequities result from differences in material living conditions.	Health inequities can be reduced by improving material living conditions.	Ensure that community development and participatory research enable people to gain control over their health.	There is the assumption that governmental authorities are receptive to and will act upon community voices and research findings.
4. Health inequities result from differences in material living conditions that are a function of group membership.	Health inequities can be reduced by improving the material living conditions of particular disadvantaged groups.	Targeted development and research activities among disadvantaged groups improve their material living conditions.	There is the assumption that governmental authorities are receptive to such activities and anticipated outcomes.
5. Health inequities result from differences in material living conditions shaped by public policy.	Health inequities can be reduced by advocating for healthy public policy that reduces disadvantage.	Analyze how public policy decisions impact health (i.e., health impact analysis).	There is the assumption that governments will create public policy on the basis of its effects upon health.
6. Health inequities result from differences in material living conditions that are shaped by economic and political structures and their justifying ideologies.	Health inequities can be reduced by influencing the societal structures that create and justify health inequities.	Analyzing how the political economy of a nation creates inequities identifies avenues for social and political action.	Require health promotion to engage in building social and political movements that will reduce health inequities.
7. Health inequities result from the power and influence of those who create and benefit from health inequities.	Health inequities can be reduced by increasing the power and influence of those who experience these inequities.	Critical analysis empowers the disadvantaged to gain an understanding of and a means of increasing their influence and power.	Require health promotion to engage in building social and political movements that increase the power of the disadvantaged.

The medical and public health concern with medical (e.g., high sugar and "bad" cholesterol levels, etc.) and behavioural (e.g., poor diet, lack of physical activity, and tobacco and excessive alcohol use) risk factors is so prevalent as to dominate professional thinking, media coverage (Hayes et al., 2007), and public understandings about the mainsprings of health and the causes of illness (Canadian Population Health Initiative, 2004b). Many government and health agency documents discuss broader approaches to reducing health inequities, but these have had little penetration into medical and public health activity and media and public awareness (Raphael, 2008b).

Unlike Approach 1, which stresses provision and improvement of services, this approach has many negative aspects. First, medical and behavioural risk factors account for relatively little of the health inequities that exist in Canada. Second, it assumes that individuals are capable of "making healthy lifestyle choices" such that individuals who fail to do so are responsible for their own adverse health outcomes (Labonté & Penfold, 1981). Third, programs show rather little evidence of effectiveness among the most vulnerable and may increase health inequities as "healthy living" messaging is more likely to be taken up by the already advantaged (Jarvis & Wardle, 2003). Investing in the approach may further disenable vulnerable populations and the health promoters administering these programs.

Approach 3: Health Inequities and Differences in Material Living Conditions

Living conditions operate through material, psychological, and behavioural pathways to "get under the skin" to shape health. Society's structures, such as employment and working conditions, and neighbourhood characteristics produce health inequities across the lifespan. Health inequities can be reduced by levelling up the living conditions experienced by the less well-off.

How do health promoters implement this approach? In Canada, it frequently involves community development, participatory, or action research (Minkler, 2005). The idea is that when community members uncover the factors that shape their health—and, in the case of disadvantaged communities, cause health inequities—governmental and other societal authorities will act upon this knowledge to improve the situation (Raphael, Steinmetz & Renwick, 1999).

All of this assumes that governmental and other authorities are receptive to the information that comes from such activities. This has become increasingly questionable over the past two decades as Canadian governments have: (1) reduced provision of supports and services to the population; and (2) demonstrated less willingness to create public policy to reduce health inequities (Bryant, Raphael, Schrecker & Labonté, 2011).

Approach 4: Health Inequities, Material Living Conditions, and Group Membership

Health promoters recognize that health inequities are frequently a function of class, gender, and race. Therefore, community development, and participatory and action research becomes focused on disadvantaged or marginalized individuals. Again, the key idea is that uncovering factors that shape health and cause health inequities will lead authorities to act upon this knowledge.

Approach 5: Health Inequities Result from Differences in Material Living Conditions Shaped by Public Policy

This analysis considers that the primary means of reducing health inequities is through public policy action. This approach is clearly endorsed by the World Health Organization's recent social determinants report (CSDH, 2008).

As an illustration of this approach, the presence of health inequities is shaped by access (or lack thereof) to material resources such as income, housing, food, and educational and employment opportunities, among others. These resources are related to parents' employment security, wages, and the quality of their working conditions and availability of quality, regulated child care, all of which are shaped by public policy decisions (Raphael, 2009a).

Raising these issues is uncommon among health promoters. The health promotion activity most consistent with this approach is health impact assessment (HIA) (Scott-Samuel, Birley & Ardern, 2001). The health promotion organization analyzes the effects a proposed public policy will have on existing health inequities. This process is similar to that of environmental assessment. Prior to the construction of a bridge or tunnel, an environmental assessment is done to identify the impacts—both positive and negative—on local flora and fauna. A health impact assessment would determine the probable impacts of, say, the reduction of affordable recreational services upon the health of local residents. Opportunities to do just this arise rather often in Canada.

Hardly a day goes by without a public policy issue arising at either the municipal/regional, provincial, or federal level that has health inequities implications: minimum wages, social assistance rates, recreation fees, labour laws, public transportation, education, child care, and just about every other social determinant of health. HIA is rarely, if ever, seen in Canada. Why this is so is considered in the following section.

Approach 6: Health Inequities Are Shaped by Economic and Political Structures and Their Justifying Ideologies

It seems reasonable that health promoters would carry out HIA of proposed policies to inform public policy-making. This view is consistent with the belief (pluralism) that public policy decisions are made on the basis of evidence (Brooks & Miljan, 2003). Pluralism is the belief that public policy decisions are made on the basis of weighing the pros and cons of policy advice contributed by a wide range of societal sectors (e.g., business, labour, and civil society). In this model, information of all kinds is valued and policy options are informed by such data. Health promotion knowledge production, dissemination, transfer, and exchange in the service of reducing health inequities is part of this approach.

How, then, can we explain the last two decades of government policy-making in Canada, which have widened the social inequalities that create health inequities, as well as the lack of any significant health impact assessment of public policies on the part of health promoters, their agencies, and institutions?

The alternative explanation (the materialist) is that governments make decisions on the basis of existing economic and political structures of influence and power (Brooks & Miljan,

2003). In this model, policy-making is seen as being made in the interests of the wealthy and powerful rather than in the interests of all. These decisions are then justified on the basis of particular ideologies and positions, such as what is good for business is good for society. If there are resulting health inequities from such decisions, they are justified on the basis that people bring their own health problems on themselves by making poor lifestyle decisions. This analysis goes far in explaining why Canada, which is seen as a leader in creating health promotion and population concepts that have been applied in the service of reducing health inequities elsewhere, has always been somewhat of a health equity laggard. Public policy, it is argued, is not being made in the interests of the majority of Canadians but in the interests of those with more influence and power.

These economic and political approaches to creating public policy that either creates or reduces health inequities differ from one jurisdiction to another. Sweden, Norway, and Finland have placed the reduction of health inequities high on their public policy agenda; nations such as Canada and the US, rather less so (Raphael & Bryant, 2006b). Health promoters and their agencies are embedded within these differing economic and political structures.

Three distinct types of welfare states have been identified: social democratic (e.g., Sweden, Norway, Denmark, and Finland); liberal (e.g., the US, the UK, Canada, and Ireland); and conservative (e.g., France, Germany, Netherlands, and Belgium, among others) (Esping-Andersen, 1990). Canadian sociologists add a fourth Latin welfare state that includes Italy, Portugal, and Spain (Saint-Arnaud & Bernard, 2003).

The approach suggests that differences in political and economic structures and processes (political economy)—themselves a result of historical traditions and governance by specific political parties over time—determine the living conditions Canadians experience. Two important examples of factors shown to create health inequities—income inequality and poverty rates—illustrate the power of such an analysis (see figures 14.5 and 14.6).

The liberal political economies (shaded dark) have the highest income inequality and poverty rates, while the social democratic nations (unshaded) have the lowest. The Latin undeveloped welfare states (dotted) show many similarities with the liberal states. Even the conservative welfare states (lightly shaded) appear to deal better with these important determinants of health inequities than Canada does. Since the dominant inspiration of liberal political economies is to minimize governmental intervention in the operation of its central institution—the market—it should not be surprising that Canada and its liberal partners fall well behind other nations in addressing health inequities (Raphael & Bryant, 2006a). Instead, emphasis is on facilitating the operation of the economic system, which tends to benefit the wealthy and powerful. This health promotion analysis broadens the health promotion role beyond simply identifying public policy implications to one of attempting to influence the political and economic structures that shape such policy.

Health promoters must recognize that the implementation of health promoting public policies that strengthen the social determinants of health will require shifts in existing economic and political structures. This will require the building of social and political movements that will increase the influence of those whose health is threatened by existing public policies. The

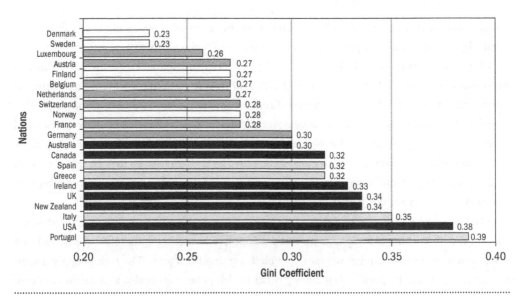

FIGURE 14.5: Income Inequality among Selected OECD Nations, Mid-2000s

Source: Organisation for Economic Co-operation and Development. (2008). *Growing unequal: Income distribution and poverty in OECD nations*. Paris: Organisation for Economic Co-operation and Development.p. 25.

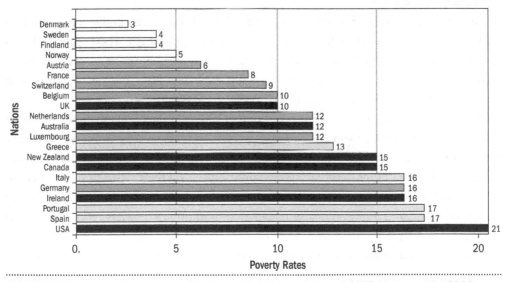

FIGURE 14.6: Poverty Rates among Families with Children, Selected OECD Nations, Mid-2000s

Source: Organisation for Economic Co-operation and Development. (2008). *Growing unequal: Income distribution and poverty in OECD nations*. Page 133. Paris: OECD.

means of doing so involves educating and engaging the public in the political process to force fundamental changes in how society works and resources are distributed.

The institution of new public policies that support health will gradually change these existing structures. As citizens come to appreciate how these public policies are supporting their health and well-being, there will be fundamental changes in the operation of society (i.e., economic and political structures) that will institutionalize these changes. Indeed, such transformation through public policy change is at the heart of every credible analysis of the means by which health inequities can be reduced (see Raphael, 2009b).

Why, then, is there such lack of public policy analysis and advocacy on the part of health promoters in Canada? I suggest that in the case of health promoters who are government employees or who work for government-funded agencies, there is a perception of professional and personal danger in criticizing governmental authorities who pay their salaries and determine their opportunities for advancement. In the case of health promoters engaged by other institutions, the reluctance to engage in public policy discussions may be based on lack of understanding of the social determinants of health and health inequities or a perception that such activities are not part of their mandate or role.

The fear of governmental blow-back among governmental and government-funded agencies is rather disturbing as it suggests we really do not live in such a democratic society, and that earnest, sincere people can get into real trouble for doing their jobs. The lack of appreciation for the role that public policy plays among other health promoters is also a cause for concern. How to deal with these barriers is discussed in later sections.

Approach 7: Health Inequities Result from Those Who Create and Benefit from Health Inequities

In this final approach the individuals and groups who—through their undue influence upon governments—create and benefit from health inequities are identified. These individuals and groups lobby for shifting the tax structures to favour the corporate sector and the wealthy, reducing public expenditures, controlling wages and employment benefits, and relaxing labour standards and protections. These are all factors that create health inequities.

Who exactly are these villains and how can their undue influence upon public policy be resisted? Langille (2009) identifies business associations, conservative think tanks, citizen front institutions, and conservative lobbyists. What form might these counterbalances take? Langille and others propose educating the public and using their strength in numbers to promote public policy to oppose this agenda. Efforts can occur in the workplace through greater union organization and increasing public recognition of the class-related forces that shape public policy.

Activities can also occur in the electoral and parliamentary arena by electing political parties that favour action to reduce health inequities. It is clear that social democratic parties are more receptive to and successful at implementing public policies that reduce social inequalities and health inequities (Navarro & Shi, 2002). If this is the case, the recent 2011 elevation of the New Democratic Party in Canada to the Official Opposition in Ottawa is a very positive development.

Health Promotion Dilemmas

If health inequities are a result of political and economic structures and the public policies that flow from such structures, generating knowledge and disseminating information about the sources of health inequities and the means of reducing them are a necessary but not sufficient condition.

There are three ways health promoters can help reduce health inequities, and these are focused on education and knowledge transmission (Raphael, 2008a). These will not by themselves lead to public policy to reduce health inequities, but will assist others engaged in public policy advocacy.

Education and Knowledge Transmission

The Canadian public remains woefully uninformed about health inequities and their sources. In addition to the constant barrage of "healthy living" messages, Canadians are subject to continuous messaging as to the benefits of a business-oriented, laissez-faire approach to governance. What this messaging has not included are the societal effects of this approach: increasing income and wealth inequality, persistent poverty, and growing health inequities.

Telling the solid facts: At a minimum, health promoters can carry out and publicize the findings from analyses of the causes of health inequities. A public-oriented document, *Social Determinants of Health: The Canadian Facts* (http://thecanadianfacts.org) can assist in this task.

There are numerous health inequity-related policy areas in which health promoters could engage: reducing poverty and housing and food insecurity, improving employment and working conditions, and fostering early child development and others. My short list of afflictions where significant health inequities are related to these living conditions include coronary heart disease, Type 2 diabetes, arthritis, stroke, many forms of cancer, respiratory disease, HIV/AIDS, Alzheimer's disease, asthma, injuries, death from injuries, mental illness, suicide, emergency room visits, school dropout, delinquency and crime, unemployment, alienation, distress, and depression.

Telling stories: Health promoters can shift public, professional, and policy-makers' focus from the dominant biomedical and lifestyle health paradigms to a broader public policy perspective by collecting and presenting stories about the impact that living conditions—and the public policy decisions that influence these—have on people's lives. Ethnographic and qualitative approaches to individual and community health produce vivid illustrations of the importance of these issues for people's health and well-being (Popay & Williams, 1994). There is some indication that policy-makers—and certainly the media—may be responsive to such forms of evidence.

There is increasing recognition of the importance of community-based action, such as community needs assessment, that applies these approaches. Such activities can be a rich source of insights about the mainsprings of health inequities and the means of influencing public policy. Such a perspective allows community members to provide their own critical reflections on society, power, and inequality. At a minimum, these approaches allow the voices of those most influenced by the public policy decisions that create health inequities to be heard and hold out the possibility of their concerns being translated into political activity on their part and policy action on the part of health and government officials.

Providing support for policy action: The final role is the most important, but potentially the most difficult: supporting policy action in support of health. And implicit in such a course of action is recognizing the important role that politics play in these activities.

Numerous public health units and health-promotion agencies have taken up the task of speaking out about public policy choices and their effects upon health inequities. Sometimes these units and agencies work in partnership with community organizations to raise these important health equity issues. These examples should spur other agencies to take up this task.

Professional Association and Agency Network Action

For health promoters and their agencies who feel vulnerable about raising these issues in their workplace, avenues of action are possible through professional associations and agency networks. Professional associations, such as the Canadian Public Health Association (CPHA) and provincial/territorial health associations, can raise the profile of health inequities and their impact on Canadian society. The Registered Nurses Association of Ontario, the Canadian Nurses Association, and the Association of Ontario Health Centres and the British Columbia Healthy Living Alliance have all produced clearly stated policy documents that raise the issue of health inequities and the importance of applying public policy analysis and action to reduce them (Raphael, 2010).

Political Engagement

Health promoters are also citizens who can vote and support particular political parties between and during political campaigns. Canadians are not a particularly politicized people, and there is no reason to think that health promoters are much different than the average Canadian (Schellenberg, 2004). The relevance of addressing health inequities to their employment goals—better health for all—should serve as a spur to increase such participation among health promoters.

Conclusions

Health promotion approaches that acknowledge the importance of public policy activity for reducing health inequities may be the best means of accomplishing this goal. There are significant barriers to such action in Canada. It may be necessary to elect specific political parties and modify economic and political structures to effect the reduction of health inequities (Raphael, 2007a).

Such transformations will result in more equitable distribution of income and wealth, which will reduce the profound social inequalities that spawn health inequities. Strong programs that support children, families, and women, and economies that support full employment are required (Raphael, 2007b).

My analysis indicates that health promotion activities operate within the confines of the dominant political and economic discourses of Canadian society. In Canada, governmental withdrawal from intervening in the operation of the economic marketplace has made concern with reducing health inequities not only unpopular among governing circles but actually threatening to agency funding and individual health promoters' career prospects.

Despite the barriers to addressing health inequities in Canada, the best means of reducing health inequities involve health promoters and their agencies and organizations navigating the difficult task of informing citizens about the political and economic forces that shape the health of a society.

Establishing an environment in which health promoters can do this would be an important first step in reducing health inequities in Canada. This would provide a solid base for public policy activity in reducing health inequities. Without this base and the public policy activity that would flow from it, significant reduction in health inequities in Canada seems unlikely.

Note

1. An inequality in health is simply a recognition that some measurable difference in health exists. An inequity in health is a moral statement that this difference is unfair and unjust and needs to be addressed.

References

Braveman, P. & Gruskin, S. (2003). Defining equity in health. *Journal of Epidemiology and Community Health, 57,* 254–258.

Brooks, S. & Miljan, L. (2003). Theories of public policy. In S. Brooks & L. Miljan (Eds.), *Public policy in Canada: An introduction* (pp. 22–49). Toronto: Oxford University Press.

Bryant, T., Raphael, D., Schrecker, T. & Labonté, R. (2011). Canada: A land of missed opportunity for addressing the social determinants of health. *Health Policy, 101*(1), 44–58.

Canadian Population Health Initiative. (2004a). *Improving the health of Canadians.* Ottawa: CPHI.

Canadian Population Health Initiative. (2004b). *Select highlights on public views of the determinants of health.* Ottawa: CPHI.

Canadian Population Health Initiative. (2008). *Reducing gaps in health: A focus on socio-economic status in urban Canada.* Ottawa: CPHI.

Commission on the Social Determinants of Health (CSDH). (2008). *Closing the gap in a generation: Health equity through action on the social determinants of health.* Geneva: World Health Organization.

Dahlgren, G. & Whitehead, M. (2006). *Leveling up (Part 2): A discussion paper on European strategies for tackling social inequities in health.* Copenhagen: WHO Regional Office for Europe.

Esping-Andersen, G. (1990). *The three worlds of welfare capitalism.* Princeton: Princeton University Press.

Faelker, T., Pickett, W. & Brison, R.J. (2000). Socioeconomic differences in childhood injury: A population-based epidemiologic study in Ontario, Canada. *Injury Prevention, 6,* 203–208.

Grabb, E. (2007). *Theories of social inequality* (5th ed.). Toronto: Harcourt Canada.

Hayes, M., Ross, I., Gasherc, M., Gutstein, D., Dunn, J. & Hackett, R. (2007). Telling stories: News media, health literacy, and public policy in Canada. *Social Science and Medicine, 54,* 445–457.

Jarvis, M.J. & Wardle, J. (2003). Social patterning of individual health behaviours: The case of cigarette smoking. In M.G. Marmot & R.G. Wilkinson (Eds.), *Social determinants of health* (2nd ed.) (pp. 224–237). Oxford: Oxford University Press.

Labonté, R. & Penfold, S. (1981). Canadian perspectives in health promotion: A critique. *Health Education, 19,* 4–9.

Langille, D. (2009). Follow the money: How business and politics shape our health. In D. Raphael (Ed.), *Social determinants of health: Canadian perspectives* (2nd ed.) (pp. 305–317). Toronto: Canadian Scholars' Press Inc.

Legowski, B. & McKay, L. (2000). *Health beyond health care: Twenty-five years of federal health policy development.* CPRN Discussion Paper no. H04. Ottawa: Canadian Policy Research Networks.

Mikkonen, J. & Raphael, D. (2010). *Social determinants of health: The Canadian facts.* Toronto: York University School of Health Policy and Management. Retrieved from http://thecanadianfacts.org/

Minkler, M. (2005). Community-based research partnerships: Challenges and opportunities. *Journal of Urban Health, 82*(Suppl. 2), ii3–ii12.

Muntaner, C., Lynch, J. & Davey Smith, G. (2000). Social capital and the third way in public health. *Critical Public Health, 10*(2), 107–124.

Navarro, V. & Shi, L. (2002). The political context of social inequalities and health. In V. Navarro (Ed.), *The political economy of social inequalities: Consequences for health and quality of life* (pp. 403–418). Amityville: Baywood.

Organisation for Economic Co-operation and Development. (2008). *Growing unequal: Income distribution and poverty in OECD nations.* Paris: OECD.

Popay, J. & Williams, G.H. (Eds.). (1994). *Researching the people's health.* London: Routledge.

Raphael, D. (2007a). The politics of poverty. In D. Raphael (Ed.), *Poverty and policy in Canada: Implications for health and quality of life* (pp. 303–334). Toronto: Canadian Scholars' Press Inc.

Raphael, D. (2007b). Who is poor in Canada? In D. Raphael (Ed.), *Poverty and policy in Canada: Implications for health and quality of life* (pp. 59–84). Toronto: Canadian Scholars' Press Inc.

Raphael, D. (2008a). Getting serious about health: New directions for Canadian public health researchers and workers. *Promotion and Education, 15,* 15–20.

Raphael, D. (2008b). Grasping at straws: A recent history of health promotion in Canada. *Critical Public Health, 18*(4), 483–495.

Raphael, D. (Ed.). (2009a). *Social determinants of health: Canadian perspectives* (2nd ed.). Toronto: Canadian Scholars' Press Inc.

Raphael, D. (2009b). Reducing social and health inequalities requires building social and political movements. *Humanity and Society, 33*(1/2), 145–165.

Raphael, D. (2010). *About Canada: Health and illness.* Halifax: Fernwood Publishing.

Raphael, D. & Bryant, T. (2006a). Maintaining population health in a period of welfare state decline: Political economy as the missing dimension in health promotion theory and practice. *Promotion and Education, 13*(4), 12–18.

Raphael, D. & Bryant, T. (2006b). The state's role in promoting population health: Public health concerns in Canada, USA, UK, and Sweden. *Health Policy, 78,* 39–55.

Raphael, D., Labonté, R. et al. (2006). Income and health research in Canada: Needs, gaps, and opportunities. *Canadian Journal of Public Health, 97*(Suppl. 3), s16–s23.

Raphael, D., Macdonald, J., Labonté, R., Colman, R., Hayward, K. & Torgerson, R. (2004). Researching income and income distribution as a determinant of health in Canada: Gaps between theoretical knowledge, research practice, and policy implementation. *Health Policy, 72,* 217–232.

Raphael, D., Steinmetz, B. & Renwick, R. (1999). The community quality of life project: A health promotion approach to understanding communities. *Health Promotion International, 14,* 197–210.

Saint-Arnaud, S. & Bernard, P. (2003). Convergence or resilience? A hierarchical cluster analysis of the welfare regimes in advanced countries. *Current Sociology, 51*(5), 499–527.

Schellenberg, G. (2004). *2003 General Social Survey on Social Engagement, cycle 17: An overview of findings.* Ottawa: Statistics Canada.

Scott-Samuel, A., Birley, M. & Ardern, K. (2001). *The Merseyside guidelines for health impact assessment.* Liverpool: International Health Impact Assessment Consortium.

Whitehead, M. & Dahlgren, G. (2006). *Concepts and principles for tackling social inequities in health: Leveling up, part 1.* Copenhagen: WHO Regional Office for Europe.

Wilkins, R. (2007). *Mortality by neighbourhood income in urban Canada from 1971 to 2001.* Ottawa: Statistics Canada, Health Analysis and Measurement Group.

Wilkins, R., Houle, C., Berthelot, J.-M. & Ross, D.P. (2000). The changing health status of Canada's children. *ISUMA, 1*(2), 57–63.

Wilkinson, R.G. & Pickett, K. (2009). *The spirit level: Why more equal societies almost always do better.* London: Allen Lane.

World Health Organization. (1986). *Ottawa Charter for Health Promotion.* Geneva: World Health Organization European Office.

Critical Thinking Questions

1. Review the health-related stories in your local newspaper over the next few weeks. If you based your understanding of health inequities on these stories, what would be your views of what makes some people healthy and others ill?

2. What evidence is available concerning the extent of health inequities in your jurisdiction? What are the current indicators of the incidence of poverty, homelessness, and food bank use in your area? Have conditions been improving or declining?

3. To what extent have other health-related courses you have taken addressed issues of health inequities? What could be done to increase your discipline's emphasis on health inequities?

4. What could be done to improve the public's understanding of the importance of tackling health inequities? What should be the role of your local public health unit or health care agencies?

5. What are some of the personal and professional dilemmas health promoters face in applying the more sophisticated approaches described in this chapter? How can these problems be overcome?

Resources

Further Readings

Bryant, T., Raphael, D. & Rioux, M. (Eds.). (2010). *Staying alive: Critical perspectives on health, illness, and health care* (2nd ed.). Toronto: Canadian Scholars' Press Inc.

This volume emphasizes the political economy of health and contains chapters on the social determinants of health and health inequities associated with social class, gender, and race.

Davey Smith, G. (2003). *Health inequalities: Life-course approaches.* Bristol: Policy Press.

This book provides an overview of the social and economic factors that are now known to be the most powerful determinants of population health in modern nations.

Graham, H. (2007). *Unequal lives: Health and socioeconomic inequalities.* New York: Open University Press.

This is an excellent overview of how public policy comes to shape the living conditions that lead to health inequities. By reviewing the various approaches to addressing health inequities, it identifies strengths of a public policy approach.

Raphael, D. (2009). *Social determinants of health: Canadian perspectives* (2nd ed.). Toronto: Canadian Scholars' Press Inc.

This book summarizes how socio-economic factors affect the health of Canadians, surveys the current state of 12 social determinants of health across Canada, and provides an analysis of how these determinants affect Canadians' health.

Whitehead, M. (2007). A typology of actions to tackle social inequalities in health. *Journal of Epidemiology and Community Health, 61,* 473–478.

This article outlines some of the ways by which health inequities can be remedied. More extensive presentations are provided by Whitehead and Dahlgren (2006) and Dahlgren and Whitehead (2006).

Relevant Websites

Canadian Public Health Association, CPHA Policy Statements

http://www.cpha.ca/en/programs/policy.aspx

These reports and statements situate the CPHA as having been in the forefront of identifying the sources of health inequities and outlining means of reducing them.

Chief Public Health Officer's Reports on the State of Public Health in Canada

http://www.phac-aspc.gc.ca/publicat/cpho-acsp/index-eng.php

These reports provide the evidence concerning the profound health inequities among the Canadian population.

Portal for Action on Health Equity

http://www.health-inequalities.eu/

This resource is identified as "a tool to promote health equity amongst different socio-economic groups in the European Union." It contains information on policies and interventions to promote health equity by action on the socio-economic determinants of health.

Wellesley Institute

http://www.wellesleyinstitute.com/

The Wellesley Institute focuses on developing research and community-based policy solutions to problems of urban health and health inequities.

World Health Organization: Social Determinants of Health

http://www.who.int/social_determinants/en

The WHO established the CSDH to provide advice on how to reduce persisting and widening inequities in health. See especially its final report, *Closing the Gap in a Generation: Health Equity through Action on the Social Determinants of Health.*

CHAPTER 15

Ethical Dilemmas in Health Promotion Practice

Raymond Massé and Bryn Williams-Jones

Introduction

Hardly anyone will question the positive contributions of public health policies and health promotion programs to the improvement of a population's health. At first glance, goals such as the promotion of healthy lifestyles and public awareness of "at-risk" behaviours may appear sufficient to justify the ethical acceptability of health promotion interventions. But a moment's reflection makes it clear that there are many challenging questions that arise throughout the development and application of health promotion programs and policies.

BOX 15.1:

Challenging Questions for Health Promotion

1. What if the goal of promoting or protecting the common good infringes on individual civil liberties or shared values of minority cultural communities?
2. How far should we go in presenting positive (even moralizing) health information campaigns in the name of protecting public health without unduly stigmatizing people or making them feel guilty for their non-compliance?
3. Are there tensions or conflicts between the goals (and practices) of health promotion and fundamental social values such as autonomy, responsibility, social justice, or beneficence?
4. What are the consequences of the social construction of health as an ultimate social good?

Health promotion is an inherently value-laden enterprise and one that can lead to major ethical dilemmas. Ethical reflection on the part of health promotion professionals is thus essential in order to understand and negotiate the potentially conflicting fundamental values and interests of the diverse stakeholders (e.g., professionals, policy-makers, and citizens) involved in health promotion.

Health Promotion as a Normative and Acculturative Enterprise

Health promotion is, by its very nature, a normative and an acculturative enterprise. It is normative because it proposes or recommends norms about what is considered good health, what is acceptable or unacceptable risk, and what is a healthy physical and social environment.

But since lifestyles and health-related behaviours and environments are grounded in cultural values and social norms, health promotion is also an acculturative enterprise—that is, it is culture transforming. Put together, the normative and acculturative aspects of health promotion make it a deeply value-laden endeavour.

Health promotion is a socially embodied "value field"; its mission is to promote a sanitary culture, one that locates health at the top of a hierarchy of cultural values and social goals. Some commentators suggest that health promotion (and public health more generally) is a new morality, or even an alternative strategy of religious control of deviance in modern societies. For Petersen and Lupton (1996), health promotion is a form of "secular religion" in the context of which the new priests (health promotion professionals) define impenetrable avenues (for the citizen uninitiated in the epidemiology of risk) of health protection via the identification of secular sins (voluntary exposure to risk factors, refusal to modify at-risk behaviour). In this view, health promotion professionals behave more like proselytizing missionaries preaching an ideology than neutral and impartial scientists who are the legitimate experts and protectors of public health.

But ethical issues do not arise only with the use of coercive measures and paternalistic interventions. Many people are convinced that diseases are often self-inflicted, the product of one's own bad lifestyles or imprudent behaviours. This popular understanding can contribute to a moralizing public discourse that places the burden of responsibility on individuals for their illness, despite the overwhelming evidence that risk factors external to an individual's control can have an enormous impact on his or her health. Health promotion often takes a more subtle approach; citizens are encouraged to internalize health norms and to conform voluntarily to sanitary recommendations in order to construct a "civilized self." In such a context, health promotion can be seen as a pedagogic enterprise used for legitimizing the practices of control over individuals' lifestyles choices. One of the important ethical challenges in health promotion, then, is to examine and evaluate the legitimacy of socio-cultural constructions of blame and moral judgments that may be attributed to "at-risk" groups.

Thus, regardless of the laudable nature and ethical objectives of health promotion (i.e., protecting the public health and the public good), the nature and the range of means used for attaining these objectives may create important ethical challenges. Health promotion cannot simply take its own moral worth for granted. Much work needs to be done in order for this profession and field of practice to establish its moral credibility (Sindal, 2002), a credibility, we suggest, that must be founded on well-reasoned and argued principles. The existence and recognition of ethical questions or challenges should not, however, become an excuse for inaction. The normative and acculturating characteristics of health promotion activities are inherent in the mission of public health; they should be accepted, but also analyzed critically. Ethics, then, lies in the reflection and evaluation of the best balance between the means and the goals of health promotion. But ethical issues do not arise only with the use of coercive measures and paternalistic interventions. Many people are convinced that diseases are often self-inflicted, the product of one's own bad lifestyles or imprudent behaviours. This popular perception can contribute to a moralizing public discourse that places the burden of responsibility on individuals for their illness, despite the overwhelming evidence that risk factors external to an individual's control can have an enormous impact on his or her health (Leichter, 2003). This chapter will identify some of these ethical issues or challenges and suggest key components of an analytical framework for determining the ethical acceptability of health promotion interventions.

What Is an "Ethics" of Health Promotion?

Ethics in health promotion is not simply individual opinion or the blind following of norma-tive rules or professional codes of ethics. Nor should ethics be seen as simply an empirical description of what people (the majority) think or believe, e.g., derived from opinion surveys; simply because something "is" does not mean that it is "good." Ethics in health promotion necessarily involves applying a critical, analytic gaze to a particular program or policy. This may mean deconstructing complex situations to show the various interests and values that are present, but that may not be obvious; or it may mean complicating apparently simple situa-tions and challenging "obvious" solutions.

Ethical questions often arise when socially recognized fundamental cultural values are infringed. Examples include the infringement on smokers' individual autonomy and right to smoke so as to respect non-smokers' right to a smoke-free public space; cyclists' right not to wear helmets versus regulations requiring helmets in order to protect cyclists' safety; the promotion of breastfeeding and the moralizing of mothers who do not seem to prioritize the health of their babies; or the protection of women's rights in a campaign against domestic violence that targets a particular ethnic population, despite the risk of stigmatization. Virtually any health promotion program will impinge upon or entail some degree of infringement of at least one of the fundamental values recognized by Canadian society. In such a situation, ethics is about performing a context-sensitive and realistic analysis of the best approach.

The terms "ethics" and "morality" are sometimes treated as synonymous in public and professional discourse. We take "morality" to be the set of shared social values, judgments, or beliefs about right and wrong behaviour. There are as many moralities as there are social, ethnic, or religious subgroups and communities. In order to be culture- and context-sensitive, a health promotion ethics has to show some flexibility. But for reasons of equity and social justice, health promotion ethics should also be founded on principles that could be applied to all Canadians. Ethics must go beyond local moralities; it is a critical discourse on particular moralities (popular, institutional, or professional), the goal of which is to ask if norms or rules are relevant or appropriate to a particular context. But what are health promotion profession-als to do when values, norms, or interests conflict? Are there underlying principles or guides to action that people can agree on to resolve a particular conflict or dilemma? These are the questions at the heart of ethics; they necessarily go beyond a discussion of what "is" in order to ask what "should be." For our purposes, then, ethics is an applied and analytic endeavour. It is very often about asking the right questions in challenging situations and less so about giving the right answers. In some cases, there may be no right answer or solution—the task may be to pick the best of various imperfect or even "bad" options.

But ethics should not be seen as solely within the domain of experts who know the answers. Health promotion professionals have responsibilities that necessarily involve ethical reflection. It would be unethical for these professionals to simply transfer the task of ethical analysis to external experts and so absolve their own responsibility to evaluate and weigh the impact of their interventions. It is critical for professionals to develop the requisite knowledge and skills in ethical reflection so that ethics becomes integral to their practice and the performance of their professional responsibilities.

Health Promotion as Value Laden

The values underlying health promotion programs need to be made explicit if professionals want to be conscious of the ethical issues raised by their practice (Massé, 2003; Ritchie, 2006). The job of thinking ethically begins with identifying problems and describing a situation with an "ethical language"; that is, it is useful to name the values and principles at stake (held by various actors or stakeholders), and identify the conflicts (of values, interests) or dilemmas involved. Both Seedhouse (1997) and Guttman (2000) remind us that in spite of the preoccupation of professionals for grounding their interventions on scientifically validated epidemiological, administrative, or evaluative data, the process is still one that is profoundly influenced by fundamental values, even if these values are rarely made explicit.

Implicit values such as respect for autonomy, social justice, responsibility, non-maleficence, the common good, liberty, anti-paternalism, and many others profoundly orient the choice of criteria that define the priority accorded to specific public health problems, the nature of intervention strategies, the content of prevention messages, the modalities of putting health promotion interventions into action, and even the choice of the criteria to evaluate the efficacy of intervention programs. For example, in programs promoting teenagers' safe sexuality, choosing intermediate objectives such as the promotion of self-esteem or empowerment presuppose the valorization of individualism, autonomy, and personal responsibility. The choice of objectives is not only based on evidence regarding risk factors or the efficacy of programs as demonstrated by rigorous evaluative research. The values conveyed by professionals constitute only one of the determinants of the choice of strategies of intervention. The problem is not that such values are integral to or part of an intervention; the ethical issues arise when professionals and policy-makers ignore this fact and act as if the intervention is objective and value-neutral.

Ethical Dilemmas of Health Promotion Interventions

In the past decade, many authors have sought to address the numerous ethical issues raised by health promotion interventions (e.g., Seedhouse, 2001; Buchanan, 2000; Massé, 2003; Holland, 2007). We will identify, as examples, some domains in which the ethical acceptability of health promotion interventions is questioned because it may interfere with fundamental cultural values or ethical principles.

Autonomy and Information Communication

Respect for autonomy, individual liberty, and private life is very important to most North American and European societies. An ethical framework should then recognize that these values are at the foundations of modern Western societies. In so doing, this reminds us to be careful about how persuasive or coercive measures are used in advancing laudable goals of promoting public health. The weighing and arbitration of individual rights and collective interests has always been a major ethical challenge for health promotion (Holland, 2007).

One of the fundamental principles of Western clinical or medical ethics is respect for individual autonomy, most often translated as a requirement for individual informed consent. But the application of this requirement becomes problematic when it is the consent of populations or communities that is at stake. Some of the ethical challenges that arise include:

- The communication of environmental risks in the case of pollution. Professionals agree that transparency of information is primordial. However, a press communiqué, a study into the impact of the risks, or a simple evaluation of the perception of risks might generate a great deal of uneasiness. The ethical dilemma results from the confrontation of two values: the right of citizens to make autonomous choices based on appropriate information, and the responsibility of professionals to not needlessly generate harmful anxiety (non-maleficence). There is a conflict between a "right to know" and a "duty to inform."

- Knowing that a public understanding of "risk" (mostly a binary notion of presence vs. absence) differs substantially from a public health understanding (statistical notion of relative risk), the challenge is then to determine how far health promotion should go in explaining the intricacies and nuances of health risks so that the information can be well understood by the population before taking action. Is there a limit to the quantity and quality of information that can be transmitted effectively and ultimately understood by a target population? And at what point can health promotion feel morally authorized to exert pressure in favour of the adoption of a particular healthy lifestyle?

- In a context where groups or communities stand to benefit from health promotion interventions—or, alternatively, suffer the consequences—should respect for autonomy be considered only with regard to individuals? For example, would it be more ethical to obtain, prior to embarking on health promotion interventions, the authorization of representatives of hemophiliac groups, the gay community, and the managers of local unions or leaders of ethnic communities? And, if so, on what basis should we recognize certain communities and not others (i.e., how do we define "community"?), or identify the credible spokespeople who are entitled to speak for these heterogeneous groups?

Self-Determination, Paternalism, and Empowerment

Health promotion has long been seen as fundamentally paternalistic in nature. In the name of protecting the public good, public health institutions have deployed coercive methods such as prohibitions of certain behaviours (e.g., smoking indoors), mandatory participation (e.g., in vaccination, fluoridation), or aggressive health promotion campaigns. While effective in many contexts, such paternalistic interventions also, to various degrees, impinge upon or limit individual liberties. So another ethical issue for health promotion is the appropriate use of soft and hard paternalist methods. If health promotion usually considers hard paternalism (coercive interventions to counter voluntarily and consciously assumed behaviours) as an infringement on ethical principles (e.g., respect for autonomy, privacy), soft paternalism (where individuals are strongly encouraged to adopt behaviours that they believe are good for them) can be seen as inherent, unavoidable, and easily justifiable components of health promotion programs (even if sometimes they are less effective in their application).

The empowerment approach appears to some professionals as a solution to this issue. By focusing on empowering individuals and communities instead of simply telling them what to do, health promotion campaigns would be more respectful of individuals. Once empowered, people would be more likely to listen to health advice and make autonomous decisions that are objectively good for their health. Nonetheless, while empowering people and communities may be laudable as an effective means of respecting autonomy, it may be simply impractical or ineffective in some circumstances. If an intervention is empowering but of limited effectiveness at a population level, are more paternalistic (e.g., directive, moralizing) interventions then ethically justified?

Beyond the issue of efficiency, can empowerment be seen as another mode of paternalism? If the goal of an empowerment-based intervention is to transform the at-risk individual into a "responsible" actor through voluntary health education and information campaigns, is it still possible to talk about voluntary participation? Or is empowerment simply an "ethical cleansing agent" of health promotion interventions, a means of making soft paternalist approaches more palatable (Duncan & Cribb, 1996)? Some authors would argue that it is always public health institutions that promote health as a supreme social good (Holland, 2007) and that define the acceptable limits of risk exposure. Empowerment may raise other ethical issues if it is seen as an end (i.e., that of making people responsible for their health) instead of as a means to reach ends defined by others (i.e., promoting public health). And if empowerment of communities is mostly a bottom-up approach that is respectful of communities' own priorities, it should nonetheless be harmonized with top-down policies in order to protect the interests of minority groups in the socio-culturally heterogeneous "bottom population" (Braunack-Mayer & Louise, 2008).

BOX 15.2:

Questioning Paternalism

1. What are the limits on or justifications for the use of emotive marketing?
2. How, when, and to what extent can health promotion campaigns play on people's beliefs, emotions, or ignorance in order to promote a particular healthy behaviour or discourage an unhealthy behaviour?
3. What happens when the intervention goes against strongly held spiritual, religious, moral, or political beliefs, or when the "scientific facts" simply do not convince?
4. When does legitimate health promotion become health marketing or even manipulative propaganda?

Social Labelling, Stigmatization, and the Challenges to Social Justice

Health promotion should respect the principle of justice when it comes to interventions among individuals and target populations. Equity in access to health promotion interventions is a central concern. But the reality is that some people, often those who are already the most vulnerable, will remain on the margins and not benefit from even the most well-intentioned health promotion campaigns (Frohlich & Potvin, 2008). Ethical issues may also be raised if some social subgroups or some communities do not have access to a given health promotion program. It is generally agreed that health promotion services should not be offered based on a person's effort (e.g., the degree of participation, implication, or collaboration of the individual with the programs) or merit (e.g., the person's "social value" or contribution to society). As well, infringement on the value of social justice may occur if some groups benefit from health promotion while others bear the burden of risks and costs associated with particular interventions. That burden is often in terms of social labelling, discrimination, and stigmatization of the groups targeted (e.g., those who refuse vaccination, smokers, mothers who refuse breastfeeding, and the overweight population).

Uncertainty in Epidemiology, Program Evaluation, and the Limits of Instrumental Reason

Principles of justice, beneficence, or autonomy are not absolute; they must be balanced with, among others, considerations of the consequences of particular interventions for individuals and populations. It is thus important to both maximize the possible benefits for a population while also limiting the harms or negative consequences for certain individuals or subgroups. The utilitarian approach, which prioritizes the maximization of goods or benefits (i.e., "the greatest good for the greatest number"), is central to health promotion interventions. In taking the health of the population as its key focus, it would be arguably unethical for health promotion interventions to not seek to promote the greatest health benefit for the greatest number of people with the least negative impact.

However, an ethics of health promotion must be aware that a focus on (positive) consequences of an intervention cannot be the only or even the main ethical principle. Specifically, health promotion should never be reduced to cost-effectiveness analyses for two main reasons grounded in two illusions related to instrumental reason.

- The "scientific certainty illusion" suggests that scientific methods (e.g., epidemiology, quantitative evaluation design) are infallible in risk factor monitoring or the measurement of program efficacy. Health promotion professionals must recognize that the modern citizen-consumer is exposed to a wealth of contradictory epidemiological research results and often divergent preventive messages. Thus, health promotion interventions that lack critical reflexivity toward the fragility of scientific knowledge will raise both important technical and ethical issues.

- The "rationality illusion" rests on the postulate that all human beings are rational and self-interested, and so naturally dedicated to the maximization of their positive health state through the management of individual lifestyles and behaviours. This illusion ignores the role of alternative forms of rationality (Massé, 1997), or the fact that even the most rational people will at times behave emotionally or irrationally. This illusion also presupposes that a particular (i.e., dominant, scientific) definition of "health" is the only one that is legitimate, something that ignores the possible diversity of views that may arise in the context of Canada's increasingly multicultural society. Yet a strong rejection of this illusion could lead to a dangerous ethical relativism whereby all values, in all contexts, are considered equal, thus undermining the possibility of applying broad ethical principles across the population (Kline & Huff, 2007).

In developing an intervention to promote or prevent a certain behaviour or policy, we need to ask why, how, and for whom the intervention is designed. First and foremost, this involves considering the risks and benefits for the various stakeholders involved, and analyzing whose interests (and what type) are at stake. Second, it means recognizing the limits of the "natural" instrumental reason of individuals and communities, and thus requires a critical gaze on the naive utilitarian view of health promotion (Holland, 2007). Third, it is essential to recognize that some alternatives may be suboptimal in terms of outcomes, but may nonetheless be more ethically justifiable.

An Ethical Framework for Health Promotion

Due to the complexity and diversity of issues/challenges at stake in health promotion as illustrated above, it is essential that health promotion professionals have relevant and practical ethical guidelines and methodologies. In this section, we describe some key elements of a "tool box" for ethical reflection that are complementary to a broader "professional ethics" for those working in health promotion.

Since the 1970s, the ethical analysis of health promotion programs has been strongly influenced by what has been called the "principlist approach," initially developed for clinical or medical ethics. According to this ethical framework, a health promotion intervention can be considered ethically acceptable if it respects a list of fundamental principles that are derived from the main ethical theories (liberalism, utilitarianism, Kantian deontology, virtue theory, etc.), are embedded in a "common morality," and respect universal values such as those expressed in the Universal Declaration of Human Rights. The most popular version of principlism is that developed by Tom Beauchamp and James Childress in their *Principles of Biomedical Ethics* (Beauchamp & Childress, 2009). According to this theory and methodology, an ethical analysis should balance the respect of four *prima facie* principles (autonomy, justice, beneficence, and non-maleficence), none of which are absolute or predominant.

In this approach, ethical analysis involves a three-step process. First, theoretical principles must be specified; that is, following an in-depth analysis of the nature, context, and facts related to the program or intervention under study, the respective potential contributions of the four principles should be defined. Second, the relative importance of each of these principles must be weighed in light of the case analyzed. Third, the ethical analysis must arbitrate between these principles considering that any health promotion (or biomedical) intervention cannot fully respect each of these principles. The best stance involves not a black or white posture, but difficult choices over which principles will have to be limited in their scope or application in the specific case.

The major contribution of principlism is arguably its pragmatic methodological approach, which relies on relatively intuitive rules of thumb. In recognizing the limits of these four principles (and the principlist approach more generally), as well as the need for specific principles adapted to the population orientation of health promotion, many researchers (Holland, 2007; Buchanan, 2000; Upsur, 2002; Guttman, 2000; Massé, 2003) have suggested other ethical frameworks and lists of principles that are specifically adapted to health promotion programs and policies. Other principles and/or fundamental values suggested include: utility, public good, fairness, proportionality, solidarity, shared responsibility, and precaution.

Some have criticized principlism for its lack of theoretical foundation, its rationalistic abstraction, the relativism of these principles, and the risk of mechanical and automatic application in a checklist approach (Clouser & Gert, 1990). This last critique is partially true since many health professionals are prone to taking shortcuts through the complex and context-sensitive analytic method suggested by Beauchamp and Childress. However, if effort is made to identify fundamental principles adapted to the population approach of health promotion, then principlism provides three important assets to a health promotion ethics: (1) principlism rejects absolutist approaches that would give one specific principle (e.g., autonomy) an absolute or priority value over others; (2) the principles are secular and allow one to transcend religious specificity in targeting fundamental universal values; and (3) this approach recognizes that ethics is not a science of truth or of morality, but a reflexive and evaluative process that often involves weighing or arbitration between a list of equally fundamental values or principles.

Professional Ethics in Health Promotion

Finally, health promotion professionals also have ethical obligations and responsibilities related to their position of authority as agents of the state, and their power—in some circumstances—to force or restrict certain behaviours or policies. In general, health promotion professionals are called upon to exercise their abilities in a competent, professional manner; to develop policies, programs, and interventions that are based on the best available evidence; to be respectful of the rights, interests, and values of individuals in the community; and to advocate for disenfranchised or vulnerable individuals or communities. Such principles are laudable and, taken at face value, unproblematic. However, it may be difficult to apply such principles in practice; in some cases, equally important principles may be in tension or even conflict.

Alongside their duty to protect the public and behave in a trustworthy manner, health promotion professionals also have a responsibility to their employer (and ultimately to the state) to follow the orders of their superiors and to execute the tasks that they are given. In some contexts, health promotion professionals may be uncomfortable performing, or even disagree completely with, a particular intervention, yet be obligated to participate, e.g., the

2009–2010 vaccination campaign for H1N1 "swine flu" influenza. To what extent can these professionals opt out on moral (or scientific) grounds? Should they have the right to be "conscientious objectors" or would the failure to follow orders be grounds for sanction or dismissal?

To deal with these questions, health promotion professionals draw upon diverse sources of ethical guidance that include, for example, professional codes of ethics, institutional or national ethics policies, as well as personal moral or spiritual convictions. A number of ethical frameworks or codes have been advanced, such as the 2002 American Public Health Association's *Code of Ethics for Public Health Practice*. While the *Ottawa Charter* may be seen as a cornerstone in the ethics of health promotion (Mittlemark, 2007), it is not in and of itself a code of ethics. The International Union for Health Promotion and Education (IUHPE) is (in 2010) engaged in exploring the need for an international code of ethics for health promotion (see http://vhpo.net/). Debate on the pertinence of such a professional code of ethics is certainly important in order to define the duties and limits of health promotion research and practice. However, a codification of ethical professional practices should not mask the need for an in-depth analysis of the mission and underlying fundamental values, language, and even relevance of health promotion. Professional ethics is not about simply following the rules and guidelines; and, while necessary, an ethical health promotion cannot be contained in a professional code of ethics or standards of good practice.

The diversity of health issues, actors, disciplines, methodologies, or political orientation militate for a common platform to define acceptable practices in health promotion. But it is not at all clear whether that platform should be a formal code of ethics (Sindal, 2002) or a global ethical framework based on guiding values or principles that leave institutions and professionals with the responsibility to develop a self-reflective ethical posture. We suggest that a professional ethics for health promotion should include, but not be restricted to, a set of practical tools to guide professionals and help them identify and manage the challenging issues or questions that arise in their daily practice. Beyond these practical tools, however, a professional ethics for health promotion should include conceptual tools designed to help professionals analyze the global impacts of health promotion on society and culture. That is, this ethics should combine: (1) an analytic applied ethics, e.g., based on the evaluation and arbitration of a list of key principles, with (2) a "critical ethics" (Cribb, 2005) that is based on a critical consciousness about the social context of health and an ethical reflexivity that incorporates a critical gaze regarding the intended and unintended effects on society of the values in which health promotion interventions are grounded.

Conclusion

Health promotion may work for health as an ultimate common good and base its actions on the best available science and evidence base, yet it will still involve many challenging ethical issues and dilemmas. One of the main issues of concern is to determine when and how fundamental values of health promotion necessitate giving priority to the needs of the population over those of the individual (Parker, Gould & Fleming, 2007). It has been suggested above that neither an ethics framework for health promotion nor a professional code of ethics can give black or white answers to the challenging questions at stake. Ethics in health promotion necessarily involves the evaluation and weighing of principles and fundamental values in order to design programs and interventions that can promote health while minimizing infringements on individual and collective common goods other than health. A central question that must continually be asked is: How far should the society go in the promotion of healthy behaviours and habits, and what should be the proper level of reflexivity on the part of the health promotion professionals?

Since health promotion evolves in the context of a very broad set of social changes, we shall follow Alan Cribb's call for a new "social reflexivity" that involves "a pervasive and growing self-consciousness about the social construction of our health experiences and practices" (Cribb, 2005, p. xi). However, if the associated challenging ethical issues are to be properly addressed, then health promotion professionals have to become actively engaged in the process of ethical reflection. Of particular importance is an in-depth and critical analysis of the goals of health promotion. Health promotion professionals must reflect on their imperative and desire to act in the name of the public good, balancing this with a precautionary attitude that recognizes the indeterminacy of much scientific evidence. In our view, an ethics for health promotion professionals should thus include an ethical reflexivity that provides nuance to formal professional responsibilities and obligations, and a healthy skepticism about the social and cultural legitimacy of health promotion interventions.

References

Beauchamp, T.L. & Childress, J.F. (2009). *Principles of biomedical ethics* (6th ed.). New York: Oxford University Press.

Braunack-Mayer, A. & Louise, J. (2008). The ethics of community empowerment: Tensions in health promotion theory and practice. *Promotion and Education, XV*(3), 5–8.

Buchanan, D.R. (2000). *An ethics for health promotion: Rethinking the sources of human wellbeing.* New York: Oxford University Press.

Clouser, K.G. & Gert, B. (1990). A critique of principlism. *Journal of Medicine and Philosophy, 15*(2), 219–236.

Cribb, A. (2005). *Setting healthcare ethics in social context.* Oxford: Clarendon Press.

Cribb, A. & Duncan, P. (2002). *Health promotion and professional ethics.* Oxford: Blackwell Science.

Duncan, P. & Cribb, A. (1996). Helping people change. An ethical approach? *Health Education Research, 11*(3), 339–348.

Frohlich, K. & Potvin, L. (2008). The inequality paradox: The population approach and vulnerable populations. *American Journal of Public Health, 98*(2), 216–221.

Guttman, N. (2000). *Public health communication interventions: Values and ethical dilemmas.* Thousand Oaks: Sage Publications.

Holland, S. (2007). *Public health ethics.* Cambridge: Polity Press.

Kline, M.V. & Huff, R.M. (Eds.). (2007). *Health promotion in multicultural populations: A handbook for practitioners and students* (2nd ed.). Thousand Oaks: Sage Publications.

Leichter, H.M. (2003). "Evil habits" and "personal choices": Assigning responsibility for health in the 20th century. *The Milbank Quarterly, 81*(4), 603–626.

Massé, R. (1997). Les mirages de la rationalité des savoirs ethnomédicaux. *Anthropologie et Sociétés*, *21*(1), 53–72.

Massé, R. (2003). *Éthique et santé publique: Enjeux, valeurs, et normativité.* Quebec: Les Presses de l'Université Laval.

Mittelmark, M.B. (2007). Setting an ethical agenda for health promotion. *Health Promotion International*, *23*(1), 78–85.

Parker, E.A., Gould, T. & Fleming, M.-L. (2007). Ethics in health promotion—Reflections in practice. *Health Promotion Journal of Australia*, *18*(1), 69–72.

Peterson, A. & Lupton, D. (1996). *The new public health: Health and self in the age of risk.* Thousand Oaks: Sage Publications.

Ritchie, J. (2006). Values in health promotion. *Health Promotion Journal of Australia*, *17*(2), 83.

Seedhouse, D. (1997). *Health promotion: Philosophy, prejudice, and practice.* New York: Wiley.

Seedhouse, D. (2001). Health promotion's ethical challenge. *Health Promotion Journal of Australia*, *1*(2), 135–138.

Sindal, C. (2002). Does health promotion need a code of ethics? *Health Promotion International Journal*, *17*(3), 201–203.

Upsur, R.E.F. (2002). Principles for the justification of public health intervention. *Canadian Journal of Public Health*, *93*(2), 101–103.

Critical Thinking Questions

1. What are the limits of paternalistic health promotion interventions? Specifically, how far can one legitimately go in using marketing tactics to name a particular behaviour as "good" or "bad" and so influence or even manipulate people to respond to the health promotion advice "for their own good"?

2. What is the acceptable level of risk associated with targeting social subgroups or communities in health promotion interventions?

3. If the ethical acceptability of a given program or intervention is based on a list of ethics principles grounded in a "common morality," how can we take into consideration the divergent understanding of these principles and values by local minorities, such as ethnic or religious groups?

4. How should health promotion professionals deal with voluntary health risk-takers (e.g., smokers, heavy drinkers), and with corresponding policies that aim to fairly allocate scarce resources (e.g., access to health interventions)?

5. Would it be ethical to ban health promotion campaigns because they infringe key principles or fundamental values? If so, in which cases, and for which principles or values?

Resources

Further Readings

Buchanan, D.R. (2000). *An ethics for health promotion: Rethinking the sources of human wellbeing.* New York: Oxford University Press.

> The author explains why health promotion is inescapably a moral and political endeavour. He suggests that its realization will be best achieved by promoting autonomy and responsibility by putting into practice the use of practical reason.

Coleman, C., Bouësseau, M. & Reis, A. (2008). The contribution of ethics to public health. *Bulletin of the World Health Organization, 86*(8), 578–579.

The authors situate the origins of public health ethics in bioethics, and then map out six major areas or issues in public health that are in pressing need of ethical reflection.

Public Health Leadership Society. (2002). *Principles of the ethical practice of public health, version 2.2.* Retrieved from: http://phls.org/CMSuploads/Principles-of-the-Ethical-Practice-of-PH-Version-2.2-68496.pdf

This is an example of a code of ethics for public health professionals, developed for the US context.

Relevant Websites

Population Health Ethics: Annotated Bibliography

http://www.cihr-irsc.gc.ca/e/40740.html#1

Population Health Ethics, a comprehensive annotated bibliography of key texts in population health ethics by H.L. Greenwood and N. Edwards, covers theoretical foundations and principles, ethical frameworks, and selected cases.

Public Health Ethics

http://phe.oxfordjournals.org/

Public Health Ethics is a key international journal on ethics of public health and health promotion.

CHAPTER 16

Two Roles of Evaluation in Transforming Health Promotion Practice

Louise Potvin and Carmelle Goldberg

Introduction

This chapter is about the meanings and roles of evaluation in the context of health promotion. More precisely, we argue that an important, and often neglected, role for evaluation is to support the transformation of practices in health promotion. To do so, we consider definitions of evaluation, the particularities of evaluation in the context of health promotion interventions, and the importance of evaluation for health promotion practice. Using Canadian examples, we then explore two major reasons why health promotion should be evaluated: (1) to increase the effectiveness of health promotion intervention; and (2) to support innovative practices.

What Is Evaluation?

There are many definitions of evaluation. In its simplest form, evaluation is the critical appraisal of human actions in context. It is a value-laden feedback response to action. In its most sophisticated form, evaluation research: (1) spans several years, if not decades; (2) mobilizes a large amount of human and material resources to design and implement a complex system of activities to define, gather, analyze, and interpret a huge quantity of data; and, finally, (3) produces knowledge about numerous aspects of interventions. The knowledge produced by such evaluations potentially influences the practice of thousands of professionals and ultimately the health of hundreds of thousands of people.

Mark, Henry, and Julnes (2000) provide one of the most encompassing definitions of evaluation: "Evaluation assists sense making about policies and programs through the conduct of systematic inquiry that describes and explains the policies' and programs' operations, effects, justifications, and social implications" (p. 3). Compared to most, this definition avoids falling into the trap of pitting against one another various forms of evaluations based on their object, purpose, or method. Especially in health promotion, evaluations often deploy a variety of methods to address a number of stakeholders' issues regarding various program components.

Following a similar argument, the WHO-EURO working group on health promotion evaluation also proposed a very broad definition: "evaluation is the systematic examination and assessment of features of a programme or other intervention in order to produce knowledge that different stakeholders can use for a variety of purposes" (Rootman, Goodstadt, Potvin & Springett, 2001, p. 26). Thus, whenever the object of inquiry is an intervention or one aspect of it, whenever the method of enquiry is systematic, and whenever the purpose is to produce information that can be used by a variety of social actors, we think it is proper to identify such activity as evaluation.

What Is Evaluated in Health Promotion?

Evaluation is about interventions. It is thus important to have a clear understanding of what an intervention is in the context of health promotion. The verb "to intervene" contains the Latin verb *venire*, which means "to come," and the prefix *inter-*, which means "in between." Literally, to intervene is to come in between, to disturb the natural order of things. An intervention implies an action from external actors who have the power to mobilize and deploy resources in the pursuit of specific results (Couturier, 2005). Interventions are planned and coordinated actions, or systems of action (Potvin & Bisset, 2008) to achieve projected changes. They form the core of a practice, understood as skills learned, reproduced, and improved by professionals through their actions. "Intervention" is a generic term that encompasses diverse modalities of planned actions.

As seen throughout this book, there are many definitions of health promotion and they all, as Rootman et al. (2001) pointed out, "involve a set of actions, focused on the individual or environment, which through increasing control, ultimately leads to improved health or well-being" (p. 13). Clearly, at the core of health promotion is the idea of intervention.

As also seen in several chapters of this book, the field of health promotion is characterized by a tension between perspectives that emphasize changes in individuals and those that target environmental social conditions. According to Rootman et al. (2001), this tension is the main divider between existing definitions of health promotion. The implications of this divide in terms of approach and forms of interventions are seldom discussed. However, the emerging field of population health intervention research is developing a strong argument in favour of distinguishing evaluation of interventions that aim at changing the distribution of health and its determinants in a population from evaluation of interventions that target individual changes (Hawe & Potvin, 2009).

In the rest of this chapter, we will concentrate our discussion on the evaluation of complex multi-level health promotion interventions that involve systems of action planned and implemented at a collective level and this for two reasons. First, the prominent evaluation tradition in the health sector, represented by clinical epidemiology, is well equipped to address evaluation issues of interventions targeting individual changes, but its usefulness and relevance for evaluating health promotion strategies that call for collective action is much more limited (Potvin & Chabot, 2002). Second, as Potvin, Gendron, Bilodeau, and Chabot (2005) indicate, defining a practice that advocates collective strategies of actions represents a major innovation of the *Ottawa Charter* for the health sector. This issue has been seldom discussed with regard to evaluation.

This chapter will also restrict its focus to the most common form of health promotion interventions: programs. Although programs can be designed for a variety of purposes, including developing individual skills, we will focus our attention on those programs that imply a composite and multifaceted package of activities as promoted in three of the *Ottawa Charter* strategies of action: creating supportive environment, strengthening community actions, and reorienting health services.

What Is a Program?

Although health promotion literature is replete with terms such as "programs," "projects," "initiatives," "activities," and "interventions," there have been very few attempts to identify common and unique characteristics of the realities defined by those terms. Very often these labels are used interchangeably or they are used in reference to various levels of organization of actions in composite interventions. One reason for this confusion is that the reality circumscribed by these terms is necessarily complex and its delineation necessarily related to a specific context. Judging whether something or someone belongs to a program greatly depends on the particular viewpoint of the individual making the judgment. If programs are systems of action, then, as in any system, the borders that distinguish what constitutes the system and what makes up the environment is somewhat arbitrary and depends on the analyst's viewpoint (Potvin, Bilodeau & Gendron, 2008).

In a school program aimed at increasing children's resilience, for example, a teacher trained and deeply involved in leading classroom resilience-enhancement activities may perceive that many elements in her school and her broader environment are parts of the program, such as the school social worker who runs teachers' resilience workshops, the local health centre that provides documentation, and the school physical activity teacher who develops "feel good with your body" activities. This view contrasts with that of children's parents, who know about the program only through their child, and who may perceive only the teacher and the documents they receive periodically as the program's components. So what is to be considered as being part of a program needs to be defined and agreed upon because programs are not a given. They are the product of social activity that result from people establishing relationships in order to work together to address common problems (Davies, 2004, 2005; Durland & Frederick, 2006; Williams & Imam, 2007).

Most often, programs are represented by the problematic situation they address, the objectives pursued, the resources mobilized, the services and activities produced, the expected results, and the chain of events necessary for the program to yield those results (Potvin, Haddad & Frohlich, 2001). Such representations are often referred to as program logic models (Cooksy, Gill & Kelly, 2001). It is very rare for the existing relationships between relevant program actors to be represented as part of the program. Indeed, most representations portray programs as technical procedures, independent of the social identity of people involved in it. In response to this problem, the network metaphor is being used increasingly to characterize "program" wherein program implementation is conceived as operating connections between previously unconnected entities (Hawe, Shiell & Riley, 2009; Bisset, Daniel & Potvin, 2009) through a series of events that bring in new actors that slowly transform the program (Bisset & Potvin 2007).

The Problem of Values in Health Promotion Programs

The *Ottawa Charter* (World Health Organization, 1986) identifies key values and principles that form the core of the health promotion agenda (McQueen, 2001). Many of these values and principles of action call for a strong integration of programs into the social reality of the milieu in which they are implemented. Furthermore, values such as participation, empowerment, and intersectoral collaboration can be actualized only by positioning programs, program participants, and program context in a network of reciprocal relationships. It is within such networks that health promotion programs germinate and come to life. Those values that are inherent to health promotion need to be accounted for by evaluation. Health promotion evaluators have been very innovative in developing evaluation practices that help align values in health promotion with the rigour of the scientific process that underlines evaluation (Potvin & McQueen, 2008).

Health promotion programs based on those values involve a strong integration into local context (Poland, Frohlich & Cargo, 2008), and therefore can hardly be elaborated outside of this context and then imported and tested. Such programs need to evolve within their social context, constantly adapting and negotiating practices imported from effective programs. Through this process it is not only the social context and life trajectories of those who interact with the program that get transformed, but also the program itself (Potvin, Haddad & Frohlich, 2001). Values underlying health promotion are at odds with a conception of program participants as passive subjects who need intervention through programs. On the contrary, these values imply that programs are better conceptualized as reconfigurations of existing contextual elements to adapt to new practices suggested by programs, practices that are themselves adapted to fit better the characteristics of the context. "Documenting the events that marked the evolution of this relational system and constructing a coherent narrative to interpret the system's dynamism is as crucial for understanding health promotion intervention as is the 'evidence' about its efficacy" (Potvin & Chabot, 2002).

Why Evaluate Health Promotion Programs?

Following Mark et al. (2000) above, evaluation is about making sense of what happens in programs. Since programs are a defining modality for health promotion practice, it follows that evaluation is central for the transformation of health promotion practice. In this section we discuss two crucial roles for evaluation with regard to health promotion practices. One is to increase the effectiveness of interventions; this role has been widely advocated by professional associations in attempts to increase the relevance of health promotion for policy-makers (International Union for Health Promotion & Education, 1999;, Briss & Harris, 2005). The other role is to support the development and diffusion of innovative practices (Bilodeau, Chamberland & White, 2002).

Evaluation to Increase the Effectiveness of Health Promotion Interventions

To play this role, evaluation tries to attribute a result to an intervention, i.e., establish causal links between program and outcomes. Causal claims are usually achieved by holding constant everything but the intervention under study, in an effort to isolate the causal mechanism of interest (Campbell, 1984). Because this can never be totally achieved outside of the laboratory, evaluation researchers use strategies and methods that emulate laboratory conditions. This experimentalist approach to evaluation found two main traditions in health promotion evaluation: clinical epidemiology and social sciences quasi-experimental designs.

Clinical Epidemiology

Strongly anchored in experimental medicine, clinical epidemiology is associated with a strong stream of experimental evaluation research facilitated by the fact that medical clinics and hospitals are highly institutionalized settings where power and decisions are concentrated among clinicians. Because of this, clinicians and evaluators can and do exercise a high level of control over two fundamental aspects of the experimental situation: patients' random assignment and treatment standardization. Because most of the early evaluation studies of prevention interventions were developed in clinical settings, these two aspects rapidly became customary features for quality evaluation. The limitations of the experimentalist tradition for evaluating prevention interventions, however, were soon experienced.

As early as the 1970s the Multiple Risk Factor Intervention Trial (MRFIT) study assigned 12,866 healthy male volunteers to three modalities of clinical preventive services. Randomization worked and study groups ended up being statistically equivalent. The three preventive treatments were successfully implemented in 20 clinics throughout the US. Interestingly, though, the power of this trial was greatly diminished by the fact that many subjects who had been randomly assigned to either the low-intensity prevention intervention or to the usual care groups sought and were given high-intensity preventive interventions outside of trial clinics (Ockene, Hymowitz, Lagus & Shaten, 1991). So, even in clinical settings where randomization can be implemented, conclusions from efficacy trials are limited by the availability of interventions obtained through other means.

Social Science Quasi-experimental Designs

The quasi-experimentalist stream of evaluation developed by Campbell, Cook, and their students (Shadish, Cook & Leviton, 1991) has also been very influential for defining a paradigm for the evaluation of health education and health promotion programs. Taking the randomized control trial as the gold standard for establishing causal relations between treatments and observed effects, quasi-experimentalists characterized alternative weaker research designs in terms of their capacity to control for plausible rival hypotheses and advocated for their proper use in evaluation research.

Unfortunately, very early in the development of the field of evaluation, numerous quasi-experimental evaluation projects failed to produce the expected straightforward results that would fuel rational decisions (Pawson & Tilley, 1997). In the field of public health, quasi-experimental evaluations of very important projects such as the Minnesota Heart Health were unable to show that the reduction in cardiovascular risk factors in the experimental communities was greater than that observed in control communities (Luepker et al.,1994). Although this project showed a significant reduction of risk factor prevalence in exposed populations, this reduction was not significantly different from that observed in non-equivalent control communities.

For Campbell (1984, 1987) the problem lies within the evaluation paradigm itself. People entertain unrealistic expectations given the inherent limitations of evaluation, which has to operate outside of the well-controlled world of laboratories. The complexity of real-life situations in which programs are implemented interferes with the evaluator's capacity to control the experimental situation, thus threatening studies' internal validity (the capacity to infer a causal link between specific interventions and observed outcomes). Furthermore, because programs are social products necessarily embedded into their social contexts, external validity (the capacity to generalize results of a single evaluation to other program instantiations) is also greatly reduced. It is thus impossible for any single evaluation study to clearly establish a program causal effect.

The Difficulties for Experimentalists to Evaluate Health Promotion Programs

The experimentalist tradition does not accommodate well approximations and uncertainties in evaluating interventions. Because such uncertainties are often inherent in health promotion programs, there is much debate on the appropriateness of the experimental paradigm for evaluating health promotion (McQueen, 2001; Rychetnik, Frommer, Hawe & Shiell, 2002).

In the rare cases where practices have evolved into well-packaged and well-defined programs, they could be suitable for experimental evaluations. We agree with Hawe, Shiell, and Riley (2004) that it is not so much procedural aspects that should be used to create the intervention and control groups to be compared in experimental evaluations but the *functions* that are thought to be related to the intended effects. For these authors functions are the essential operating mechanisms that constitute interventions. For example, resources in the form of a community organizer would be a function in a community development program. Such a function could lend itself to randomization, but not the activities that are designed by this actor to suit specific community contexts in which it operates. But even in randomized trials of program functions, the complex interactions between programs and contextual factors further complicate the role of experimental evaluation. In terms of the transformation of practices, what comes out of existing syntheses is that programs with documented effectiveness are usually simple and not very well integrated within local networks of actors (Zaza et al., 2005). Even more, it appears that programs with greater fidelity between the program as planned and the program as it is implemented are less effective than programs in which activities are adapted to contextual conditions (Doak, Visscher, Renders & Seidell, 2006).

This requirement for experimental control might be detrimental for health promotion programs whose effective mechanisms are often conceptualized as residing in the interaction between programs and contextual conditions (Poland, Frohlich & Cargo, 2008). This inherent conflict between controlling for conditions and the principle that health promotion interventions should be adapted to context might contribute to the difficulty of evaluating health promotion programs and to the difficulty of finding an effect when programs are evaluated with a randomized controlled trial. Answering questions such as for whom does an intervention have an impact and under which conditions may be more appropriate for health promotion than the question of determining an intervention's effect, everything else being held constant. But we also think that there is room for other types of questions, such as: How does the intervention produce its intended effect?

Evaluation to Support Innovative Practices

This is a much less developed but potentially much more important role for evaluation in health promotion. In this section we want to emphasize that one key role of evaluation is to support the development of innovative practice. There are at least three reasons why it is so.

Why Is Supporting Innovation through Evaluation Important?

First, well-defined programs form only a small part of health promotion practice, and these well-defined programs are usually not well aligned with the innovative practices advocated for in the *Ottawa Charter* (Potvin et al., 2005). Second, to go the participatory route advocated by health promotion, practitioners have to start from the preoccupations and possibilities of the local milieus (Israel, Schulz, Parker & Becker, 1998). In those cases, at best, well-tested programs with a demonstrated effectiveness constitute only a good starting point for designing interventions that can go in totally different directions to accommodate local circumstances. Unfortunately, very few studies document those partnerships' roles and contributions to programs' effectiveness. Third, identifying a problem locally, even when its causes are scientifically known, does not mean that interventions can be readily available or designed in that context. Indeed, program components are always strongly intertwined into the broader social context through a dense network of partnerships. For many, thus, the social context is thought to be at least as important, if not more important, than the technical aspects of program delivery (Bilodeau et al., 2002). The case study in Box 16.1 illustrates this.

In real-life contexts of health promotion programs, the selection and implementation of program interventions is not simply a by-product of rational choices informed by scientific

---

BOX 16.1:

Scientific and Contextual Elements for Program Planning: The Case of the Kahnawake Schools Diabetes Prevention Project

In their analysis of the genesis of a school and community-based diabetes prevention project in an Aboriginal community, Bisset et al. (2004) found that results of epidemiological studies documenting the high prevalence of diabetes risk factors and their potential complications, along with scientific knowledge about diabetes risk factors, were only partial contributors to the planning and implementation of this program. It is through Elders' and community leaders' knowledge of the community, existing community networks, and local history that specific aspects of program goals and target populations were developed. Throughout the project, a community advisory board, which was perceived as the main project's owner (Cargo et al., 2003), played the crucial role of orienting the project to better correspond with the local values and traditional knowledge about health and wellness.

knowledge. It is strongly influenced by a continuous negotiation and adjustment process. The aim of such a process is to find convergence between: (1) scientific theoretical and empirical knowledge about the identified problem and about effective interventions; (2) people's subjective knowledge about the problem, its causes, its impact on their lives, and about their own community and its strengths; and (3) the local values and norms relevant to the situation. The outcome of this process is a socially constructed innovation where practices are continuously transformed by a dense network of social interactions constitutive of the program. This, as developed in Chapter 5, clearly requires the evaluation to serve a reflexive function that fosters program stakeholders' capacity to incorporate and act upon the knowledge provided to them (Potvin et al., 2005). One of the crucial roles of evaluation is thus to systematize and facilitate the reflexive function on programs in order to illuminate the process by which programs become local innovations and to support their transformative practices. A recent book by Michael Quinn Patton provides insight on the appropriate methods to conduct what he calls "developmental evaluation" and that essentially serves the purpose of informing the innovative features of an intervention as it is developed (Patton, 2011).

Conclusions

In this chapter we proposed that there are mainly two ways in which evaluation can support changes in health promotion practice. The first is to attempt to direct health promotion practice to specific interventions found effective in controlled experiments through evidence-based procedures. It is grounded within the experimentalist tradition, where innovations are derived from scientific knowledge and tested in controlled conditions. The viability of this evaluation approach to inform practice is, however, challenged by the assumptions underlying methodologies that systematically remove context from the evaluation inquiry.

The second way evaluation can support changes in health promotion practice is by facilitating social innovation. This approach is grounded in social science theory where innovation is created by systematizing and putting in place reflexive processes responsive to local project implementation. This approach engages practitioners in a continuous dialogue on the performance and meaning of program actions, and their interactions with the local context. The dynamic relationship fostered by this approach allows practitioners to consciously reinforce certain actions while reorienting others. This facilitates programs' adaptation by strengthening their reflexive and innovative capacity.

These are two opposite perspectives on evaluation. Both are laden with enormous methodological challenges that somehow impede their capacity to fulfill these roles, leading many stakeholders toward a narrow accountability perspective on evaluation, one that limits evaluations to the collection of routine data regarding program operations and resources. We strongly believe that this accountability approach is of limited utility in informing practice and orienting program transformation because no attention is devoted to the actions that are actually performed by the program. This is so mostly because we are conceptually and methodologically ill equipped to observe and analyze the unfolding of the social processes that involve a diversity of actors implicated in dynamic relationships at the heart of health promotion programs. This, we think, constitutes a priority for future evaluation research, in order to better understand how health promotion operates and therefore effectively induces changes in the social determinants of health.

References

Bilodeau, A., Chamberland, C. & White, D. (2002). L'innovation sociale, une condition pour accroître la qualité de l'action en partenariat dans le champ de la santé publique. *Revue canadienne d'évaluation de programme, 17*(2), 59–88.

Bisset, S.L., Cargo, M., Delormier, T., Macaulay, A.C. & Potvin, L. (2004). Legitimizing diabetes as a community health issue: A case analysis of the Kahnawake schools diabetes prevention project. *Health Promotion International, 19,* 317–326.

Bisset, S., Daniel, M. & Potvin, L. (2009). Exploring the intervention-context interface: A case from a school-based nutrition intervention. *American Journal of Evaluation, 30*(4), 554–571.

Bisset, S.L. & Potvin, L. (2007). Expanding our conceptualization of program implementation: Lessons from the genealogy of a school-based nutrition program. *Health Education Research, 22,* 737–746.

Campbell, D.T. (1984). Can we be scientific in applied social science? *Evaluation Studies Review Annual, 9,* 26–48.

Campbell, D.T. (1987). Guidelines for monitoring the scientific competence of the preventive intervention research centers: An exercise in the sociology of scientific validity. *Knowledge—Creation, Diffusion, Utilization, 8,* 389–430.

Cargo, M., Levesque, L., Macaulay, A.C., McComber, A., Desrosiers, S., Delormier, T. et al. (2003). Kahnawake schools diabetes prevention project (KSDPP) community advisory board. Community governance of the Kahnawake schools diabetes prevention project, Kahnawake Territory, Mohawk Nation, Canada. *Health Promotion International, 18,* 177–187.

Cooksy, L. J., Gill, P., & Kelly, A. (2001). The program logic model as an integrative framework for multimethod evaluation. *Evaluation and Program Planning, 24* (3), 119-128.

Couturier, Y. (2005). *La collaboration entre travailleuses sociales et infirmières: Éléments d'une théorie de l'intervention interdisciplinaire.* Paris: l'Harmattan.

Davies, R. (2004). Scale, complexity, and the representation of theories of change (Part 1). *Evaluation, 10,* 101–121.

Davies, R. (2005). Scale, complexity, and the representation of theories of change (Part 2). *Evaluation, 11,* 133–149.

Doak, C., Visscher, T., Renders, C. & Seidell, J. (2006). The prevention of overweight and obesity in children and adolescents: A review of interventions and programmes. *Obesity Reviews,* 7, 111–136.

Durland, M. & Frederick, K. (2006). *Social network analysis in program evaluation: New Directions for Evaluation 107.* San Francisco: Jossey-Bass.

Hawe, P. & Potvin, L. (2009). What is population health intervention research? *Canadian Journal of Public Health, 100*(1), I8–I14.

Hawe, P., Shiell, A. & Riley, T. (2004). Complex interventions: How "out of control" can a randomized control trial be? *British Medical Journal, 328,* 1561–1563.

Hawe, P., Shiell, A. & Riley, T. (2009). Theorising interventions as events in systems. *American Journal of Community Psychology, 43,* 267–276.

International Union for Health Promotion and Education. (1999) *The evidence of health promotion effectiveness: Shaping public health in a new Europe.* Part Two Evidence book. Brussels: European Commission.

International Union for Health Promotion and Education (IUHPE). (2009). *The evidence of health promotion effectiveness.* Paris: IUPHE.

Israel, B.A., Schulz, A.J., Parker, E.A. & Becker, A.B. (1998). Review of community-based research: Assessing partnership approaches to improve public health. *Annual Review of Public Health, 19,* 173–202.

Luepker, R.V., Murray, D.M., Jacobs, D.R. Jr. et al. (1994). Community education for cardiovascular disease prevention: Risk factor changes in the Minnesota Heart Health Program. *American Journal of Public Health, 84*(9), 1383–1393.

Mark, M., Henry, G.T. & Julnes, G. (2000). *Evaluation: An integrated framework for understanding, guiding, and improving public and non-profit policies and programs.* San Francisco: Jossey-Bass.

McQueen, D.V. (2001). Strengthening the evidence base for health promotion. *Health Promotion International, 11,* 261–268.

Ockene, J.K., Hymowitz, N., Lagus, J. & Shaten, B.J. (1991). Comparison of smoking behavior change for SI and UC study groups. MRFIT Research Group. *Preventive Medicine, 20,* 564–573.

Patton, M.Q. (2011). *Developmental evaluation: Applying complexity concepts to enhance innovation and use.* New York: Guilford Press.

Pawson, R. & Tilley, N. (1997). *Realistic evaluation.* London: Sage.

Poland, B., Frohlich, K. & Cargo, M. (2008). Context as a fundamental dimension of health promotion program evaluation. In L. Potvin & D. McQueen (Eds.), *Health promotion evaluation practices in the Americas: Values and research* (pp. 299–318). New York: Springer.

Potvin, L., Bilodeau, A. & Gendron, S. (2008). Trois défis pour l évaluation en promotion de la santé. *Promotion & Education* (Suppl. 1), 17–21.

Potvin, L. & Bisset, S.L. (2008). There is more to methodology than method. In L. Potvin & D. V. McQueen (Eds.), *Health promotion evaluation practices in the Americas: Values and research* (pp. 63–80). New York: Springer.

Potvin, L. & Chabot, P. (2002). Splendour and misery of epidemiology for evaluation of health promotion. *Revista Brasileira de Epidemiologia, 5*(Suppl. 1), 91–103.

Potvin, L., Gendron, S., Bilodeau, A. & Chabot, P. (2005). Integrating social science theory into public health practice. *American Journal of Public Health, 95,* 591–595.

Potvin, L., Haddad, S. & Frohlich, K.L. (2001). Beyond process and outcome evaluation: A comprehensive approach for evaluating health promotion programmes. In I. Rootman, M. Goodstadt, B. Hyndman, D.V. McQueen, L. Potvin, J. Springett & E. Ziglio (Eds.), *Evaluation in health promotion: Principles and perspectives* (pp. 45–62). European series no. 92. Copenhagen: WHO Regional Publications.

Potvin, L. & McQueen, D.V. (Eds.). (2008). *Health promotion evaluation practices in the Americas: Values and research.* New York: Springer.

Rootman, I., Goodstadt, M., Potvin, L. & Springett, J. (2001). A framework for health promotion evaluation. In I. Rootman, M. Goodstadt, B. Hyndman, D.V. McQueen, L. Potvin, J. Springett & E. Ziglio (Eds.), *Evaluation in health promotion: Principles and perspectives* (pp. 7–38). European series no. 92. Copenhagen: WHO Regional Publications.

Rychetnik, L., Frommer, M., Hawe, P. & Shiell, A. (2002). Criteria for evaluating evidence on public health interventions. *Journal of Epidemiology & Community Health, 56,* 119–127.

Shadish, W.R., Cook, T.D. & Leviton, L.C. (1991). *Foundations of program evaluation: Theories of practice.* Newbury Park: Sage.

Williams, B. & Imam, I. (Eds). (2007). *Systems concepts in evaluation: An expert anthology.* Point Reyes: EdgePress of Inverness.

World Health Organization. (1986). *Ottawa Charter for Health Promotion.* Retrieved from www.phac-aspc.gc.ca/ph-sp/phdd/pdf/charter.pdf

Zaza, S., Briss, P.A. & Harris, K.W. (2005). *The guide to community preventive services: What works to promote health?* New York: Oxford University Press.

Critical Thinking Questions

1. How are evaluated programs different from non-evaluated programs?
2. Who is implicated in conceptualizing and implementing the evaluation? How are the various actors represented in this process?
3. Whose interests are being served by the evaluation?
4. Who is defining evaluation questions? How are the evaluation questions contributing to social betterment?
5. How are evaluation recommendations translated into practice? Whose interests are or are not being served by this process?

Resources

Further Readings

Mark, M., Henry, G.T. & Julnes, G. (2000). *Evaluation: An integrated framework for understanding, guiding, and improving public and non-profit policies and programs.* San Francisco: Jossey-Bass.

This book offers a new approach to evaluation, one that will encourage organizations or agencies to improve their contribution to social betterment. The authors draw from three decades of evaluation practice and theory to present a framework for conceptualizing evaluation and pragmatically assessing social policies and programs.

McQueen, D.V. & Jones, C.M. (Eds.). (2007). *Global perspectives on health promotion effectiveness.* New York: Springer.

This book is a collection of essays in which authors from around the world examine issues of effectiveness with regard to health promotion. In addition to reports from the field in which various health promotion intervention strategies are critically examined, the book contains a section in which difficult issues associated with evidence-based practice in health promotion are discussed.

Pawson, R. & Tilley, N. (1997). *Realistic evaluation.* London: Sage.

The authors present a critique of traditional evaluation practice for its inability to produce straightforward results that would fuel rational decisions. They articulate a new evaluation paradigm that requires a careful blend of theory and method to understand causality in terms of underlying causal mechanisms. It is concerned with understanding causal mechanisms and the conditions under which they are activated to produce intended outcomes.

Potvin, L. & McQueen, D.V. (Eds.). (2008). *Health promotion evaluation practices in the Americas: Values and research.* New York: Springer.

This book develops the thesis that in order to be relevant for the field of health promotion, evaluation has to account for the values that characterize health promotion practice. The book first defines evaluation as a social practice and identifies how evaluation practice may interfere with health promotion values. The last section presents a collection of essays by health promotion evaluators from the three Americas reporting on the practices by which they attempt to better align the rigour of evaluation with the values of health promotion.

Rootman, I., Goodstadt, M., Hyndman, B., McQueen, D.V., Potvin, L., Springett, J. et al. (Eds.). (2001). *Evaluation in health promotion: Principles and perspectives.* European series no. 92. Copenhagen: WHO Regional Publications.

This book is one product resulting from the five-year work of the WHO-EURO Working Group on Health Promotion Evaluation, led by Irving Rootman and David McQueen. With contributors from Europe and North America, the book provides a broad overview of the challenges and opportunities for evaluation associated with health promotion.

Relevant Websites

American Evaluation Association

www.eval.org

The American Evaluation Association is an international professional association of evaluators devoted to the application and exploration of program evaluation, personnel evaluation, technology, and many other forms of evaluation. They publish the *American Journal of Evaluation*, *New Directions for Evaluation*, and *Guiding Principles for Evaluators*. Their activities include an annual conference, training opportunities, career opportunities, and much more.

Canadian Evaluation Society

www.evaluationcanada.ca

The Canadian Evaluation Society is a Canada-wide, non-profit bilingual association dedicated to the advancement of evaluation theory and practice. The society promotes leadership, knowledge, advocacy, and professional development. It does this through diverse activities, including the publication of the *Canadian Journal of Program Evaluation*, annual conferences, diverse professional development events, notification of employment and contact opportunities, and much more.

CDC Evaluation Working Group

www.cdc.gov/eval/index.htm

The CDC Evaluation Working Group was charged by the US Centers for Disease Control and Prevention with developing a framework that summarizes and organizes the basic elements of program evaluation. The working group develops resources and linkages to evaluation of health programs.

Chaire Approche communautaire et inégalités de santé

www.cacis.umontreal.ca

The Chaire has conducted multiple studies in which evaluation was supporting innovations in health promotion. This site proposes a variety of resources.

Evaluation Center, Western Michigan University

www.wmich.edu/evalctr/

The Evaluation Center, Western Michigan University, offers links to evaluation tools and resources, publications, and other important websites in the field of evaluation. It is also the site of *The Journal of Multi Disciplinary Evaluation*, edited by Michael Scriven and E. Jane Davidson, with a mission of providing news and thinking of the profession and discipline of evaluation in the world.

CHAPTER 17

Perspectives on Health Promotion from Different Areas of Practice

Sophie Dupéré, Robert Perreault, Marcia Hills, Clémence Dallaire, Judith Burgess, Kadija Perreault, Donna Anderson, Pamela Ponic, Wendy Frisby, Louise St-Pierre, Anika Mendell, Larry Hershfield, Lise Renaud, Yanick Villedieu, Diane Morin, and Serge Dumont

Introduction

Sophie Dupéré

The first image that usually comes into a layperson's mind when we talk about health promotion is a health professional, usually a doctor or a nurse, who gives advice to a patient on how to prevent illnesses or promote health. Although health education and individual behavioural interventions are important areas of practice in health promotion, health promotion practice today goes way beyond this (see Chapter 1). Physicians and nurses are definitely key health professional groups involved in health promotion practice in Canada, but are far from being the only ones who devote time to improve the health of the population. Indeed, a recent Canadian survey concluded that "a key contextual element health promoters share is the diversity of its workforce. Those working in health promotion come from a wide range of backgrounds, are employed in a variety of settings and in some cases do not necessarily identify themselves as health promoters" (Ghassemi, 2009, p. 17).

In the second edition of our book, one chapter examined the roles of physicians and nurses in health promotion, discussed the gap between their clinical practices and their discourse, as well as the challenges of integrating health promotion into their basic training (Hills, Carrol & Vollman, 2007). In this edition, we opted to present the perspectives of a wide array of professions and practitioners involved in health promotion practice to illustrate the diversity of the workforce. We have collected short contributions that discuss the situation of current health promotion practice in the following areas of practice: medicine, nursing, nurse practitioners, rehabilitation, community development, policy-making, health communication, and journalism. A final section discusses interprofessional practice, a key element very frequently advocated in health promotion practice. Each author, selected because of his or her professional knowledge and experience, was asked to identify promising practices in the field. A few remarks are presented from the gathered material in the concluding section of the chapter, which also has some questions to stimulate critical thinking and a list of further resources.

Health Promotion as a Lab Service for Primary Care[1]

Robert Perreault

Primary care physicians acknowledge that prevention is good, but no one has time to promote it to patients. In a typical visit, not more than one minute is available to deal with prevention (Baghelai, Nelkin & Miller, 2009). There are obstacles with reimbursement and in finding ways to cue the doctor about a patient's prevention needs. Electronic medical records are best suited for the task, but are not yet widely available (Webster, 2010). Without tracking tools, few doctors remember to address prevention.

We have implemented a platform that aims to address most of the obstacles to increasing clinical prevention. A consultation with 60 primary care physicians from diverse types of clinics identified smoking cessation, nutrition, and physical activity counselling as priorities for support. An extensive literature review confirmed this to be appropriate (Voelker, 2010).

To reach beyond the first adopters, our intervention had to extend the doctor's influence and, at the same time, not burden clinic routines. We tried to work around the obstacles by creating what is essentially a new lab service. In each of Montreal's 12 autonomous health jurisdictions, we organized a clinical prevention system around three components: a nurse facilitator (Murphy-Smith, Meyer, Hitt et al., 2004) in charge of calling on doctors to introduce the prevention support services; a primary care doctor from each major clinic who acts as a public health champion (Soo, Berta & Baker, 2009); and a local Health Education Centre that offers a lifestyle work-up. This resource makes prevention and health promotion more easily accessible and the "prevention minute" can be used to refer patients to the centre.

In the waiting room, patients fill out a short questionnaire to determine their interest in talking about nutrition, physical activity, or smoking cessation. It also monitors perceived self-efficacy. The questionnaire cues the doctor to prescribe the lifestyle work-up: a web-based health risk appraisal with printed personalized recommendations followed by a motivational interview and telephone or face-to-face follow-up. A summary report is sent to the referring physician.

Does it work? We had a slow start but, in our fourth year we are seeing more and more signs of the project's integration into routine practice. Our data suggest that the centres are being used as a resource for patients with risk factors for chronic conditions. This is a shift from their original intent, which was to offer lifestyle counselling to healthy people as a primary prevention measure.

The medical community has a strong unmet need for secondary prevention, which has created a *de facto* reorientation of the centres' mission. This underlines the challenges of positioning health promotion services in the medical clinical environment.

Other obstacles include time constraints, unease at addressing lifestyle issues, difficulty going from a prescriptive mode to a motivational mode, worries about raising issues that they have no capacity to treat, and the absence of fee-for-service.

Difficulties for health system managers include working with physicians they have no authority over and assigning competent personnel to the tasks required by the program while dealing with competing demands.

Difficulties for clinical prevention support nurses include problems reaching doctors and describing a model that is not specifically clinical.

Nevertheless, the program is gaining recognition. Strategies have been put in place to make the program more appealing to physicians. These range from educational materials for physicians and nurses, to tools for patients, to updated lists of local community resources adapted to various patient profiles.

This region-wide approach seems to be showing the beginnings of an effect on the behaviour of primary care physicians. Many questions have yet to be answered and further evaluation is needed in order to determine the best fit to meet the needs of patients, physicians, and public health. Would other health professionals find prevention to be closer to their preoccupations? Alternatively, should we target the general public more directly using "demand management" strategies such as web portals and intelligent device platforms that support self-management of clinical prevention, thus helping people come better prepared for their medical visits?

In closing, your feedback would be most welcome. I may be reached at rperreau@sante-pub-mtl.qc.ca.

The Symbiotic Relationship of Nursing and Health Promotion: Promising Practices from Education, Research, and Practice

Marcia Hills and Clémence Dallaire

Nursing and health promotion share a value base that makes health promotion a gift to nursing, and nursing a guiding light for health promotion. The purpose of this section is to highlight promising practices in nursing education, practice, and research that articulate the symbiotic relationship between nursing and health promotion.

Nursing, as a discipline, has had a difficult time "growing up" mostly because of its ambiguous and difficult relationship with medicine. Often there is confusion between nursing and medicine's domains of practice. In the 1980s nursing was like an adolescent. Health promotion was one of the developments that helped launch it into early adulthood. Health promotion helped nursing reclaim its domain of practice as primarily being concerned with people and their experiences of health and healing with a focus on caring, whereas medicine's domain was on diagnosing and treating diseases with a focus on curing. There is, of course, an overlap between these disciplines. However, because nurses began to embrace a health promotion perspective, they were able to articulate core caring practices based on health promotion principles.

Many have argued that health promotion is not a discipline and while that debate is beyond the scope of this section, we argue that when a discipline is young and evolving, it relies on more mature sister disciplines to support its evolution. Health promotion and nursing share this "path."

Promising Practices in Nursing Health Promotion Education, Research, and Practice

Education

For many years, nursing was entrenched in a behavioural, medically based, disease-oriented model of education that failed to recognize nursing foundations of human caring science.

Fortunately, this is changing as nursing works more from a health promotion perspective, embracing this human caring science as the appropriate way to educate future nurses (Hills & Watson, 2011; Boykin, Touhy & Smith, 2011; Hills & Lindsey, 1994; Lewis, Rogers & Naef, 2006).

Using a health promotion framework to develop nursing programs provides a rationale for empowering and emancipatory pedagogies in a way that no education theory could have done. Education in nursing has a long history of "power over" relationships. If we are to be successful in developing curricula based on a health promotion perspective, we need to join students as partners in the learning process. In addition, it seems reasonable to expect that students who have experienced empowerment in their education would be more likely to use principles of equity and empowerment when they work with their clients (Hills & Lindsey, 1994). The health promotion concepts of equity, participation, empowerment, and collaboration are easily recognizable in most nursing curricula today. As nursing programs continue to advance their curricula from a health promotion perspective, they provide leadership and demonstrate how other disciplines could do the same (Hills & Watson, 2011).

Research

Nursing has contributed to health promotion research in many areas, but the one that stands out as exemplary is primary health care, which relates to the *Ottawa Charter*'s action area of "Reorienting Health Services." Although the uptake of primary health care (PHC) was slow during the 1970s and early 1980s, with the advent of the *Ottawa Charter* (World Health Organization, 1986), there was a major professional mobilization in nursing in relation to PHC and the new health promotion (MacDonald, 2000; Roger & Gallagher, 1985). The Canadian Nurses Association (CNA), provincial nursing associations across Canada, the Canadian Public Health Association, nursing scholars, and educators all endorsed and studied PHC as the basis of nursing practice (CNA, 1988; Clarke & Mass, 1998; Brown & Piper, 1997; Butterfield, 1990).

Practice

Many would argue that health promotion nursing is an activity that belongs solely in a community setting. However, with approximately 90 percent of nurses working in hospitals, we need to ask: What would it look like if we practise nursing from a health promotion perspective in acute care settings? Is there a role for health promotion in acute care? When you view health promotion from a philosophical perspective—that is, as a "way of being" that embraces partnerships, collaboration, equity, empowerment, and participation—there is no question that nursing, from a health promotion perspective, is critical to all nursing practice, including acute, emergency, and intensive care. As nurses begin to implement this health promotion nursing practice in these challenging settings, nurses contribute to the development of health promotion theories and practices.

Nurses who are educated from a health promotion perspective do practise nursing from this perspective in acute care settings (Hills, 1998, 2000). Studies that examined students' practice journals revealed three overall themes and several sub-themes that were consistent with health promotion. These included: the centrality of caring for the person, not the disease;

empowerment with the sub-themes of partnership, participation, and power; and, finally, the primacy of people. Nurses are continuing to push the boundaries of health promotion in all settings where nurses work, and this promising practice will contribute to the overall health promotion movement in Canada.

According to the Royal College of Nursing:

> The nursing workforce remains very much a sleeping giant. Its huge size means that nurses have enormous potential as agents of social control in promoting health and well-being. It does not take too much to imagine what the impact might be if over half a million people (plus many more nurses in the world) became empowered, assertive and articulate agents of change for better health promotion. (Royal College of Nursing, 1998, p. 12)

Nurses can also influence other disciplines to explore health promotion as a viable perspective from which to practise because they are the largest group of professionals working in the health care system, because of the passion that they display when talking about health promotion, and because of their shared value base with health promotion. This insight provides the moment of opportunity for all disciplines to recognize the synergy that health promotion provides to actually practise in collaborative, intersectoral, multidisciplinary ways.

Nurse Practitioners

Judith Burgess

Nurse Practitioners in Primary Health Care

The nurse practitioner (NP) role has been formally introduced in all Canadian provinces/ territories through enabling legislation, regulation, and education programs (Canadian Nurses Association [CNA], 2006). Legislation has given NPs the autonomy to: diagnose a disease, disorder, or condition; order and interpret diagnostic and screening tests; prescribe medications; and perform advanced clinical procedures. Provincial/territorial nursing bodies regulate NPs and set the standards, conditions, and limitations for practice. Educational programs for NPs are committed to or moving toward graduate-level designation. NPs are experienced registered nurses with additional education to offer holistic clinical care, health promotion, population health, and collaborative partnership. The aim of the NP's role is to complement physician functions of illness care through the value-added of an integrated approach (Burgess & Purkis, 2010).

Politics of the Nurse Practitioner Role

The NP role is decidedly political because it represents a new way of delivering primary health care (PHC) to clients and communities. This new PHC, referred to as integrative or comprehensive PHC (Boon et al., 2004), aligns well with the recent efforts of the World Health Organization (2008) to revitalize the Alma Ata Declaration (World Health Organization, 1978). WHO highlights four PHC reforms, all of which have applicability to the NP's role, and include: universal coverage with emphasis on access, health equity, and social justice; socially relevant and responsive health services; public policy to integrate public health with primary care; and leadership reforms to bring about inclusion and participation. Located in varied PHC settings, NPs employ flexible practice patterns to provide client-centred care and respond to community needs. The NP's role is expected to improve access for marginalized populations and address social justice issues (Browne & Tarlier, 2008), as well as catalyze a team approach in PHC (Keith & Askin, 2008). These promising practices of NPs can shift the vision and effects of PHC.

The *Ottawa Charter* (World Health Organization, 1986) was built on the Alma Ata Declaration (World Health Organization, 1978) to emphasize prerequisites for health, and identify international actions that would more effectively address the ecological interactions of biology, behaviour, and environment (Stokols, 1996). NPs as change agents are well positioned to advance health promotion actions and interventions, which have historically been taken up as issues, populations, and settings (Frohlich & Poland, 2007). The NP's role situated in community health centres (CHCs) is a promising practice that exemplifies an ecological approach in addressing health issues, at-risk populations, and social settings. With over 300 CHCs in Canada, NPs can effectively advance the health of clients, populations, and communities.

Promising Practices of Nurse Practitioners in Community Health Centres

CHCs are non-profit, community-governed, team-based organizations that provide comprehensive PHC (Canadian Alliance of Community Health Centre Associations, 2009). Quebec's centre local de services communautaires (CLSC) further combines health and social services into a one-stop shop model. Within CHCs, NP practice emulates the *Ottawa Charter*'s actions to enable, advocate, and mediate (World Health Organization, 1986). NPs provide direct clinical services, focus on health issues such as chronic diseases, and offer lifestyle education and counselling, thereby enabling clients to have more control over their individual health status. NPs are often linked to such at-risk populations as Aboriginal peoples, new immigrants/refugees, marginalized youth, the homeless, and frail seniors, and in advocating for improved social conditions for disenfranchised groups, NPs have notable impact on population health status. They also have a mediating presence in bridging intersectoral collaborations and bringing together community stakeholders to attend to problematic social settings and environmental conditions that affect health status. In the CHC model, the promising practice of NPs is to enable, advocate, and mediate in an ecological model of care and thus address individual, population, and environmental dimensions of health.

Health Promotion Practice in Rehabilitation in Canada

Kadija Perreault and Donna Anderson

In 1996, Renwick, Brown, Rootman, and Nagler stated that rehabilitation had just started integrating health promotion. Fifteen years later, we explored the subject by searching the literature and contacting key informants.

Rehabilitation "aims to enable people with health conditions experiencing or likely to experience disability to achieve and maintain optimal functioning in interaction with the environment" (Stucki, Cieza & Melvin, 2007, p. 282). It is practised in health, education, labour, and social affairs. In the health sector alone, it involves professionals such as occupational therapists, physiotherapists, speech-language pathologists, nurses, doctors, social workers, and psychologists.

Many authors and some professional groups (e.g., the Canadian Physiotherapy Association) have advocated incorporating health promotion principles and practices in rehabilitation. For O'Neill and Stirling (2006), health promotion can be applied at any stage of a health problem, including rehabilitation. Rimmer (1999) conceptualized health promotion as an extension of the rehabilitation continuum into one's environment. Brown, Renwick, and Nagler (1996) stated that quality of life is health promotion and rehabilitation's common outcome. Still, conceptual links between the two are scarcely addressed.

On a practical level, health promotion lacks integration in rehabilitation. For instance, searching the Canadian Best Practices Portal for Health Promotion (http://cbpp-pcpe.phac-aspc. gc.ca/) for "rehabilitation" provided three results, none of them Canadian-based. A search in the Database of International Rehabilitation Research (http://cirrie.buffalo.edu/search/index.php) for "health promotion" and "Canada" yielded only 27 results. In addition, many papers discuss health promotion for people with disabilities, but don't make explicit links with rehabilitation.

Based on our knowledge and contact with informants, we contend there are nonetheless many health promotion practices in rehabilitation in Canada, e.g., health education and physical activity for people with disabilities. However, such practices are under-documented, not easily accessed, nor explicitly labelled as "health promotion." We highlight two practices. The first, Traité santé, is the Quebec City–region rehabilitation program aiming to improve quality of life. It contains individual and group-based activities relating to physical activity, nutrition, smoking cessation, psychosocial issues, sexuality, and spirituality. The program clearly defines rehabilitation along a continuum with prevention, and its main activities and objectives can be linked with health promotion. Furthermore, interventions are based on theories of behaviour change. The second, Quebec's Stand up!, a province-wide, 12-week falls-prevention program for seniors, is implemented by rehabilitation professionals in community-based organizations. The program includes home and group exercises, and information/discussion sessions. The objectives include increasing balance and strength, developing abilities to reduce the risk of falls in the home, and adopting safe behaviours and active lifestyles. Yet, health promotion was not clearly conceptualized in these two practices, as is true for the majority of practices we identified. Hence, we wonder to what extent they actually share common assumptions and values with health promotion.

But what could explain the lack of explicit integration of health promotion in rehabilitation? An underlying issue may be their different definitions of health (Brandon, 1985). Many rehabilitation professionals, although encouraged to take on a broader definition of health, continue to define it as the absence of disease (Grönblom-Lundstrom, 2001). For these fields to come together, rehabilitation would have to embrace a broader definition of health. Including health promotion in rehabilitation may require professionals to assume new roles beyond the traditional one-on-one clinician. For example, Majnemer (2009) envisions rehabilitation professionals advocating for policy change to facilitate participation of children with disabilities. Meanwhile, brief appointments in outpatient settings may leave little time for health promotion (Stuifbergen & Rogers, 1997). Also, some Canadian rehabilitation professionals may not see health promotion as their responsibility or know how to integrate it in their practice (Davis & Chesbro, 2003). To our knowledge, health promotion has only recently been integrated into rehabilitation professionals' basic training in Canada. But even if health promotion is present in many Canadian rehabilitation-related programs (e.g., University of Manitoba and Université Laval), to what extent is it covered and integrated into practice?

Overall, although practices exist, explicitly defined and conceptualized health promotion practices appear limited in rehabilitation in Canada. There is certainly a need to further explore links between both fields.

Improving Access to Recreation for Low-Income Women: A Community Development Approach to Health Promotion

Pamela Ponic and Wendy Frisby

Community development (CD) is a dynamic process in which community members combine their skills, knowledge, and resources to collectively take action to address social, economic, and health issues of common concern (Adams, Witten & Conway, 2009). The practice of CD is long-standing, yet the term "community" is itself contested. While most often defined by static categories of geography, identity, or social cause, Walter (2005) depicts communities as multidimensional to illustrate how "people and organizations, consciousness, actions, and context are integrally related with one another forming the whole that is community" (p. 68). Historically, CD is grounded in values of democracy, equity, and inclusion, such that it is initiated by and benefits community members (Leishner, 2004). As well as addressing the issues at hand, CD can foster skill-building and decision-making power within communities. Yet CD is not a neutral process; it is infused with inequitable power relations and shaped by varying and sometimes competing social, economic, and political conditions (Frisby, Reid & Ponic, 2007). These forces can make CD very challenging in practice. Consciously navigating and reflecting on power imbalances and contexts is central because it is these very inequities that need to be redressed to promote health, particularly for members of marginalized social groups (see Chapter 11—the reflexive practitioner). Community-level health promotion is a foundational strategy outlined in the *Ottawa Charter* because of its potential for individual, organizational, and social change (Chappell et al., 2006). The following example illustrates the promise of CD for health promotion, and the tensions and complexities associated with conducting it across power and other differences (e.g., race, class, gender, and health status).

Promising Practice: Women Organizing Activities for Women

Women Organizing Activities for Women (WOAW) was a health promotion initiative designed to improve low-income women's access to local recreation. Recreation was provided through a community-development strategy whereby the women involved in WOAW, with the support of local service providers and academic researchers, decided upon and organized recreational activities that would address some of their core health issues. WOAW strove to organize itself such that women were "empowered, respected, and connected" across their diversity, all of which are core community-development values. This approach stands in contrast to traditional top-down and user-pay public recreation programming, which often excludes poor women from participation (Taylor & Frisby, in press).

WOAW evolved from a workshop designed to facilitate community discussion about how low-income women could access recreation to promote their health. Over 85 diverse women and service providers enthusiastically participated, and the women confirmed the importance of recreation in addressing their key barriers to health, which they identified as social isolation, stress, and physical inactivity. WOAW existed for six years, and members organized and attended hundreds of social, physical, educational, and political activities of their choice. The women contributed their organizing and management skills; service providers contributed access to facilities and local resources; and the researchers provided funding, academic knowledge, and facilitation. WOAW operated under feminist organizing principles, including a non-hierarchical structure, consensus decision-making, and shared leadership (Frisby, Reid & Ponic, 2007). For nearly all WOAW activities, transportation and child care were provided. Members reported that their participation in WOAW reduced their stress and enhanced their social support and activity levels, all of which helped them better cope with their health issues (Ponic, 2007). Importantly, they also stated that it was WOAW's collaborative CD process, as much as the activities themselves, that promoted their health.

Alongside WOAW's successes, there were many challenges common in CD practice. Numerous conflicts emerged among the membership, typically regarding issues of inclusion and exclusion. These conflicts perpetuated traditional power relations and thus flew in the face of the values from which we were attempting to operate. Further, resources diminished over time, particularly as neo-liberal governments cut social services and the service providers had to withdraw their participation. In the end, these problems resulted in WOAW's demise, despite some members' attempts to keep it alive. This example illustrates that CD is a long-term endeavour that requires time, resources, and a willingness to embrace complexity. Navigating the tensions and power differences is essential so as not to recreate patterns of exclusion and marginalization that perpetuate the very health issues that CD is attempting to redress.

Policy-making in Health Promotion

Louise St-Pierre and Anika Mendell

Influencing policy-making in order to foster healthy public policy requires health promoters to develop new knowledge and skills, work in an intersectoral manner, and use appropriate tools. Health impact assessment (HIA) is a promising practice to help accomplish these goals. Indeed, this tool allows health promoters to participate in the policy-making process and to collaborate with actors outside the health sector, and can be used at local or higher levels of government. Below, we present HIA and its links to the policy-making process, and provide a Canadian example of HIA.

What Is HIA?

Health impact assessment is a five-step, prospective process to evaluate the potential health effects of a policy proposal from outside the health sector. The first step, *screening*, establishes whether an HIA is warranted and determines the level of analysis (rapid versus in-depth) of the HIA. The next step, *scoping*, consists of planning the HIA and determining the information and resources that will be required. *Appraisal* is the actual HIA. It consists of collecting and analyzing information. During the *reporting* step, results are shared with stakeholders in a written report that contains recommendations. Finally, the last step, *evaluation and monitoring*, is an opportunity to determine the effects of the HIA.

A Health Promotion Tool

HIA stems from two sources: Environmental impact assessment (EIA) and health promotion (Kemm, Parry & Palmer, 2004). The values and principles of HIA (democracy, equity, citizen participation, empowerment, ethical use of evidence, and intersectoral action) (Quigley et al., 2006) originate from health promotion. Indeed, the practice of HIA reflects the orientations of the *Ottawa Charter for Health Promotion* (World Health Organization, 1986), most particularly in its potential to build healthy public policy and create supportive environments.

This tool is based on a perspective that values both quantitative and qualitative methods, giving importance to "scientific knowledge" and to "civic science." It is rooted in a holistic model of health (see Dahlgren & Whitehead, 1991) that considers a wide range of health determinants, particularly the social determinants. Concern for health equity is also embedded in HIA as the appraisal must assess not only the impact but the distribution of these effects on different subgroups of the population. A major benefit of the HIA process is that it creates opportunity for intersectoral action, bringing together public health experts, policy-makers, and citizens to discuss how a proposal may impact the determinants of health and how to mitigate the negative impacts and maximize the positive effects.

The Policy-Making Perspective

The principal aim of HIA is to clarify for decision-makers the various ways in which policies influence health and to ensure that health considerations are not overlooked. As such, HIA could be considered as a policy analysis tool (Putters, 2005). Furthermore, since HIA provides health information tailored to one specific situation under consideration by decision-makers (before the final decision is made), it has the potential to shape policy.

A Canadian Example

Used widely in Europe, HIA is beginning to be applied in Canada. One recent HIA took place in the region of Montérégie, Quebec. The regional public health authority, along with the local health centre and three municipalities, undertook three HIA projects with the objective of implementing HIA as a decision-making tool at the municipal level.

One of the projects to be assessed was the development of a domestic waste-management plant, which would transform domestic waste into compost. Six potential risk factors arose during the *screening* stage. Among them was housing affordability due to the expected increase in municipal taxes. In fact, the report demonstrated that one-third of city households already devote more than 30 percent of their income to housing, and stated that this change might put pressure on households to reduce their expenses on essential goods. These results provided an opportunity to discuss health inequalities with decision-makers and to underline the importance of the cumulative effects of municipal decisions on disadvantaged groups.

HIA certainly has limitations. For one, it is difficult to document its effect on health. What has been shown, however, is that HIA provides a structured approach that leads to a better understanding of the effects of policy on health, while promoting intersectoral action and strengthening the decision-making process (Wismar et al., 2007). For this reason, HIA is used internationally, and various public health organizations in Canada consider it to be a key strategy in working toward healthy public policy.

Promising Practices in Health Communication

Larry Hershfield and Lise Renaud [2]

What Is It?

Health communication is the study and the use of different communication strategies (e.g., interpersonal, mass media) to inform and influence the individual and collective decisions conducive to the improvement of health (Caron-Bouchard & Renaud, 2001). There are many different ways of classifying and organizing health communication. For example, Maibach and Holtgrave (1995) suggested several types of health communication. These include:

- *social marketing*, which traditionally focuses on changing individual behaviour by increasing perceived benefits relative to cost
- *risk communication and behavioural decision-making*, which considers various types of risk, and determines what individual and collective action is preferable
- *media advocacy*, which is the practice of working with mass media to advance healthy public policy
- *entertainment education*, which leverages the benefits of entertainment media in terms of reach and attention (such as soap operas) with embedded pro-health messages
- *interactive decision-support systems*, which provide people with tools that help them to make informed decisions

Societal technology trends are greatly influencing the field of health communication. For example, the rapid increase in Internet use has significantly shaped the way many Canadians learn about health issues and has expanded their options for ways to engage others on these issues.

Underlying the use of these new technologies is a set of skills called e-health literacy, which expands traditional concepts of literacy to include skills in computer use, science, and media awareness, along with basic reading, writing, and computation skills (Norman & Skinner, 2006).

One might also add the more recently described type of health communication, namely, communication for social change or communication to promote social development (Waisbord, 2001), which combines specific health changes with broader health promotion values such as increased connectivity, social capital, capacity, and empowerment.

Another way of looking at health communication is through different theoretical and research traditions of communication. These include rhetorical, semiotic, cybernetic, socio-cultural, critical, and other disciplines. The reader is encouraged to refer to Babrow and Mattson's chapter in the *Handbook of Health Communication* (2003) for further illumination.

Finally, perhaps the most practical way to define or describe a health communication effort is to locate it at a particular ecological level (i.e., individual, network, organizational, societal) (Flora, Maibach & Maccoby, 1989). Each level focuses on a unique purpose and certain types of audiences.

Is It Effective?

Researchers generally agree that well-planned and executed health communication campaigns can be effective in increasing awareness, changing attitudes, and changing behaviours in the short term. For example, Snyder et al.'s (2004) unique work on meta-analysis of mediated health communication campaigns found that short-term health behaviour changes in the 5–9 percent range might result from exposure to mass media campaigns. Although effects are typically modest in size, they can translate into a significant public health impact because they reach large numbers of people directly and indirectly.

There are many guides (see, for instance, Abroms & Maibach, 2008) available on how to design a good health communication campaign, but unifying features include an emphasis on audience research, application of suitable theoretical models, and adequate resources to ensure sufficient reach and frequency of messages.

The health communication practitioner must understand and apply theories of change, such as how to address issues of self-efficacy through communication (at various levels of intervention), as well as issues related to message effects themselves (such variables as vividness, source credibility, one-sided or two-sided arguments).

Also, it is also widely accepted that a well-designed campaign is most effective in the context of multiple strategies.

Example of Well-Designed Individual-Level Canadian Health Communication Efforts

In 2005, a 12-week health promotion campaign in Quebec introduced a multimedia communication strategy in which a website was used to supply information and to serve as an accompaniment to support individual engagement with the campaign (Renaud & Caron-Bouchard, 2010). The *Défi Santé 5/30* or 5/30 Health Challenge was intended to reinforce behaviours related to healthy eating and the regular practice of physical activity. This communications strategy offered the public the ability to personally engage in a "health challenge" by setting objectives to attain over the course of the campaign. The campaign's media use and impact were evaluated using a telephone survey (n = 609), discussion groups with individuals (n = 102) who had been exposed to the campaign, and with health professionals (n = 32).

The *Défi Santé 5/30* demonstrated that a website using virtual, media-based, interpersonal and technical accompaniment can contribute to behavioural change: 94 percent modified their fruit and vegetable consumption; 80 percent completed their physical activities objectives. It also supported the findings from the literature that certain characteristics can contribute to the development of motivation and fidelity in users, including: specific objectives of the site; content; architecture and usage techniques; media convergence and contribution of partners; and an accompaniment approach that is at once virtual, media-based, and interpersonal while also using contributions from health professionals. Non-facilitating factors were also noted: technical and socio-cultural accessibility, and ethics and constraints related to the participation of health professionals.

In conclusion, health communication supports a broad variety of health promotion approaches and goals.

Promoting Health through Health Information: The Evolving Role of the Journalist

Yanick Villedieu

For a long time, journalists dealing with health issues in media for the general public had as their only source experts, mainly physicians and researchers in the field. Health information was thus almost exclusively about medicine and its wonders.

However, the medical model began to be challenged during the 1970s. *A New Perspective on the Health of Canadians*, published in 1974, suggested a broader view of health and its determinants, a view that sees medical services as only one element of a broader health field (see Chapter 1). At the same time, Ivan Illich (1975) published a book called *Medical Nemesis*, which came as a bombshell in which he questioned the correlation between the intensity of the medical act and the frequency of healing. From then on, health information was no longer exclusively the point of view of experts in curative medicine.

The challenge to the classical medical paradigm continued in the 1980–1990s. With the emergence of HIV/AIDS and the politicization of health issues, a newcomer, namely, the patient, inserted himself between the expert and the journalist. This new patient questions, inquires, criticizes, insists on having answers, takes action, organizes powerful community groups, and becomes an activist. Sometimes as expert as the expert, these patients influence research priorities, request new services, and take positions in the media. The doctor-patient relationship changes: the patient no longer wants to be subjected to the knowledge and decisions of a powerful physician; on the contrary, he or she wants to take part in the management of his or her illness. This kind of relation to the medical world developed by HIV/AIDS patients then extended to other illnesses, from breast cancer to psychiatric disorders or diabetes. Health and medical information naturally followed this evolution and, more and more, the patient has a word in the media.

The end of 1990s has seen the emergence of a new player on the health information scene: the Internet. A large number of health and medical sites appear on the web. They are followed by blogs, Facebook, Twitter, and the others. Rarely has a new technology spread this fast. According to the Internet World Stats website, 266 million North Americans (or 77.4 percent of the population) were "Internet users" on June 30, 2010 (http://www.internetworldstats. com/stats2.htm). A survey from Yahoo, published in September 2010, showed that 62 percent of Quebecers find health-related information on the Internet (Web Montréal, 2010). And they have a lot to read: typing "treatment for breast cancer" on Google in December 2010 generated 1.3 million hits in French in 0.37 of a second and over 3 million hits in English in 0.24 of a second! Today, health and medical information is no longer limited to traditional media, in which the journalist reports the point of view of experts and patients. This information is also developed by new non-conventional media.

People quickly discover that there is a lot on the web in terms of health and medicine. There are excellent sites, well designed and credible, providing scientifically sound information; most of the time, these sites are created by universities, governments, or other solid institutions. However, there are also sites and blogs produced by self-proclaimed experts, by the supporters of phoney theories, if not by charlatans. These sites and blogs frequently spread scientifically questionable information while pretending to reveal "the real truth" that classical science "hides" from the general public. As was noticeable during the fall of 2009, when the H1N1 flu pandemic was expected, the web and its tools of instantaneous communication offered such people considerable power to disseminate their ideas. The recent claim of a new "miracle treatment" for multiple sclerosis (by unblocking veins that drain the blood in the brain) is another example of questionable medical information, which, when passed on and amplified on the web, attracts desperate and certainly naive patients.

So, the web has drastically changed the rules in terms of spreading and circulating information. It also greatly changes the way a journalist now works. The health and medicine journalist no longer deals only with experts and patients. He or she now has access to a phenomenal amount of scientific articles, reports, studies, and press releases. Access to that much information is certainly a good thing, but there are also pernicious effects. Since the information has to be treated more and more rapidly, not to say instantaneously, the journalist runs the risk of providing only a superficial perspective, forgetting nuances or giving excessive importance to news of little significance, while highlighting the surprising or the unusual, and may be gradually pushed into the trap of sensationalism.

At a time when the non-conventional media become increasingly popular while traditional media are pressured by newcomers and new practices in the information field, journalists in health and medicine must rigorously check the facts, stick to reliable sources, put the information in perspective, and not create false hopes in patients or populations.

A good example of that is the "flu desk," created by Radio-Canada's Information Service during the so called "flu vaccine crisis" in November 2009. This desk, rapidly nicknamed "quarantine's bureau" by colleagues in the newsroom, gathered journalists from television, radio, and web services, including two scientific and medical reporters, who attended each morning the main production meeting of the information service of the Radio-Canada's French network, where decisions were made about the coverage of the crisis. Essentially, we were checking facts and sources before going on air. From my point of view and according to some comments from colleagues, the flu desk, which operated approximately from 6 a.m. to 6 p.m. over three weeks, provided scientifically and medically sound information to the public.

What if novelty would just maintain the classical methods and tenets of sound and ethical journalism?

Interprofessional Collaboration

Diane Morin and Serge Dumont

In order to establish a basis for a common comprehension of interprofessional collaboration (IPC) in relation to health promotion (HP), we will first present a definition of IPC and then discuss how IPC is embedded in the larger and more complex reality of intersectoral collaboration. Finally, arguments on why the *P* in IPC should be the target of more attention will be addressed.

Interprofessional Collaboration (IPC): What Are We Talking about?

The growing complexity of factors that influence health and illness require health profession-als from diverse professions to work together in a collaborative manner. IPC is defined by D'Amour et al. (2005) as a set of relationships and interactions that enable health profession-als to pool their expertise and share their knowledge and experience in a concerted effort to deliver health services for the greater good. IPC's definition also evolves in relation to four major groups of factors: (1) the nature and the importance of problems for which people have to work together (e.g., HP programs, policy development); (2) the way collaboration is viewed within a given context (e.g., values, beliefs, experience); (3) the type of stakeholders involved (e.g., health-related or social work professionals, administrators, patients, families); and, finally, (4) the type of organization within which they work (e.g., NGO, hospital, com-munity care centre). However, very little is known about the specific contribution of IPC to better health outcomes in relation to the important role that patients, families, and com-munities play in HP processes.

Nevertheless, a recent synthesis review supports the view that IPC is associated with posi-tive outcomes for patients, clients, providers, and the health system (Barrett et al., 2007). More specifically, this seems to be the case when it is fostered and supported on the basis of servicing geographic populations or population health programs driven by health models. Also, studies examining IPC as a variable associated with positive outcomes in health care created such interest in the 1990s and early 2000s in Canada, the US, and Europe that interprofessional, collaborative, patient-centred care was formerly put on national research agendas. Finally, although IPC is not the only variable leading to health benefits, it is considered among a top five associated in multi-collinear relationships with enhanced outcomes. The other four variables are: (1) the presence and use of evidence-based practice; (2) access to services (Pineault et al., 2005); (3) continuity of care (Haggerty et al., 2003); and (4) synergy (Irvine et al., 2002; Jones & Barry, 2010).

Health Promotion as a Precursor in Collaboration Schemes

Since the release of the *Ottawa Charter* (World Health Organization, 1986), collaboration between the health, community, and policy sectors is widely accepted as a means to promote better states of well-being. Therefore, the health sector recognizes the influence of health determinants other than those directly related to health and health care (Wilkinson & Marmot, 2004) and also recognizes that, through IPC and intersectoral collaboration, HP can achieve its goals in more effective, efficient, and sustainable ways (Kreisel & von Schirnding, 1998; World Health Organization, 1998)—for example, in interventions employing multiple actions at multiple levels (individual, family, community, social, policy), as is the case with suicide prevention or domestic violence; interventions requiring intersectoral collaboration (public, private, volunteer), such as the promotion of healthy aging; or those targeting inter-organizational partnerships that require engagement or participation in planning and decision-making, such as the promotion of better nutrition in schools, law enforcement regarding drinking and driving, pandemic preparedness and response, or preparedness for coping with a major crisis or disaster.

An example of how IPC is important to HP can certainly be viewed in secondary prevention for patients throughout their cancer journey, for example. Working together means that health professionals consult their colleagues about the services needed by their patients, about who will provide them and, depending on the nature of the health issue and the availability of resources, what adjustments need to be made to ensure that the care pathway is as efficient as possible.

Interprofessional Collaboration and the Disciplines

We believe that the discipline in which one works not only shapes thoughts and ideas, it also shapes actions. We also think that professional identity derives from one's discipline as well as from the sector in which one works. If this is indeed the case, we are persuaded that in order to improve IPC, greater attention has to be paid to how professional identity develops and consolidates through interprofessional education. Barrett et al. (2007), along with D'Amour and Oandasan (2005), also state that IPC should be studied in relation to interprofessional education as it is still unclear how the ability to work with others to attain a shared goal develops either in action or through education. The latter is certainly of great interest for schools of nursing, medicine, dentistry, pharmacy, and social work, and institutions whose curriculum includes rehabilitation, community development, and health systems management or communication sciences.

Finally, one should remember that IPC is not a new phenomenon in HP. From an early stage it was considered essential because partners involved in HP schemes embrace the vision that they need to share and combine their best resources in order to pursue common goals. Also, it is not because there are needs for collaboration in HP programs that the people involved in day-to-day collaborative schemes really know how to initiate, promote, or conduct IPC successfully. Strategies to improve IPC include exposure to systematic methods of education and teaching of interprofessional collaboration, either in joint curricula or in team settings (Barrett et al., 2007). Finally, in order to support policy, community, and individual efforts in favour of IPC, more scientific work enabling a broader comprehension of IPC in view of the specific complexity of HP should be encouraged (CIHC, 2009).

Conclusion

Sophie Dupéré

This chapter aimed to illustrate the diversity of the workforce and breadth of health promotion practice in Canada. As we saw in Chapter 14, health promotion is not considered a distinct profession or a specialized field of practice in Canada. Health promotion activities are carried out by various professionals and agencies from diverse sectors, health promotion frequently constituting a part, not all, of their function. We collected short reflections on health promotion from the perspectives of a few key professions and practice areas. Although many important voices are missing, each of the five key action areas identified in the *Ottawa Charter* (World Health Organization, 1986) that are considered to be integral to health promotion practice have been covered by the authors:

1. *Building healthy public policy*—St-Pierre and Mendell proposed health impact assessment (HIA) as a promising tool to put health on the agenda of policy-makers in all sectors.
2. *Creating supportive environments* and the importance of adopting an ecological approach to health have been emphasized by some authors (e.g., Burgess).
3. *Strengthening community action* by empowering and enabling communities to improve their health is particularly well developed by Ponic and Frisby.
4. *Developing personal skills* through information, health education, and counselling is also discussed by many of the authors (e.g., R. Perreault; K. Perreault & Anderson; Hershfield & Renaud).
5. *Reorienting the health services toward a stronger health promotion direction*, beyond its responsibility for providing clinical and curative services, has also been discussed, particularly by Burgess, who highlights the promising role of NPs in strengthening primary health care.

The range of ways in which contributors of this chapter undertook their task was broad and there was great diversity in terms of styles and content. Despite this diversity, we note a few common issues across the contributions, particularly on the situation of health promotion in the respective fields of practice. Whereas health promotion has strong and long relationships with certain fields of practice, such as nursing, community development, and health communication, its integration in some fields has been more recent (e.g., rehabilitation) and more difficult, notably in the medical clinical environment, as discussed by R. Perreault. Furthermore, many pointed out similar challenges and obstacles to health promotion practice in their field of practice, such as: the challenge to integrate health promotion into clinical practice and acute care settings because of time constraints, reimbursement mechanisms, inadequate tools, and competing demands; competing social, economic, and political conditions; power imbalances; the rapid rise of social technology; the funding of health promotion activities and neo-liberal government cuts in social and health programs. A few authors also raised the difficulty of evaluating effectiveness and the practice, which remains under-documented.

Several of the authors identified key elements for effective health promotion actions, including: political commitment and leadership; the ecological approach and the combination of strategies operating at multiple levels of structural, community, and individual determinants; bottom-up and participatory approaches; values-based approaches aimed toward empowerment, equity, inclusion, and democracy; time, funding, and the willingness to embrace complexity. A few authors also stressed the importance of interprofessional and intersectoral collaboration.

Apart from presenting some of the diversity of the Canadian health promotion workforce, this chapter and the examples that are cited provide some useful guidance to health promotion practitioners who are interested in learning more about a practice in a specific field.

Notes

1. This project is funded by Montreal's Health and Welfare Agency.
2. The authors would like to thank François Lagarde, Cameron Norman, Jodi Thesenvitz, Gilles Paradis, and Mauricio Gomez for their contributions to the section.

References

Abroms, L. & Maibach, E. (2008). The effectiveness of mass communication to change public behaviour. *Annual Review of Public Health, 29*, 219–234.

Adams, J., Witten, K. & Conway, K. (2009). Community development as health promotion: Evaluating a complex locality-based project in New Zealand. *Community Development Journal, 44*(2), 140–157.

Babrow, A. & Mattson, M. (2003). Theorizing about health communication. In T. Thompson, A. Dorsey, R. Parrott & K. Miller (Eds.), *Handbook of health communication* (pp. 35–63). Mahwah: Lawrence Erlbaum Associates.

Baghelai, M.S., Nelkin, V.S. & Miller, T.R. (2009). *Health risk appraisals in primary care: Current knowledge and potential applications to improve preventive services and chronic care.* Rockville: Final Report—Agency for Healthcare Research & Quality. Retrieved from: http://www.ahrq.gov/clinic/enviroscan/enviroscan.pdf

Barrett, J., Curan, V., Glynn, L. & Godwin, M. (2007). *CHSRF synthesis: Interprofessional collaboration and quality primary healthcare.* Ottawa: CHSRF.

Boon, H., Verhoef, M., O'Hara, D. & Findlay, B. (2004). From parallel practice to integrative health care: A conceptual framework. *BMC Health Services Research, 4*(1), 15. See: http://www.biomedcentral.com/bmchealthservres/4 or http://www.biomedcentral.com/1472-6963/4/15

Boykin, A., Touhy, T. & Smith, M. (2011). *Evolution of a caring-based college of nursing.* In M. Hills & J. Watson, *Creating a caring curriculum: An emancipatory pedagogy for Nursing* 157–184. New York: Springer.

Brandon, J.E. (1985). Health promotion and wellness in rehabilitation services. *Journal of Rehabilitation* (October–November–December), 54–58.

Brown, I., Renwick, R. & Nagler, M. (1996). The centrality of quality of life in health promotion and rehabilitation. In R. Renwick, I. Brown & M. Nagler (Eds.), *Quality of life in health promotion and rehabilitation* (pp. 3–13). Thousand Oaks: Sage Publications.

Brown, P. & Piper, S. (1997). Nursing and the health of the nation: Schism or symbiosis? *Journal of Advanced Nursing, 15,* 297–301.

Browne, A. & Tarlier, D. (2008). Examining the potential of nurse practitioners from a critical social justice perspective. *Nursing Inquiry, 15*(2), 83–93.

Burgess, J. & Purkis, M. (2010). The power and politics of collaboration in nurse practitioner role development. *Nursing Inquiry, 17*(4), 297–308.

Butterfield, P. (1990). Thinking upstream: Nurturing a conceptual understanding of the social context of health behavior. *Advances in Nursing Science, 12*(2), 1–8.

Canadian Alliance of Community Health Centre Associations. (2009). *Community health centres: An integrated approach to strengthening communities, and improving the health and wellbeing of vulnerable Canadians and their families.* Retrieved from: http://www.cachca.ca/resources/documents/CACHCA-FederalrolereCHCdevelopment_000.pdf

Canadian Interprofessional Health Collaborative (CIHC). (2009). *Program evaluation for interprofessional education: A mapping of evaluation strategies of the 20 IECPCP projects.* Vancouver: College of Health Disciplines.

Canadian Nurses Association (CNA). (1988). *Health for all Canadians: A call for health care reform.* Ottawa: CNA.

Canadian Nurses Association (CNA). (2006). *Nurse practitioners: The time is now.* Retrieved from: http://www.cna-nurses.ca/CNA/documents/pdf/publications/cnpi/tech-report/section1/01_Integrated_Report.pdf

Caron-Bouchard, M. & Renaud, L. (2001). *Guide pratique pour mieux réussir vos communications médiatiques en promotion de la santé* (2nd ed.). Quebec: Institut national de santé publique du Québec.

Chappell, N., Funk, L., Carson, A., Mackenzie, P. & Stanwick, R. (2006). Multilevel community health promotion: How can we make it work? *Communication Development Journal, 41*(3), 352–356.

Clarke, H. & Mass, H. (1998). Comox Valley Nursing Centre: From collaboration to empowerment. *Public Health Nursing, 15*(3), 216–224.

Dahlgren, G. & Whitehead, M. (1991). *Policies and strategies to promote social equity in health.* Stockholm: Institute of Future Studies. Retrieved from: http://ideas.repec.org/p/hhs/ifswps/2007_014.html

D'Amour, D., Ferrada-Videla, M., San Martin-Rodriguez, L. & Beaulieu, M.D. (2005). The conceptual basis for interprofessional collaboration: Core concepts and theoretical framework. *Journal of Interprofessional Care, 19*(2) (Supp. 1), 116–131.

D'Amour, D. & Oandasan, I. (2005). Interprofessionality as the field of interprofessional practice and interprofessional education: An emerging concept. *Journal of Interprofessional Care, 1,* 8–20.

Davis, L.A. & Chesbro, S.B. (2003). Integrating health promotion, patient education, and adult education principles with the older adult: A perspective for rehabilitation professionals. *Journal of Allied Health, 32*(2), 106–109.

Flora, J., Maibach, E. & Maccoby, N. (1989). The role of media across four levels of health promotion intervention. *Annual Review of Public Health, 10,* 181–201.

Frisby, W., Reid, C. & Ponic, P. (2007). Leveling the playing field: Promoting the health of poor women through a community development approach to recreation. In K. Young & P. White (Eds.), *Sport and gender in Canada* (pp. 121–136). Don Mills: Oxford University Press.

Frohlich, K. & Poland, B. (2007). Points of intervention in health promotion practice. In M. O'Neill, A. Pederson, S. Dupéré & I. Rootman (Eds.), *Health promotion in Canada: Critical perspectives* (2nd ed.) (pp. 46–60). Toronto: Canadian Scholars' Press Inc.

Ghassemi, M. (2009). *Development of pan-Canadian discipline-specific competencies for health promoters: Summary report consultation results.* Health Promotion Ontario. Retrieved from: http://hpo. squarespace.com/storage/HP%20Competencies%20Consultation%20Summary%20Report%20 March%202009.pdf

Grönblom-Lundstrom, L. (2001). *Rehabilitation in light of different theories of health: Outcome for patients with low-back complaints—a theoretical discussion.* Umeå: Umeå University.

Haggerty, J.L., Reid, R.J., Freeman, G.K., Starfield, B.H., Adair, C.E. & McKendry, R. (2003). Continuity of care: A multidisciplinary review. *British Medical Journal, 327*, 1219–1221.

Hills, M. (1998). Student experiences of nursing health promotion practice in hospital settings. *Nursing Inquiry, 5*, 164–173.

Hills, M. (2000). Perspectives on learning and practicing health promotion in hospitals: Nursing students' stories. In L. Young & V. Hayes (Eds.), *Transforming health promotion practice* (pp. 229–240). Philadelphia: F.A. Davis.

Hills, M., Carrol, S. & Vollman, A. (2007). Health promotion and health professions in Canada: Toward a shared vision. In M. O'Neill et al. (Eds.), *Health promotion in Canada* (2nd ed.) (pp. 330–346). Toronto: Canadian Scholars' Press Inc.

Hills, M. & Lindsey, L. (1994). Health promotion: A viable curriculum framework for nursing education. *Nursing Outlook, 42*, 158–163.

Hills, M. & Watson, J. (2011). *Creating a caring curriculum: An emancipatory pedagogy for nursing.* New York: Springer.

Illich, I. (1975). *Medical nemesis: The expropriation of health.* London: Calder & Boyars.

Irvine, D., Baker, G., Murray, M., Bohnen, J., Zahn, C., Sidani, S. & Carryer J. (2002). Achieving clinical improvement: An interdisciplinary intervention. *Health Care Management Review, 27*(4), 42–56.

Jones, J. & Barry, M.M. (2010). *Developing a scale to measure synergy in health promotion partnerships.* Health Service Executive (HSE) West. Retrieved from http://hdl.handle.net/10147/94574

Keith, K. & Askin, D. (2008). Effective collaboration: The key to better health care. *Journal of Nursing Leadership, 21*(2), 51–61.

Kemm, J., Parry, J. & Palmer, S. (Eds.). (2004). *Health impact assessment.* Oxford: Oxford University Press.

Kreisel, W. & von Schirnding, Y. (1998). Intersectoral action for health: A cornerstone for health for all in the 21st century. *World Health Statistics Quarterly, 51*(1), 75–78.

Lalonde, M. (2004). *A new perspective on the health of Canadians.* Ottawa: Government of Canada.

Leishner, C. (2004). *Building healthy communities: The process.* Prince George: Northern Family Health Society.

Lewis, S., Rogers, M. & Naef, R. (2006). Caring-human science philosophy in nursing education: Beyond the curriculum revolution. *International Journal of Human Caring, 10*(4), 31–37.

McDonald, M. (2002). Health promotion: *Historical, philosophical, and theoretical perspectives. In* L.Young, *& V.Hayes (Eds.), Transforming health promotion practice: Concepts, issues and applications (pp. 22–45). Philadelphia, PA: F. A. Davis and Co.*

Maibach, E. & Holtgrave, D. (1995). Advances in public health communication. *Annual Review of Public Health, 16*, 219–238.

Majnemer, A. (2009). Promoting participation in leisure activities: Expanding role for pediatric therapists. *Physical & Occupational Therapy in Pediatrics, 29*(1), 1–5.

Murphy-Smith, M., Meyer, B., Hitt, J., Taylor-Seehafer, M.A. & Tyler, D.O. (2004). Put prevention into practice implementation model: Translating practice into theory. *Journal of Public Health Management & Practice, 10*(2), 109–115.

Norman, C.D. & Skinner, H. (2006). eHealth literacy: Essential skills for consumer health in a networked world. *Journal of Medical Internet Research, 8*(2) e9. Retrieved from http://www.ncbi.nlm. nih.gov/pmc/articles/PMC1550701/

O'Neill, M. & Stirling, A. (2006). Travailler à promouvoir la santé ou travailler en promotion de la santé? In M. O'Neill, S. Dupéré, A. Pederson & I. Rootman (Eds.), *Promotion de la santé au Canada et au Québec, perspectives critiques* (pp. 42–61). Quebec: Presses de l'Université Laval.

Parker, J. (2005). The art and science of nursing. In J. Daly, S. Speedy, D. Jackson, V. Lambert & C. Lambert, *Professional nursing: Concepts, issues, and challenges* (pp. 51–68). New York: Springer Publishing Company.

Pineault, R., Tousignant, P., Roberge, D., Lamarche, P., Reinharz, D., Larouche, D., Beaulne, G. & Lesage, D. (2005). *Collectif de recherche sur l'organisation des services de santé de première ligne au Québec.* Montreal: Direction de santé publique et Agence de développement de réseaux locaux de services de santé et de services sociaux de Montréal.

Ponic, P. (2007). *Embracing complexity in community-based health promotion: Inclusion, power, and women's health.* Unpublished doctoral dissertation, University of British Columbia, Vancouver.

Putters, K. (2005). HIA, the next step: Defining models and roles. *Environmental Impact Assessment Review, 25*(7–8), 693–701.

Quigley, R., den Broeder, L., Furu, P., Bond, A., Cave, B. & Bos, R. (2006). *Health impact assessment: International best practice principles.* Special Publication Series no. 5. Fargo: International Association for Impact Assessment. Retrieved from: http://www.iaia.org/publicdocuments/special-publications/SP5.pdf

Renaud, L. & Caron-Bouchard, M. (2010). L'impact d'un site internet dans une campagne de promotion de la santé; Le Défi Santé 5/30. In L. Renaud (Ed.), *Les médias et la santé: de l émergence à l'appropriation des normes sociales* (pp. 203–220). Quebec: Presses de l'Université du Québec.

Rimmer, J.H. (1999). Health promotion for people with disabilities: The emerging paradigm shift from disability prevention to prevention of secondary conditions. *Physical Therapy, 79*(5), 495–502.

Roger, G. & Gallagher, S. (1985). The move toward primary health care in Canada: Community health nursing from 1985 to 1995. In M. Stewart (Ed.), *Community nursing: Promoting Canadians' health* (pp. 37–58). Toronto: W.B. Saunders.

Royal College of Nursing (RCN). (1998). *Imagining the future: Nursing in the new millennium.* London: RCN.

Snyder, L., Hamilton, M., Mitchell, E., Kiwanuka-Tondo, J., Fleming-Milici, F. & Proctor, D. (2004). A meta-analysis of the effect of mediated health communication campaigns on behavior change in the United States. *Journal of Health Communication, 9*(Suppl. 1), 71–96.

Soo, S., Berta, W. & Baker, G.R. (2009). Role of champions in the implementation of patient safety practice change. *Health Care Quarterly, 12*(Special Issue), 123–128.

Stokols, D. (1996). Translating social ecological theory into guidelines for community health promotion. *American Journal of Health Promotion, 10*, 282–298.

Stucki, G., Cieza, A. & Melvin, J. (2007). The International Classification of Functioning, Disability, and Health (ICF): A unifying model for the conceptual description of the rehabilitation strategy. *Journal of Rehabilitation Medicine, 39*(4), 279–285.

Stuifbergen, A.K. & Rogers, S. (1997). Health promotion: An essential component of rehabilitation for persons with chronic disabling conditions. *Advances in Nursing Science, 19*(4), 1–20.

Taylor, J. & Frisby, W. (in press). Addressing inadequate leisure access policies through citizen engagement. In D. Reid, H. Mair & S. Arai (Eds.), *Decentering work: Critical perspectives on leisure, development, and social change.* Calgary: University of Calgary Press.

Voelker, R. (2010). Surgeon general's prevention priorities dovetail with health care reform law. *JAMA, 303*, 2123–2124.

Waisbord, S. (2001). *Family tree of theories, methodologies, and strategies in development communication: Convergences and differences.* Retrieved from: http://www.comminit.com/en/node/1547

Walter, C. (2005). Community building practice: A conceptual framework. In M. Minkler (Ed.), *Community organizing & community building for health* (2nd ed.) (pp. 66–78). New Brunswick: Rutgers University Press.

Web Montréal. (2010). *Internet a changé positivement la vie des Québécois et des Canadiens.* Référencement Web Montréal. Retrieved from: http://referencement-web-montreal.com/2010/09/internet-a-change-positivement-la-vie-des-quebecois-et-des-canadiens/

Webster, P.C. (2010). National standards for electronic health records remain remote. *Canadian Medical Association Journal, 182,* 888–889.

Wilkinson, R. & Marmot, M. (2004) *Les déterminants sociaux de la santé: les faits* (2nd ed.). Genève: OMS/Europe.

Wismar, M., Blau, J., Ernst, K. & Figueras, J. (Ed.). (2007). *The effectiveness of health impact assessment: Scope and limitations of supporting decision-making in Europe.* European Observatory on Health Systems and Policies. WHO Regional Office for Europe. Retrieved from: http://www.euro.who.int/__data/assets/pdf_file/0003/98283/E90794.pdf

World Health Organization. (1978). *Primary health care: Report of the international conference on primary health care.* Alma-Ata, USSR. Geneva: WHO.

World Health Organization. (1986). *Ottawa Charter for Health Promotion.* Ottawa: Canadian Public Health Association.

World Health Organization. (1998). *Health promotion glossary.* Geneva: WHO.

World Health Organization. (2008). *The world health report: Primary health care now more than ever.* Retrieved from: http://www.who.int/whr/2008/en/index.html

Critical Thinking Questions

1. From the various examples cited by the authors, choose a promising practice that you find particularly interesting and explain why.

2. Do you think the diversity of the Canadian health promotion workforce is a strength or a weakness? Why?

3. Do you think interprofessional collaboration is an important issue in health promotion? Why or why not?

4. Do you agree with the authors on the strategies suggested to improve interprofessional collaboration? Why or why not?

5. Is there a discipline or a field of practice that is more central in health promotion? If so, explain why.

Resources

Further Readings

Agence de la santé et des services sociaux de la Capitale-Nationale. (2007). *Cadre de référence Traité santé: Programme régional de réadaptation pour la personne atteinte de maladies chroniques.* Retrieved from: http://www.rrsss03.gouv.qc.ca/pdf/CadreRefTraiteSante.pdf

This document is the frame of reference of the Traité santé program, and offers a very detailed description of the program's basis and content.

Brown, I., Renwick, R. & Nagler, M. (1996). The centrality of quality of life in health promotion and rehabilitation. In R. Renwick, I. Brown & M. Nagler (Eds.), *Quality of life in health promotion and rehabilitation* (pp. 3–13). Thousand Oaks: Sage Publications.

Although published a while back, this is a comprehensive book on health promotion and rehabilitation.

Minkler, M. (Ed.). (2005). *Community organizing and community building for health* (2nd ed.). New Brunswick: Rutgers University Press.

A thorough text covering the historical, theoretical, and practical aspects of conducting community-based practices for health.

Oandasan, I. & Reeves S. (2005). Key elements for interprofessional education. Part 1: The learner, the educator, and the learning context. *Journal of Interprofessional Care, Suppl. 1,* 21–38.

This article, although mainly oriented toward education and training, nevertheless highlights the current international status of interprofessional collaboration, presents factors that facilitate collaborative practice, and identifies actions that can be applied to improve health outcomes in the health promotion continuum.

Provost, S., Pineault, R., Levesque, J.-F., Groulx, S., Baron, G., Roberge, D. & Hamel, M. (2010). Does receiving clinical preventive services vary across different types of primary healthcare organizations? Evidence from a population-based survey. *Healthcare Policy, 6*(2), 67–83.

One of the first population-based surveys that deals with the determinants of preventive services in primary care.

WHO. (2010). *Framework for action on interprofessional education and collaborative practice.* Geneva: Division of Health Promotion, Education and Communications (HPR) and Health Education and Health Promotion Unit (HEP)

A recent and useful WHO framework in relation to interprofessional education and collaborative practice.

Relevant Websites

Canadian Alliance of Community Health Centre Associations

http://www.cachca.ca

This site provides information about the Canadian Alliance of Community Health Centre Associations (CACHCA), including history, objectives and values, and defining characteristics of a community health centre (CHC). The site also provides CHC locations across Canada, up-to-date news information, and relevant resources and links.

Canadian Health Services Research Foundation/Canadian Institutes of Health Research Advanced Practice Nursing Chair

http://www.apnnursingchair.mcmaster.ca

This website documents the chair's activities and is a depository for scholarly publications, data collection tool kits, and other related resources.

Canadian Nurses Association

http://www.cna-aiic.ca/CNA/practice/advanced/initiative/default_e.aspx

This site is the home of the Canadian Nurses Association and is also the repository for the Canadian Nurse Practitioner Initiative and a rich library of publications and tool kit resources for NPs and PHC. The site provides information about nursing ethics, standards and best practices, leadership, and patient safety.

Communication Initiative

http://www.comminit.com/en/about-global.html

The Communication Initiative network is an online space for building global bridges between the people and organizations engaged in supporting communication as a fundamental strategy for economic and social development and change. The website includes an extensive selection of publications, research, and discussion platforms.

Community Development and Health Network

http://www.cdhn.org

The Community Development and Health Network is an Ireland-based, member-led organization that aims to make a significant contribution to ending health inequalities by using a community development approach. This website is an excellent example of the scope of community development for health in practice.

Database of International Rehabilitation Research

http://cirrie.buffalo.edu/search/index.php

The Database of International Rehabilitation Research of the Centre for International Rehabilitation Research Information & Exchange for research conducted outside of the US can be searched in English, French, and Spanish.

Health Communication Unit

www.thcu.ca

Founded in 1993, and now located within Public Health Ontario (also known as the Ontario Agency for Health Protection and Promotion), the Health Communication Unit provides training and support to health promotion practitioners in Ontario. THCU offers provincial and regional workshops, as well as webinars, tailored consultations, and quality resource materials. THCU's free online resource database contains capacity-building health promotion resources, including checklists, workbooks, learning communities, educational opportunities, and comprehensive online planning tools.

HIA Connect

www.hiaconnect.edu.au

The site is maintained by the Centre for Health Equity Training, Research, and Evaluation, part of the University of New South Wales. It is one of the most comprehensive websites on HIA. Its newsletters and HIA blog allow people to track the evolution of knowledge and HIA practice worldwide. In addition, this site deals specifically with the impact on health inequalities.

National Collaborating Centre for Healthy Public Policy

http://www.ncchpp.ca/en/

This site gives updated information on the practice of HIA in Canada and abroad, and provides public health actors with more general knowledge to support their practice related to the development of healthy public policy.

On Social Marketing and Social Change

http://socialmarketing.blogs.com

R. Craig Lefebvre (2007) describes himself as an architect and designer of public health and social change programs. His searchable blog is a rich source of resources and commentary about current health communication trends and activities.

Prescription for Health—Promoting Healthy Behaviors in Primary Care

www.prescriptionforhealth.org

Through innovation grants, Prescription for Health helps primary care clinicians aid their patients in addressing risk behaviours.

Stand up!

http://www.santepub-mtl.qc.ca/programmechute/standup.html

This website of the Stand up! program includes a program description, the required training and material to offer the program, as well as related publications.

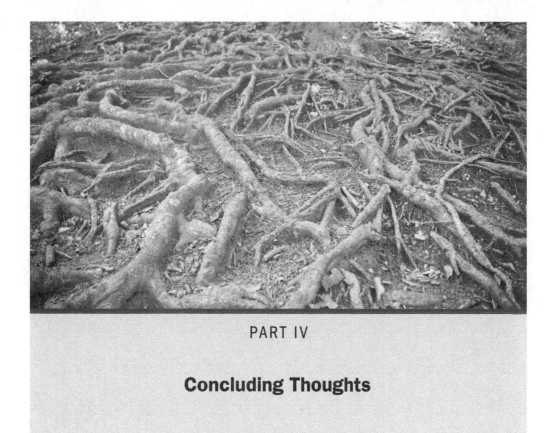

PART IV

Concluding Thoughts

This final section of the book includes a chapter by the editors and an Afterword by Ilona Kickbusch, who also made a significant contribution to the first two editions of the book.

In Chapter 18 we reflect on the developments in health promotion in Canada as a whole through the same sociological and historical lenses adopted in the previous editions of this book. We first discuss the main forces that shape current health promotion practice at the macro level in Canada and globally. We then put forward what we mean by a "promising practice," and why we chose to use this term instead of "best practice" or "evidence-based practice," as well as suggest the characteristics of good practice in health promotion, drawing on examples provided throughout the book. Finally, after considering the evolution of the field since the release of the second edition of this book in 2007, we offer our views on how we think it will develop over the next five years or so, suggesting that it will continue to evolve through paths that were impossible to even imagine 25 years ago when the *Ottawa Charter for Health Promotion* was proclaimed.

In the Afterword, Ilona Kickbusch revisits some of the central messages of the *Ottawa Charter* and considers what became of them in terms of what she called "the rhizome effect" in the second edition of this book. Specifically, she focuses on the following four messages:

(1) the goal of healthy public policy "to move health high on the political agenda"; (2) the challenge of the socio-ecological approach to health, which postulates the "inextricable links between people and their environment"; (3) the notion of "making the healthier choice the easier choice"; and (4) the challenge to go "beyond healthy life-styles to well-being." Among other things, she notes that these four messages represent foresight that is still relevant today. She optimistically concludes that there is a great opportunity to revitalize the health promotion agenda by linking it with the broader social agenda.

CHAPTER 18

Twenty-Five Years of Developing the Roots of Health Promotion in Canada:
Striking a Balance

Michel O'Neill, Ann Pederson, Sophie Dupéré, and Irving Rootman

Introduction

The signature event in the history of health promotion in Canada was, without doubt, the release of the *Ottawa Charter for Health Promotion* in 1986. In the 25 years since, the field of health promotion has been quite resilient, despite difficult moments, and has taken directions that were not necessarily ones that could have been foreseen. In describing the many paths health promotion has taken, it is helpful to employ the metaphor of the contrast between the ways that trees and rhizomes grow, as suggested by Ilona Kickbusch in the second edition of the book. She argued (Kickbusch, 2007) that globally, since the *Ottawa Charter*, health promotion had developed not so much like a tree with strong vertical, visible infrastructure in governments, universities, and other institutions, but like a rhizome.

As noted in Chapter 1, Kickbusch defined a rhizome as a "system that has many roots, that is connected and heterogenic; it does not respect territory but expands continuously ..." (Kickbusch, 2007, p. 363). It spreads horizontally, a bit anarchically and invisibly, but nevertheless successfully infiltrates and influences its environment. In 2007, we argued that if health promotion had the characteristics of both the tree and the rhizome, it might have a stronger impact on the health of populations (Dupéré et al., 2007). Today, Kickbusch reminds us anew (see the Afterword) that health promotion—in the broadest sense of the *Ottawa Charter*—has affected almost every corner of modern and postmodern societies. Yet we remain curious about its specific impact in Canada, its structure, and the balance of its growth pattern: Which metaphor continues to describe it the best?

Our aim in this chapter is to reflect on the developments in health promotion in Canada as a whole through the same sociological and historical lenses we adopted in the previous editions of this book. First, in order to help practitioners reflect on their work, we look at what we consider to be the main forces that shape current health promotion practice at the macro level, here and abroad. Secondly, after discussing what we mean by a "promising practice" and why we chose to use this term instead of "best practice" or "evidence-based practice," we try to single out the characteristics of good practice in health promotion, drawing on examples provided throughout the book. Finally, after considering the evolution of the field since the release of the second edition of this book in 2007, we offer our views on how it is likely to develop over the next five years or so.

What Shapes Health Promotion Practice in Canada?

There are a variety of factors that influence health promotion practice, but we have long argued that the overall state of the political economy is a key determinant, not only of the health status of populations, but also of the type and number of interventions, including health promotion ones, that practitioners will be able to enact. By the political economy we are referring to the way in which the economy evolves and how it relates to the decisions made by governments (the state). We see no reason to abandon this argument, given the field's recent developments. Two chapters of this book are especially useful for this purpose. Chapter 6 by Labonté and Chapter 14 by Raphael offer many concrete examples of how the political economy impacts on the health of populations and the practice of health promotion at the global level and in Canada respectively.

The picture they offer is not very encouraging. As Labonté mentioned, the global political economy is in a difficult situation. The 2008 global fiscal crisis and its aftermath have seen massive wealth transfer from the poorer and middle classes to the wealthier classes across the globe, in order to save banks and the financial system. This process has led to yet another series of severe reductions in governmental social expenditures in many countries, with the measures to control the processes that generated the crisis (e.g., the end of banking secrecy) not yet implemented in any significant way.

As described by Raphael in Chapter 14 and elsewhere (Raphael, 2008), the Canadian situation is not very encouraging either, given recent further ascendance of neo-liberal approaches to public policy-making as expressed in recent federal government policies and their impact on health and health promotion practice. Internationally, the policies put forward during the last few years (in the fields of climate change or international aid, for instance) have contributed to severely altering the country's reputation, as reflected by the denial of a seat to Canada on the United Nations Security Council in 2010. Canada is increasingly seen as a renegade country that is taking internationally marginal and very unpopular positions, as in the climate change debates, for instance. Nationally, much of the social security net developed during the welfare state era is being dismantled, and there is continued interest in the "privatization" of structures such as the pension system and even in the growth of private, for-profit health care across Canada (Ontario Health Coalition, 2008). The federal government is also shifting the way in which it enacts its role with respect to the health portfolio—limiting action to the "federal" arena and its unwillingness to "impose" on the provinces and territories—leading to a shift in the federal role and visibility in the field.

The renewed governmental interest in "prevention" and the various initiatives on "healthy living" at the national and provincial levels—e.g., for Quebec (MSSS, 2006) and for British Columbia (PHAC, 2009), as well as activities such as the push for a lifetime prevention guide for physicians—are once more putting responsibility for health on individuals, whereas the general conditions in which they are asked to act are making the task increasingly difficult for larger and larger segments of the population.[1] As Godin (2007) reminded us in Chapter 21 of the second edition, this does not mean that individuals have no responsibility for their health, and that understanding what motivates them to alter or maintain health-enhancing behaviour is not important. What it means, however, is that in the current state of the political economy, the range of choices for making "the healthiest choice the easiest choice," as advocated by Milio (1986) decades ago, is shrinking for many, if not most, Canadians.

Given this overall difficult period, Raphael and Labonté argue that even if it is potentially somewhat risky, health promotion professionals should become more political and transform their practice toward trying to influence public policies at the local, regional, national, and even global levels. Both authors provide precise suggestions about how to do so at the individual and collective levels, especially through the professional associations that health promotion workers belong to. Refining the political skills required to play these new roles is important and it is why practical tools for political analysis and intervention (O'Neill, Roch & Boyer, 2010), for health impact assessments (as discussed in Chapter 17 by St-Pierre and Mendell), as well as for sex- and gender-based analysis in health (Kelleher, 2004; Östlin, 2005), will become increasingly needed.

The single most important message of this book about what shapes the current practice of health promotion in Canada and what to do about it is this: Never forget that individual health-related behaviour is shaped by its environment, and always design interventions having in mind both the individual level (in context) and the structural level (of policies, organizations, communities, etc.), using one or more of the numerous available health promotion planning tools (e.g., Green & Kreuter, 2005; Bartholomew et al., 2011) to establish the mix appropriate for the problem at hand!

Other aspects of what constitutes good health promotion practice that were discussed in this book are detailed below.

Using Promising Practices to Transform Health Promotion Interventions

"Evidence-Based," "Best," or "Promising" Practices?

Evaluating health promotion practices in order to develop interventions based on the best possible evidence has been a concern for as long as the field has existed (Green, 1986; Abelin, Brzezinski & Carstairs, 1987; Noack & McQueen, 1988). However, since the mid-1990s, with the emergence of evidence-based practices launched by clinical epidemiology within medicine, health promotion has been forced to position itself in relation to the evidence-based movement (O'Neill, 2003). The first half of the following decade thus produced a flurry of task forces, working groups, and concerned individuals focused on how to assess the effectiveness of health promotion, the most important of which was probably a WHO working group on health promotion evaluation (Rootman et al., 2001). The challenge was to try to figure out if the evidence-based strategies proposed by the Cochrane Collaboration and other similar efforts were appropriate for health promotion (Jackson et al., 2001).

Overall, people in health promotion concluded that the usual hierarchy of evidence suggested by the Cochrane Collaboration and others, which was then heavily influenced by the biomedical view of science and held the randomized clinical trial (RCT) as the gold standard of evidence to decide if a practice was efficient or not, was not appropriate to assess health promotion interventions, especially the community-based ones (Jackson et al., 2001). Potvin and Goldberg, in Chapter 16 of this book, address why this is the case in some detail. Nevertheless, given the strong belief in evidence-based practices held by many powerful constituencies, particularly those with the mandate to allocate resources (O'Neill, 2003), the field has been forced to engage with this question in a serious and sustained manner.

In relation to the type of scientific evidence required to assess health promotion programs, there have been heated debates, leading even the Cochrane Collaboration, and especially its group on public health and health promotion, to enlarge its view of what was acceptable (Armstrong, Waters & Doyle, 2008). More concretely, at the practical level, various operations to analyze actual practices all over the world have been undertaken, one of the most important being the Global Program on Health Promotion Effectiveness of the International Union for Health Promotion and Health Education (IUHPE, 2010), which has run since 2000 and has produced many publications.

It is in the wake of these efforts and reflections that in order to include a wide set of potentially useful and interesting interventions, incorporating a broadly defined vision of scientific evidence as well the values of health promotion, Canadians have developed an *Interactive Domain Model for Best Practices for Health Promotion*, a manual to work with it, which in 2005 was in its third edition (Kahan & Goodstadt, 2005), and an Internet portal, which has been operating for years (www.idmbestpractices.ca/idm.php). There are other best practices for health promotion portals in Canada (for instance, the IDM website was proposing links to five others in December 2010), some of which have a less open focus than the IDM one (see, for example, the Canadian Best Practices Portal for Health Promotion and Chronic Disease Prevention at http://cbpp-pcpe.phac-aspc.gc.ca/). As this introduces some confusion about what a "best practice" is, we have chosen in this book to use the term "promising practice" in order to maintain a wider, rather than a strictly scientific focus on practice. Our definition of a promising practice—i.e., a practice that might or might not have been evaluated enough to reach the status of "best practice," but that is nevertheless illuminating and inspiring—is thus very close to the encompassing definition of a best practice proposed on the IDM portal as shown in Box 18.1.

BOX 18.1:

What Is a "Promising Practice" in Health Promotion?

Promising practices in health promotion are those sets of processes and activities that are consistent with health promotion values, goals, and ethics; theories and beliefs; evidence, and understanding of the environment, and that are most likely to achieve health promotion goals in a given situation.

Source: Adapted from IDM. (2010). *Interactive best practices portal.* Retrieved from: http://www.idmbestpractices.ca/idm.php?content=basics-overview

Important Characteristics of Promising Practices

We therefore think that health promotion practitioners should be careful not to reinvent the wheel and should be aware of the types of interventions already available for the issue, population, or setting in which they work, as compiled on the portals mentioned above or other similar ones. But we also think that they should not refrain from being innovative and creative, and should let themselves be inspired by interventions that might not have reached the status of an "evidence-based" or a "best practice," but that show promising possibilities. In order to do so, we think that a few characteristics emerge from our definition and should be taken into account in developing any health promotion practice. This does not mean that an intervention that has all of them will automatically yield positive results for the population, nor that not having one or the other will automatically lead to failure. We nevertheless think that if a health promotion intervention is *reflexive, theory-based*, and *context-sensitive*, as well as *planned and evaluated in a participatory manner*, it is more likely to succeed. We will illustrate this below by referring to various aspects of this approach and some key examples throughout the book.

Being *reflexive* about one's practice is, put in the simplest of terms, taking the time to think about what one is doing in order to improve it. As most practitioners are overloaded and are often barely able to do what they have to do, this might sound interesting but idealistic. Several chapters of this book nevertheless advocate the benefits derived from approaching health promotion practice reflexively, be it in applying theory in practice (in Chapter 4 on intersectional theory) or in evaluating interventions (see Chapter 16). In Chapter 12, Boutilier and Mason provide several concrete tools to apply reflexivity in practice, particularly through writing, but also through drawing or using online means. We also encourage people involved in health promotion practice other than intervention work, such as policy-making, teaching, or research, to also apply reflexivity to their work. As two of us realized (O'Neill & Dupéré, 2006), even if this is unusual in the academic world, it can be a very useful endeavour in that realm as well.

In the conclusion of the second edition (Dupéré et al., 2007), we argued that *grounding practice in theory* was an important theme that had emerged at that point in time. This is why we included a whole chapter on the importance of theory in this new edition (Chapter 3). Other chapters develop this argument in particular directions: Chapter 4, for example, looks at the contributions that intersectional theory can make to understanding diversity; Chapter 5 addresses the value of ecological theory in planning interventions; and Chapter 7 explicitly discusses the contribution of social theory in understanding collective lifestyles and their impact on behaviour. Importantly, evidence that health promotion programs planned using theoretical foundations to achieve better results is growing (Godin et al., 2007; Bartholomew et al., 2011) and can be used to decide if a program should be uni- or intersectoral, targeted to a particular group or approached through a particular intervention mechanism. The capacity to select relevant theories and models and apply them adequately in practice is indeed a key competence for health promoters (Hyndman, 2009).

Dynamic exchanges among theory, research, and practice are also desirable to make health promotion more effective. Not only is a best practice likely to be grounded in theory, but the best theory is also likely to be grounded in real lessons from practice. The development of theory in health promotion should itself be practice-based (Crosby & Noar, 2010). In Chapter 16, Potvin and Goldberg, using an important body of literature and concrete examples of their own work—notably among First Nations communities—strongly argue that even if an intervention has been shown to be effective somewhere else, a health promotion intervention needs to be adapted to each new *context* where it is implemented. Too often practitioners tend to import, without sufficient critical sensitivity, interventions that have been designed in particular cultural, linguistic, or social contexts, an issue also addressed in chapters 7, 8, 9, and 11 on issues, populations, and settings. The balance between not reinventing the wheel and uncritically importing interventions, especially if they have succeeded elsewhere, calls for weighing the general and the specific/contextual. A reflexive approach can be a very useful safeguard against missing the nuances of a particular situation that are critical to shaping a project's success.

Finally, another helpful strategy to ensure that health promotion practice is useful and more likely to succeed is developing it in a *participatory* manner with the people who could benefit from it. Beyond the fact that participation is a major component of the value base of health promotion, as advocated by Kahan and Goodstadt (2005), among many others, numerous chapters of the book (chapters 4, 7, 8, 9, 11, 14, and 16 notably) provide concrete illustrations that a participatory approach to research, program development, and/or evaluation really produces results, a phenomenon for which evidence has also been accumulating for many years (Minkler & Wallerstein, 2008).

Thus, not only is the political economy a significant factor in shaping health promotion practice, but the health promotion field is now sufficiently mature that it has a set of well-documented practices, which share certain characteristics that can orient the work of health promotion practitioners.

The Current and Future Developments of Health Promotion in Canada

To conclude the chapter, we will look at the recent past of health promotion both internationally and in Canada to see what it suggests to us about the field's immediate future.

The Recent Past of Health Promotion

Internationally, perhaps the most important development since the release of the second edition of this book in 2007 has been the global economic crisis triggered by the collapse of the sub-prime mortgage market in the United States. In the first part of this conclusion we discussed how the evolution of the political economy significantly affects health promotion practice. Globally, it has begun to force countries to radically re-evaluate their commitment to social programs and activities such as health promotion, as discussed in a special issue of *Critical Public Health* in 2008 (CPH, 2008). This has been notably visible in the Euro monetary zone, where countries like Greece had to be saved from bankruptcy in 2010, and where severe public spending cuts have since occurred, leading to general strikes and significant social unrest (a situation that is likely to continue for several years).

On the other hand, an interesting countervailing development was the release in 2008 of the report of the World Health Organization's Commission on the Social Determinants of Health (CSDH, 2008). This report called on countries to increase their efforts to address inequities associated with the social determinants of health by various means, including health promotion. It remains to be seen whether the economic environment will overshadow any serious attempts to enhance commitments to health promotion activities. Nevertheless, the commission's report and WHO's pursuit of its series of global health promotion conferences, with the seventh held in Nairobi in 2009, have inspired people working in the field around the world.

At the opening ceremony of the twentieth world conference of the International Union for Health Promotion and Health Education (IUHPE), held in Geneva in July 2010, the Director of WHO, Dr. Chan, described herself as a strong ally of the field and renewed the commitment of her organization to health promotion with an enthusiasm not seen in many years. At that conference—where the Canadian contingent was the third largest; where many key conference activities and events were organized or presented by Canadians; and where there was a growing recognition of the importance of building a bridge between the health promotion agenda and the sustainability agenda, which has been advocated for years by Canadian health promotion leaders like Hancock—the international visibility and leadership of Canada was still strong.

Within Canada, in addition to an increased emphasis on inequities in health due in part to the WHO report—in which Canada participated significantly, both institutionally and through the contributions of several individuals—there have been a few other changes that have occurred since the nineteenth IUHPE world conference in Vancouver in 2007. Some have been addressed by Raphael in the special issue of *Critical Public Health*, referred to above (Raphael, 2008). Given the context of the political economy in the country already noted, Raphael suggests we might be "grasping at straws"—that is, "trying to find reasons to feel hopeful about a bad situation" (Raphael, 2008, p. 483). There are indeed reasons to worry about the development of the field as a tree in recent years. However, if we keep in mind the concept of the rhizome, the picture looks more promising.

On the one hand, there have been some significant changes in the infrastructure for health promotion research and training. One such change is the closing of some of the university-based centres that were core members of the Canadian Consortium for Health Promotion Research, two of which (at the University of Toronto and then the University of Victoria) were its successive leaders. The reasons for the centres' closing appear to be different, but may reflect a reduced status for health promotion, as well as the fact that the Canadian Consortium for Health Promotion Research, which was responsible for the Vancouver IUHPE Conference, itself dissolved shortly thereafter.

The elimination of these centres and the consortium are bound to have consequences for the kind and quantity of health promotion research undertaken in Canada. For instance, there may be a reduction in health promotion participatory research, which several of the research centres were noted for, as well as a reduction in nationwide collaborative research, which for years was facilitated by the consortium (Rootman, Jackson & Hills, 2007). In addition, the dissolution of the University of Toronto's Centre for Health Promotion (see Box 18.2) led to the cancellation in 2010 of the Ontario Summer School for Health Promotion, which had run annually for 18 years. This cancellation reduces the opportunities for capacity development among health promotion practitioners in Ontario, the province with the largest infrastructure for health promotion in the country.

BOX 18.2:

Centre for Health Promotion 1990–2009

Suzanne Jackson

When the Centre for Health Promotion (CHP) at the University of Toronto was created in 1990, health promotion was "in the limelight" in Canada under federal and provincial government leadership (Jackson & Riley, 2007). In its first decade under the leadership of Irv Rootman, the CHP started the North York Community Health Promotion Research Unit, the Ontario Tobacco Research Unit, the Health Communication Unit, the annual Health Promotion Summer School series, received WHO Collaborating Centre status, chaired the Canadian Consortium for Health Promotion Research (CCHPR), and received the Ron Draper Award from the Canadian Public Health Association and a Healthy University of Toronto award. These initiatives focused on building capacity in practice, evaluation, and research, and promoted health promotion practice. For most of this decade, health promotion in Canada was "behind the scenes," where the emphasis had shifted to local sectors and universities (Jackson & Riley, 2007). The CHP played a role in encouraging the engagement of many different disciplines and players, in training and capacity-building, and provided a beacon for those facing obstacles in the field.

   After SARS and the revitalization of the public health sector in Canada, health promotion was positioned as a fundamental element of public health and "restaged" from 2003 to 2007 with a greater profile nationally. During this time, the CHP was led by Suzanne Jackson and played a role via its partnerships in putting mental health promotion on the Canadian agenda, in being the Canadian Health Network Affiliate in Health Promotion, and in continuing to play a role globally through its support of WHO international conferences and PAHO regional initiatives to promote health promotion evaluation. Since 2007, health promotion has gone behind the scenes again, but this time, the universities did not take up the leadership mantle. Along with other members of the former CCHPR, the CHP closed its doors in 2009. The deep roots that were nurtured so well for 20 years by CHP in many organizations and individuals will have to find a way to flourish without the touchstone of a recognized health promotion champion such as the CHP. Previously, when health promotion went underground, it seemed to be necessary to have a set of strong leaders outside governments to keep the field alive. Whether the CHP really built lasting roots remains to be seen.

On the other hand, it has become apparent over the last three years that despite this rather grim general climate, health promotion concepts, values, theories, and practices continue to be diffused widely. Some academic research centres, like the Atlantic Health Promotion Research Centre and the Centre for Health Promotion Studies in Alberta, have indeed survived and are continuing their important work. Significant recent reports, like the ones for a subcommittee of the Canadian Senate (Keon, 2009) or by the Health Council of Canada (2010), continue to reaffirm the value of working at the level of the political economy if governments really want to promote the health of human populations in this decade (see Box 18.3).

BOX 18.3:

A Healthier Canada Is Not Just the Responsibility of Health Ministries

Blake Poland

A report released in December 2010 by the Health Council of Canada declares that unless governments change their approach to addressing the needs of poorer and socially disadvantaged Canadians, we are destined to continue paying handsomely for the consequent demands on our health care system. Created by the 2003 First Ministers' Accord on Health Care Renewal, the Health Council of Canada is an independent national agency that reports on the progress of health care renewal in Canada.

The report, entitled *Stepping It up: Moving the Focus from Health Care in Canada to a Healthier Canada*, indicates that health disparities play a significant role in health system costs. It states that ongoing spending on acute care and programs that encourage a healthy lifestyle is not enough to improve the overall health of Canadians, particularly those who live in or close to poverty. Significantly, a "whole-of-government" approach is advocated, and key informants with a wealth of experience at various levels of government canvassed for the report offer sanguine advice and insights on how to move forward on intersectoral action. The report underscores the need for a "seismic shift" in how politicians and governments think about health, calling for a better balance between investing in an acute care system and investing in the factors that materially affect our health.

Penned by none other than noted social justice author Dennis Raphael, and steered by an Expert Panel that was a veritable who's who of health promotion in Canada, the report's conclusions are hardly a surprise. Nevertheless, in the context of accelerating program cuts brought on by economic recession and political conservatism, and continued lack of media attention to non-medical determinants of health, it is clear that this is a message that still needs to be heard.

However, history shows that knowledge is rarely sufficient on its own to trigger social change. Whether politicians hear the report's message depends on Canadians demanding action. Fortunately, the public intuitively knows that prevention matters, that poverty kills, and that health care—while vital and universally valued—is more about restoring health compromised by other factors than it is about prevention and ensuring the vitality of the population. On the other hand, shifting the debate from collaborative service provision to the creation of a guaranteed annual income—to take one example of how we could "step it up"—will not be easy, though at least one municipality in Canada has already passed such legislation. One thing is clear: Health is as political as it ever was, and the message is urgent.

As noted in Chapter 8, a good example of a "whole of government" initiative is the Healthy Living Alliance in British Columbia, which was funded by ActNow BC and which adopted approaches from health promotion, including paying attention to inequities in health and empowering citizens (PHAC, 2009). Health promotion has also become more integrated into public health, as exemplified by the fact that one of the ongoing committees of the Public Health Agency of Canada's expert committee structure has been a population health promotion committee, which is chaired by Trevor Hancock, a long-term leader in health promotion in Canada and internationally. There are also signs of the integration of health promotion into health care practice, as discussed in several sections of Chapter 17 of this book.

Finally, on the research and training side of things, the fact that the University of British Columbia changed the name of its Health Promotion Institute to Population Health Promotion may reflect a continued shift in a direction in which both health promotion and population health have found their respective niches. The thriving health promotion developments at the Université de Montréal (see Box 18.4), where there was never a structure as formal as in the centres mentioned above, is a good example of how the rhizome remains probably the best metaphor to understand the developments of the field in the near future.

BOX 18.4:

Health Promotion at Université de Montréal: The Legacy of an Option in a Graduate Training Program

Louise Potvin, Lise Gauvin, Katherine L. Frohlich, and Lucie Richard

The health promotion label was used for the first time at Université de Montréal as one of the five options developed in 1988 for its PhD program in community health. At that time, only two researchers were specifically attached to the health promotion option. Given our PhD was then the only doctoral training program in community or public health in Quebec, its health promotion option attracted students from a variety of disciplinary backgrounds coming from several countries. A critical mass of researchers and research projects built up in the following years, with two immediate paybacks. First, partnerships were created with practitioners and policy-makers in departments of community health and other public health agencies in the Montreal area, which yielded academic and practice benefits. Secondly, these partnerships led to several successful applications on requests for proposals aimed at capacity-building in health promotion across Canada, thereby strengthening health promotion research within public health research centres in the area, notably the Groupe de recherche interdisciplinaire en santé at Université de Montréal.

Currently, 20 years later and even if it was never formalized into a specific centre or unit, health promotion is a thriving stream of research and training within the Université de Montréal's new School of Public Health and its various research units. Our research expertise on social inequalities in health and on health promotion evaluation, our work on urban environments and health and on healthy public policy, as well as our strong interdisciplinary and theoretical focus that puts the *Ottawa Charter*'s vision into our academic practice, are nationally and internationally recognized. Over 40 students have successfully completed their PhD in community or public health within the health promotion option, and 25 are currently enrolled in it (www.medsp.umontreal.ca/doctorat/index.asp).

In addition, two research chairs were awarded to health promotion researchers of our group: one by the Canadian Health Services Research Foundation (www.cacis.umontreal.ca) and the other by the Institute of Population and Public Health (IPPH) of the Canadian Institutes of Health Research (www.chumtl.qc.ca/crchum/chercheurs/chercheurs-liste/gauvin-l.fr.html).

Finally, the Léa-Roback Research Centre on Social Inequalities in Health (www.centrelearoback.ca), which is housed in the Montreal Region Department of Public Health (www.santepub-mtl.qc.ca), is one of the seven Canadian research development centres funded by the IPPH and is another example of the contribution over the years of Université de Montréal and its partners to research and training in health promotion in Canada.

Health Promotion in Canada over the Next Five Years: The New Paths of the Rhizome

What does this recent evolution of the field indicate to us for the near future? Our general impression is that we will see more of the same of what has been happening over the last few years. Health promotion is not likely to disappear in Canada over the next five years, but it is also not likely to get a much higher profile. Despite many alarming signals, it does not seem that globally and in Canada, unless natural or social catastrophes increase significantly in magnitude, important changes will happen in how we humans behave toward each other and toward the environment that sustains us.

What this means for the practice of health promotion in Canada is that the field in the academic or governmental worlds will still be in an era of retrenchment, continuing to argue for structural changes, but caught up in the day-to-day business of trying to improve individual health behaviour through "active living" types of programs. If during the period covered by the first edition of this book (1974–1994), governments, especially the federal one, were the key leaders of health promotion, and academics were the leaders during the period of the second edition (1994–2007), it might very well be that practitioners and the market (consumers) will lead the field in the years to come. We have already begun to observe this in the period covered by this third edition (2007–2011), notably in the fact that several of the early pioneers have either retired or withdrawn from this world and the younger generations involved in the field may do so in settings other than the academic or the governmental one.

These generations, especially the "C generation" (people now aged between 15 and 25) who have lived all their lives with computers and the Internet), are evolving in a different universe than the older ones, largely defined by the new instantaneous and interactive ways of communicating that computers, cellphones, and other social media have made possible. In this universe, the market is already far ahead of most governmental and academic health promotion in offering all kinds of human healthy lifestyle coaches, as well as an even more impressive set of electronic devices to monitor your own health, alter your own behaviour, or even organize demonstrations.

If this proves true, the rhizome will indeed develop through paths that were impossible to even imagine 25 years ago, when the *Ottawa Charter* was proclaimed. This raises many issues, notably the fact that the "digital divide" between those who are computer literate and those who are not will increasingly become, for health promotion, one to attend to with a lot of energy. The good news, though, is that the new generations of health promoters are better trained than ever and will surely find their ways to promote the values of the field even if it turns out to be through paths that will seem novel to those who have been involved in it to date. Indeed, who would have thought that the libertarian children of the 1960s and 1970s would invade the state and use governmental institutions at the local, national, and even international levels to promote their agenda of social justice and equity? So we might be increasingly surprised by the means through which the children of the 1990s and the 2000s will take up the leadership of health promotion here and abroad, the next five years being very interesting to observe in this respect.

Conclusion

Being a human endeavour, the field of health promotion has continued and will continue to take on—locally, nationally, and globally—the colours of the societies that produce it.

Despite the fears that the *Ottawa Charter* would lose its status and profile and be replaced by the *Bangkok Charter*,[2] Canada still has a very significant international reputation in the field, though this may be somewhat exaggerated, given what is currently happening in the country. Finally, the changing of the guard mentioned above will most likely affect our team as well, and the fourth edition of the book will surely be led by the younger members of our team, most likely without the older ones. We are all looking forward to it!

Notes

1. Some argue that the renewed interest in prevention reflects a shift toward libertarian market values and neo-liberal values of personal responsibility for health. There is an increased emphasis on the need for individuals to take care of their own health to contain growing government costs in health care expenditures (Pauly, MacKinnon & Varcoe, 2009).
2. See the interesting debate on this held in 2005. Retrieved from: http://rhpeo.net/reviews/2005/index.htm#Anchor-Ottawa-35882

References

Abelin, T., Brzezinski, Z.J. & Carstairs, V. (Eds.). (1987). *Measurement in health promotion and protection.* WHO Regional Publications, European series, no. 22. Copenhagen: World Health Organization.

Armstrong, R., Waters, E. & Doyle, J. (2008). Reviews in public health and health promotion. In J. Higgins & S. Green (Eds.), *Cochrane handbook for systematic reviews of interventions* (pp. 593–607). London: Wiley-Blackwell.

Bartholomew, L.K., Parcel, G., Kok, G. & Gottlieb, N. (2011). *Planning a health promotion program: An intervention mapping approach* (3rd ed.). San Francisco: Jossey-Bass.

CPH. (2008). *Critical public health.* Special issue on *Health Promotion, 18*(4), 431–540.

Crosby, R. & Noar, S.M. (2010). Theory development in health promotion: Are we there yet? *Journal of Behavioral Medicine, 33*(4), 259–263.

CSDH. (2008). *Closing the gap in a generation: Health equity through action on the social determinants of health.* Geneva: World Health Organization.

Dupéré, S., Ridde, V., Carroll, S., O Neill, M., Rootman, I. & Pederson, A. (2007). Conclusion: The rhizome and the tree. In M. O'Neill et al. (Eds.), *Health promotion in Canada* (2nd ed.) (pp. 363–366). Toronto: Canadian Scholars' Press Inc.

Godin, G. (2007). Has the individual vanished from Canadian health promotion? In M. O'Neill et al. (Eds.), *Health promotion in Canada* (2nd ed.) (pp. 371–387). Toronto: Canadian Scholars' Press Inc.

Godin, G., Gagnon, H., Alary, M. & Lévis, J.-J. (2007). The degree of planning: An indicator of the potential success of health education programs. *Promotion and Education, 14*(3), 138–142.

Green, L.W. (1986). *Measurement and evaluation in health education and health promotion.* Palo Alto: Mayfield.

Green, L.W. & Kreuter, M.W. (2005). *Health program planning: An educational and ecological approach* (4th ed.). New York: McGraw-Hill.

Health Council of Canada. (2010). *Stepping it up: Moving the focus from health care in Canada to a healthier Canada.* Toronto: Health Council of Canada.

Hyndman, B. (2009). Towards the development of skills-based health promotion competencies: The Canadian experience. *Global Health Promotion, 9*(2), 51–55.

IDM. (2010). *Interactive best practices portal.* Retrieved from: http://www.idmbestpractices.ca/idm.php?content=basics-overview

IUHPE. (2010). *The global program on health promotion effectiveness.* Retrieved from: http://www.iuhpe. org/index.html?page=510&lang=en

Jackson, S., Edward, R., Kahan, B. & Goodstadt, M. (2001). *An assessment of the methods and concepts used to synthesize the evidence of effectiveness in health promotion: A review of 17 initiatives.* Toronto: Canadian Consortium for Health Promotion Research.

Jackson, S.F. & Riley, B.L. (2007). Health Promotion in Canada 1986-2006. *Promotion and Education, XIV(4)*, pp. 194-198.

Kahan, B. & Goodstadt, M. (2005). *IDM manual for using the interactive domain model approach to best practices in health promotion* (3rd ed.). Toronto: Centre for Health Promotion, University of Toronto.

Kelleher, H. (2004). Why build a health promotion evidence base about gender? *Health Promotion International, 19*(3), 277–279.

Keon, W. (2009). *A healthy, productive Canada: A determinant of health approach.* Ottawa: Senate Sub-committee on Population Health.

Kickbusch, I. (2007). Health promotion: Not a tree but a rhizome. In M. O'Neill et al. (Eds.), *Health promotion in Canada* (2nd ed.) (pp. 371–387). Toronto: Canadian Scholars' Press Inc.

Milio, N. (1986). *Promoting health through public policy* (2nd ed.). Ottawa: Canadian Public Health Association.

Minkler, M. & Wallerstein, N. (Eds). (2008). *Community-based participatory research for health* (2nd ed.), San Francisco: Jossey-Bass.

MSSS. (2006). *Investir pour l'avenir: Plan d action gouvernemental de promotion des saines habitudes de vie et de prévention des problèmes reliés au poids.* Quebec: Ministère de la santé et des services sociaux du Québec.

Noack, H. & McQueen, D. (Eds.). (1988). Special issue on health promotion indicators. *Health Promotion International, 3*(1), 1–125.

O'Neill, M. (2003). Pourquoi se préoccupe-t-on tant des données probantes en promotion de la santé? *SPM International Journal of Public Health, 48*(5), 317–326.

O'Neill, M. & Dupéré, S. (2006). Du carré à la spirale: Réflexions sur quelques années de participation au comité AVEC du Collectif pour un Québec sans pauvreté. *The Canadian Journal of Program Evaluation, 21*(3), 227–234.

O'Neill, M., Roch, G. & Boyer, M. (2010). *Petit manuel d analyse et d intervention politique en santé.* Quebec: Presses de l Université Laval.

Ontario Health Coalition. (2008). *Eroding public medicare: Lessons and consequences of for-profit health care across Canada.* Privatization reports, Ontario. Retrieved from: http://www.web.net/~ohc/ Eroding%20Public%20Medicare.pdf

Östlin, P. (2005). *What evidence is there about the effects of health care reforms on gender equity, particularly in health?* Retrieved from: http://www.euro.who.int/__data/assets/pdf_file/0015/73230/E87674.pdf

Pauly, B., MacKinnon, K. & Varcoe, C. (2009). Revisiting "Who gets care? Health equity as an arena for nursing action." *Advances in Nursing Science, 32*(2), 118–127.

PHAC. (2009). *Mobilizing intersectoral action to promote health: The case of ActNowBC in British Columbia.* Ottawa: Public Health Agency of Canada.

Raphael, D. (2008). Grasping at straws: A recent history of health promotion in Canada. *Critical Public Health, 18*(4), 483–495.

Rootman, I., Goodstadt, M., Hyndman, B., McQueen, D., Potvin, L. & Springett, J. (Eds.). (2001). *Evaluation in health promotion: Principles and perspectives.* WHO Regional Publications, European series, no. 92. Copenhagen: World Health Organization.

Rootman, I., Jackson, S. & Hills, M. (2007). Developing knowledge for health promotion. In M. O'Neill et al. (Eds.), *Health promotion in Canada* (2nd ed.) (pp. 123–138). Toronto: Canadian Scholars' Press Inc.

Critical Thinking Questions

1. What are the key lessons that you would draw from this book about practice in health promotion?
2. What are the main forces that shape current health promotion practice at the macro level here and abroad? Do you agree that political economy is a key determinant? Can you identify other key determinants?
3. Drawing on examples offered throughout the book, what are the characteristics of a good practice in health promotion? How about a promising practice? Do you agree with the characteristics identified by the authors?
4. How would you go about predicting the future of a field of practice?
5. What do you think will be the state of health promotion practice in Canada in five years? In 25 years?

Resources

Further Readings

IUHPE. (2007). *Shaping the Future of Health Promotion: Priorities for Action*. Retrieved from: http://www.iuhpe.org/uploaded/Activities/Scientific_Affairs/SFHP_ENG.pdf

> This document presents priorities for action in health promotion for the International Union for Health Promotion and Education.

Nutbeam, D. (2008). What would the *Ottawa Charter* look like if it were written today? *Critical Public Health, 18*(4), 435–441.

> This paper by one of the international leaders in the field provides interesting insights on the current value and limits of the *Ottawa Charter*.

Poland, B. (2007). *Health promotion in Canada: Perspectives and future prospects*. Revista Brasileira em Promoçao da Saude (Brazilian Journal of Health Promotion), 20(1), 3–11.

> This paper discusses various perspectives on health promotion in Canada, as well as its future prospects.

Raphael, D. (2008). Grasping at straws: A recent history of health promotion in Canada. *Critical Public Health, 18*(4), 483–495.

> A very interesting view-point by one of the leading analysts of health related public policies in Canada.

Wills, J. & Douglas, J. (2008). Health promotion: Still going strong? *Critical Public Health, 18*(4), 431–434.

> The introduction to a special issue of the journal *Critical Public Health* devoted to the study of the situation of health promotion around the world in 2008.

Relevant Websites

Global Forum for Health Research

www.globalforumhealth.org

The Global Forum for Health Research was established in 1998 to promote health research devoted to improving the health of people in developing counties.

Global Health Watch

www.ghwatch.org

The Global Health Watch is a broad collaboration of public health experts, non-governmental organizations, civil society activists, community groups, health workers, and academics. The Global Health Watch produces an alternative World Health Report.

Interactive Best Practices Portal for Health Promotion, Public Health, and Population Health

www.idmbestpractices.ca/idm.php

This portal presents a comprehensive best practices approach to preventing illness and enhancing health, for people working in health promotion, public health, and population health.

People's Health Movement (PHM)

www.phmovement.org

The People's Health Movement has its roots in grassroots organizing. It is calling for a revitalization of the principles of the Alma-Ata Declaration of Health for All by the Year 2000. It contains a copy of *The People's Charter for Health*.

Understanding the Rhizome Effect:
Health Promotion in the Twenty-first Century

Ilona Kickbusch

Introduction

As we look forward to the future of health promotion, it can help to revisit some of the central messages of 25 years ago and consider what became of them in terms of what I call the rhizome effect. I would like to focus on four messages:

- the goal of healthy public policy "to move health high on the political agenda"
- the challenge of the socio-ecological approach to health, which postulates the "inextricable links between people and their environment"
- the notion of "making the healthier choice the easier choice"
- the challenge to go "beyond healthy life-styles to well-being"

Above all, these four messages document foresight. Each of them is linked to critical societal challenges at the beginning of the twenty-first century—the governance of health, sustainable development, individual responsibility, and the overall goal of modern societies. Health promotion must continue to make significant contributions to each of these decisive debates or it will become irrelevant, but these contributions can take on very different forms and need not always be qualified as health promotion. The goal of the *Ottawa Charter for Health Promotion* (WHO, 1986)—as expressed in its subtitle, "towards a new public health"—was to suggest innovation in public health or, in other words, to give guidance on how the health challenges at the end of the twentieth century could be addressed, not to establish a discipline.

Indeed, one measure of the success of health promotion could well be that much of health promotion thinking, as codified in the *Ottawa Charter*, is now so commonplace that it is no longer referenced back to its source. For me, an excellent example of this is the report of the Commission on Social Determinants of Health: Just by looking at the table of contents, one can see it is steeped in health promotion thinking, highlighted by the focus on "daily living conditions" and reinforced by the statement that health depends on the "conditions in which people are born, grow, live, work, and age" (CSDH, 2008, p. 1). Compare this to the *Ottawa Charter*'s phrasing: "Health is created and lived by people within the settings of their everyday life; where they learn, work, play and love" (WHO, 1986, p. 2).

The Rhizome

This is what I meant when, in my contribution to the second edition of this book (Kickbusch, 2007), I had argued that health promotion is like a rhizome. A rhizome is a root system that some plants (like lilies, orchids, ginger, and bamboo) use to spread themselves about. It is connected and heterogenic; it does not respect territory but expands continuously. From the horizontal stem of the plant, which is usually underground, rhizomes send out roots and shoots from their nodes. These seemingly unrelated individuals are actually all connected through a system that is not immediately visible. If rhizomes are broken into pieces, each piece can give rise to a new plant. According to Deleuze and Guttari (1976), modern knowledge systems are rhizomes—they oppose the idea that knowledge must grow in a tree structure from previously accepted ideas.

New thinking need not follow established patterns; knowledge must migrate into new conceptual territories resulting from unpredictable juxtapositions (see http://rhizomes.net). If health promotion is a rhizome, then its success is measured not only by the extent it has influenced how societies think about health and its determinants, but also by its ability to give rise to innovation and its capacity to respond to changes in the context by moving into new conceptual territories. Without such migration, the rhizome withers away. This is why, on the conceptual level, the constant link to social theory is so important to health promotion and, on the practical level, the network-based and participatory approach (i.e., the migration of the ideas and approaches to different settings) is constitutive for much of the rhizome effect. A challenge I would like to put forward for health promotion research is to study the rhizome effect in its various dimensions. Below I give some examples that illustrate the different levels of impact.

The Rhizome Effect 1: Health in All Policies

This is the area of health promotion that, in my view, probably shows the highest rhizome effect. Health has moved up the political agenda and has migrated into new political territories, but health promotion theory and practice have not always followed, in part because they have underestimated their rhizome effect and their level of influence. Health has become vital to overall government performance at the national level, and consequently it has moved into the centre of political and ideological debates, which is very similar to its position in the nineteenth century, another period of seminal change. The multidimensional nature of many problems, including health, needs an integrated and dynamic policy response across portfolio boundaries, new administrative forms such as "joined up government" within government, or new strategic relationships with non-state actors that are increasingly being explored.

In Europe, health promotion has shown itself as a rhizome of considerable impact and resilience, particularly in relation to healthy public policy. Healthy public policy, says the *Ottawa Charter*, "puts health on the agenda of policy makers in all sectors and at all levels, directing them to be aware of the health consequences of their decisions and to accept their responsibilities for health" (WHO, 1986, p. 2). Indeed, many of the key tenets of healthy public policy are now an integral part of the official policies of the European Union, and are well summarized in the Council Conclusions on Equity and Health in All Policies: *Solidarity in Health* (Council of the European Union, 2010). Article 9 of the European Treaty of Lisbon, which came into effect in 2009, underlines that health has to be one of the considerations when formulating European policies for the 500 million inhabitants of the EU.

In this arena health promotion has also shown its capacity to respond to context and provide innovation. Using the EU terminology of "health in all policies," the new health governance has also been the subject of the recent *Adelaide Statement on Health in All Policies—Moving towards a Shared Governance for Health and Well-being* (Adelaide Recommendations on Healthy Public Policy, 2010), underlining the need not only to make health a shared goal across all parts of government, but also to indicate how health would contribute to the achievement of other societal goals. For example, a shared societal goal such as "equity" or "well-being" would have health as one important indicator; this shift from "intersectoral action for health" to "intersectoral action for shared societal goals" is also highlighted in a major study on *Crossing Sectors* by the Public Health Agency of Canada (2007). According to the *Ottawa Charter*, it is this kind of "coordinated action that leads to health, income and social policies that foster greater equity" (WHO, 1986, p. 2). This is critical because good or bad health outcomes not only depend on the action of other sectors, but also affect the outcomes of a wide range of other sectors. Finland, as the initiator of the EU Council Conclusions on Health in All Policies (2006), will reinforce the spread of the rhizome—supported in particular by the WHO Regional Office for Europe—by hosting the 2013 Global Conference on Health Promotion with the focus on health in all policies. It is to be expected that it will move the field into new territories.

The Rhizome Effect 2: The Socio-ecological Approach

In the twenty-first century, the purpose of governance should be healthy and sustainable development. The *Ottawa Charter* called for a socio-ecological approach to health, which builds on the "inextricable links between people and their environment" (WHO, 1986, p. 2). This was taken forward in the Sundsvall Statement on Supportive Environments (1991), probably the most undervalued health promotion statement, particularly regarding its rhizome effect in the environmental and sustainable development debate. The Sundsvall Statement built not only on the *Ottawa Charter*, but also on the World Commission on Environment and Development and its report, *Our Common Future*, which provided a new understanding of the imperative of sustainable development. The Sundsvall Statement was taken to the United Nations Conference on Environment and Development (UNCED), held in Rio de Janeiro in 1992, and contributed to the formulation of the health sections of the *Earth Charter* and Agenda 21. I usually hear more mention of the Sundsvall Statement—and its rhizome effect—when I speak to colleagues from the sustainable development field than when I speak to health promotion experts.

Here, in my view, is one of the most critical areas for innovation and action of the young generation of health promoters. The opportunities for health promotion and sustainable development to join forces were already fully recognized in the *Ottawa Charter*. Both are highly challenging political and normative concepts that aim to bring about a significant paradigm shift in how societal development is understood, and both want to achieve transformative change in society and propose new governance mechanisms in different sectors and spheres of activity. Through the settings networks it has built globally—particularly the Healthy Cities network—health promotion has promoted a paradigm shift at different levels of governance. The twentieth IUHPE World Conference on Health Promotion in Geneva 2010 revisited the interface of health, equity, and sustainable development. The goal was to build a bridge between the health promotion agenda and the sustainability agenda. In many cases, the best choices for health are also the best choices for the planet, and the most ethical and environmental choices are also good for health. This needs to be taken forward in a wide number of nodes for a full rhizome effect.

Of course the socio-ecological approach has been at the base of the many "settings projects" that have been initiated through health promotion—another set of nodes of the rhizome. Their rhizome effect around the world has been significant to the extent that in a number of countries, the approach to building healthy cities, schools, hospitals, and workplaces and the like is now a standard repertoire not only in the public sector, but of private consultants. It reinforces my suspicion that the main reason for many of the problems that health promotion has faced has been its confinement to the straitjacket of the health sector. Accordingly, its rhizome effect has been greater in other sectors and at the local level than within the health sector itself.

The Rhizome Effect 3: Understanding Systemic Risk

The rhizome effect of health promotion is tangibly present in the debates around individual responsibility. Responses to the obesity epidemic show a clear understanding that obesity is not a product of individual failure but a systemic risk closely related to what has been called "obesogenic environments" (Lake, Townshend & Alvanides, 2010). A consensus (if not yet the political will) has emerged in the present debate that in order to effectively tackle the global non-communicable disease epidemic, it is necessary "to first understand the social nature of risks and their movement across the globe … risk factors for non-communicable diseases move across the planet in ways that are neither random nor idiosyncratic" (Brandt, 2007, 488). While health promoters will continue to be critical about a disease-based approach, they have clearly had a long-term impact on how successful interventions are framed for specific diseases. But despite this success, health promotion went off track. As health promotion discussed "evidence-based practice" and got caught up in the mire of the Cochrane medical mindset rather than focus on the social nature of risk, I despaired. Meanwhile, two economists were lauded as "utterly brilliant" because they described how a "sensible choice architecture" could nudge people toward best decisions without restricting their freedom of choice. I must confess I was truly upset when I read the bestseller *Nudge* (Thaler & Sunstein, 2008) because it exemplified to me all the lost opportunities of health promotion in the political arena. What Thaler and Sunstein were describing was expressed in the *Ottawa Charter* as "to make the healthier choice the easier choice" (WHO, 1986, p. 2), and it became the health promotion mantra of a consumer society. While health promoters have been termed "health fascists" because they addressed the need to regulate products harmful to health, in *Nudge* the authors propose "a very mild form of government regulation," call their approach libertarian paternalism, and are considered candidates for the Nobel Prize in Economics. One of the authors is now an adviser to the British prime minister for the newly instigated public health strategy.

The Rhizome Effect:
"Health Promotion Goes beyond Healthy Life-styles to Well-being"

Don't get me wrong—*Nudge* is a brilliant book and every health promoter should read it and can gain much from it, including self-confidence. The question that bothers me is: Why—if our agenda is out there and so many of our approaches are now accepted—do so many health promoters feel so disempowered? Where did it go wrong? I think there are several issues worth considering:

- *lack of theory:* We did not do enough theoretical work on understanding the interdependent "wicked problems" of the twenty-first century and their governance implications.
- *lack of the social:* We were not serious enough about insisting on the social underpinning of all our work—even the concept of the social determinants does not fully cover the many social dynamics we would need to consider, for example, around the notion of choice.
- *lack of arguments:* We did not argue well enough (compared, for example, with *Nudge*) that the notions of individual freedom in relation to the state, developed in the eighteenth-century Enlightenment, do not fit the consumer societies of the twenty-first century.
- *lack of sophistication:* We lack sophistication in conducting the debate on the freedom of markets, the responsibility of individuals, the protection of vulnerable groups, and the extent and nature of state intervention.
- *lack of conviction:* We do not stick to our convictions or we turn into missionaries instead of negotiators.

Worst of all, we consistently undervalued our own rhizome effect.

Conclusion

I believe there is a tremendous opportunity to revitalize the health promotion agenda as—following the financial crisis—there is an increasing societal debate about well-being and the nature of happiness. The *Ottawa Charter* indicated an agenda larger than health, and stated that "health promotion goes beyond healthy life-styles to well-being" (WHO, 1986, p. 1), but somehow we got lost along the way in the medical quagmire. In a society where many dimensions of health have become either medicalized or commodified, it is well worth linking the health promotion agenda to broader social agendas that will define the future of our societies—such as equity, sustainable development, and well-being—rather than concentrate on health. The *Ottawa Charter* stated: "Health is, therefore, seen as a resource for everyday life, not the objective of living" (WHO, 1986, p. 1). The health system has not served health promotion well. Like a true rhizome, we need to migrate to more conducive territories. There is much to gain.

References

Adelaide Recommendations on Healthy Public Policy. (1988). Retrieved from: http://www.who.int/healthpromotion/conferences/previous/adelaide/en/index.html

Adelaide Statement on Health in all Policies. (2010). Retrieved from: http://www.who.int/social_determinants/hiap_statement_who_sa_final.pdf

Brandt, A.M. (2007). *The cigarette century.* New York: Basic Books.

Commission on Social Determinants of Health (CSDH). (2008). *Closing the gap in a generation: Health equity through action on the social determinants of health.* Geneva: World Health Organization. Retrieved from: http://www.who.int/social_determinants/thecommission/finalreport/en/index.html

Council of the European Union. (2006). Council Conclusions on Health in All Policies (HiAP), Brussels: Council meeting, 30 November and 1 December.

Council of the European Union. (2010). *Council conclusions on equity and health in all policies: Solidarity in health.* Brussels: 3019th Employment, Social Policy, Health, and Consumer Affairs Council meeting, June 8. Retrieved from: http://www.consilium.europa.eu/uedocs/cms_data/docs/pressdata/en/lsa/114994.pdf

Deleuze, G. & Guttari, F. (1976). *Rhizome.* Paris: Les Editions de Minuit.

Kickbusch, I. (2007). Health promotion: Not a tree but a rhizome. In M. O'Neill et al. (Eds.), *Health promotion in Canada* (2nd ed.) (pp. 363–366). Toronto: Canadian Scholars' Press Inc.

Lake, A., Townshend, T.G. & Alvanides, S. (Eds.). (2010). *Obesogenic environments.* Mississauga: Wiley-Blackwell.

Public Health Agency of Canada (PHAC). (2007). *Crossing sectors: Experiences in intersectoral action, public policy, and health.* Ottawa: Public Health Agency of Canada. Retrieved from: http://www.phac-aspc.gc.ca/publicat/2007/cro-sec/index-eng.php

Sundsvall Statement on Supportive Environments for Health. (1991). Retrieved from: http://www.who.int/healthpromotion/conferences/previous/sundsvall/en/index.html

Thaler, R. & Sunstein, C. (2008). *Nudge: Improving decisions about health, wealth, and happiness.* Toronto: Penguin Books.

WHO. (1986). *Ottawa Charter for Health Promotion.* Ottawa: World Health Organization, Health and Welfare Canada, Canadian Public Health Association. Retrieved from: http://www.who.int/health-promotion/conferences/previous/ottawa/en/index.html

About the Contributors

Donna Anderson is a Research Associate with the Université Laval–affiliated Centre for Interdisciplinary Research in Rehabilitation and Social Integration, and is an Adjunct Professor with the School of Social Work at Université Laval. Her academic training and work experience cross health promotion and rehabilitation. Her PhD studies focused on researching psychosocial aspects of rehabilitation and quality of life among cardiac patients. Following her post-doctoral studies in health promotion, she worked at the University of Alberta's Centre for Health Promotion Studies.

Paola Ardiles is a Manager in education and population health at BC Mental Health and Addiction Services, an agency of the Provincial Health Services Authority in British Columbia. Paola collaboratively applies health promotion values and principles in research, policy, and practice in the area of mental health promotion, immigrant women's mental health, and cultural competency. Paola leads and participates in various provincial and national projects, working across sectors with multidisciplinary researchers and clinicians, policy-makers, and community service providers to promote mental well-being and address health inequities for underserved populations.

Marie Boutilier conducts research in health policy and the organizations, professionals, and the communities they serve. She has used participatory and qualitative research strategies in local communities, health services, professional organizations, and different levels of government, both in Canada and internationally. She holds a status appointment at the University of Toronto and is a principal with Mapleview Consulting.

Judith Burgess is the Director of Health Services at the University of Victoria. She is a registered nurse with expertise in primary health care, public and population health, advanced practice nursing roles, and community-based research. She has worked as a researcher, educator, manager, and leader for both the non-profit sector in community health and for the University of Victoria in campus health. She is a strong advocate for population health promotion. She completed her doctoral dissertation on the nurse practitioner role, especially in relation to health promotion.

Simon Carroll is a post-doctoral research fellow in the School of Nursing at the University of Victoria. A sociologist by training, he has had a long interest in the health promotion research field, completing his doctoral work on alternative approaches to assessing the effectiveness of complex health interventions. He is currently developing a variety of social theory approaches to assessing the effectiveness of complex public health interventions.

Clémence Dallaire is Vice-Dean of graduate studies and of research and a professor in the Faculty of Nursing at Université Laval. Her research program includes the development of policies to support nursing, nurses' contribution to the services offered in the emergency care continuum, and the organization and administration of nursing services.

Marthe Deschesnes is a researcher at the Institut national de santé publique du Québec and Assistant Professor at the Université de Montréal. She has been working in public health for more than 20 years. Her research interests include evaluation of health promotion interventions in schools, as well as studies of adolescent health behaviour. She is responsible for a research team on the evaluation of a comprehensive school health approach in Quebec.

Serge Dumont is a Professor in the Faculty of Social Sciences at Université Laval. He is the current director of the Réseau de collaboration sur les pratiques interprofessionnelles en santé (RCPI). Dr. Dumont was the recipient of a Canadian Institute of Health Research Career Award from 2000 to 2005, and co-founded the Maison Michel Sarrazin Palliative Care Research Team in 1997. He also co-founded the Université Laval–affiliated Centre for Interdisciplinary Research in Rehabilitation and Social Integration in 2000. Dr. Dumont specializes in psychosocial oncology and health services organization.

Sophie Dupéré is an Assistant Professor in the Faculty of Nursing in Université Laval. She has been involved in community health/health promotion in Canada and internationally for the last 15 years, working as a nurse, consultant, researcher, and activist. She is the co-editor of three books, one of which was the second edition of *Health Promotion in Canada*, and has written a number of articles on gender and women's health, participatory approaches, culture/ migration issues, and poverty.

Peggy Edwards is a health promotion consultant who has worked with the World Health Organization, Health Canada, and the Public Health Agency of Canada on issues related to healthy, active aging. She is the author of several seminal documents on active aging and co-author of three bestselling books on healthy aging and grandparenting. Visit her website at www.grannyvoices.com for an exciting video and companion material related to her Alan Thomas fellowship work on the Grandmothers to Grandmothers campaign.

Jim Frankish is the Director of the UBC Centre for Population Health Promotion Research and a professor in the School of Population and Public Health (Medicine), and the College for Interdisciplinary Studies at UBC. He is trained as a clinical psychologist. In the past 10 years, he has co-led more than 115 health-promotion research projects, including many graduate research studies. His current research interests include homelessness and health literacy.

Tatiana Fraser is the Executive Director of Girls Action Foundation. Throughout her career, Tatiana has contributed greatly to the expansion of all-girls leadership programs. A central focus of Ms. Fraser's work is creating a movement that is inclusive of girls and women from marginalized communities. Growing exponentially from the first summer camp for girls, Girls Action now reaches 60,000 young women and girls annually, particularly in underrepresented communities, including northern, racialized, low-income, Aboriginal, and immigrant communities. Girls Action Foundation has provided funds or training to over 100 start-up girls' programs in communities across Canada, and has created an unprecedented network of organizations dedicated to advancing girls' equality, which now counts over 210 member organizations in all regions of Canada.

Wendy Frisby is a Professor in the School of Human Kinetics and the former chair of Women's and Gender Studies at the University of British Columbia. She has been conducting feminist participatory action research in various community health promotion settings for over 15 years. She has published widely, including in non-academic settings, to promote action and policy change.

Katherine L. Frohlich is an Associate Professor in the Département de médicine sociale et préventive at the Université de Montréal and a Research Associate at the Université de Montréal Public Health Research Institute (IRSPUM). She also holds a Canadian Institutes of Health Research (CIHR) New Investigator Award. She has published widely in the areas of health promotion, social theory in public health, social inequities in health, as well as in the sociology of smoking.

Lise Gauvin is a Professor in the Department of Social and Preventive Medicine at the Université de Montréal, a researcher at the Centre de recherche du Centre Hospitalier de l'Université de Montréal, and a Research Associate at the Léa-Roback Center on Social Inequalities of Health. She has held positions at Queen's University, Concordia University, and, more recently, at Université de Montréal. She currently holds an applied public health chair dealing with neighbourhoods, lifestyle, and healthy body weight, which is supported by the Canadian Institutes of Health Research and the Centre de recherche en prevention de l'obésité and which focuses on socio-environmental determinants of involvement in physical activity, interventions to promote physical activity at the population level, and social determinants of disordered eating.

Doris Gillis is an Associate Professor in the Department of Human Nutrition at St. Francis Xavier University. Drawing on her experience in public health nutrition and adult education, she addresses research issues relevant to health literacy, food security, and maternal and child nutrition. An interest in health promotion approaches that build capacity for effecting positive change in practice and policy has grounded her involvement in a number of community-university research initiatives applying participatory approaches.

Carmelle Goldberg is a PhD candidate in the health promotion option of the PhD program in public health at Université de Montréal. She is interested in the evaluation of community development programs.

Trevor Hancock is a Professor and Senior Scholar at the School of Public Health and Social Policy at the University of Victoria. He has a long-standing interest in the links between human and ecosystem health and the health impacts of our current unsustainable system of economic activity. He was a founder of the Green Party of Canada (and was its first leader), the Canadian Association of Physicians for the Environment, and the Canadian Coalition for Green Health Care.

Larry Hershfield is a consultant whose longest term involvement has been managing the Health Communication Unit at the University of Toronto. Under this umbrella, he led the development of numerous products, events, and services, including the Online Health Program Planner. He also co-teaches a graduate course in health communication at the University of Toronto's Dalla Lana School of Public Health, and is on the editorial board of the *Journal of Health Communication*.

Marcia Hills has held a tenure-track appointment in the School of Nursing since 1989. During her time in the school, she has held many key positions, perhaps most prominent being coordinator of the Collaborative Nursing Program of BC from its inception in 1989 through to implementation in 1992. She was also the director of the Centre for Community Health Promotion Research, an interdisciplinary research centre focusing on community-based research designed to develop an evidence base to support high-functioning primary health care practice teams.

Catharine Hume has worked in the mental health field for the past 20 years. Catharine is the Vancouver site coordinator of the Mental Health Commission of Canada's At Home-Chez Soi project since 2008 and, until recently, was also Director of Grants and Community Initiatives at the Vancouver Foundation. Previously, she held a number of positions with the Canadian Mental Health Association (CMHA) at both national and provincial levels. From 2003 to 2007, Catharine was the director of policy and research in CMHA's BC division. Catharine has a Master of Health Science from the University of Toronto and a certificate in conflict resolution from the Justice Institute of British Columbia.

Ilene Hyman is an Assistant Professor in the Dalla Lana School of Public Health and a Research Associate at Cities Centre, University of Toronto. She has over 20 years of experience as a health planner, researcher, program evaluator, and policy analyst with government, academic, and community-based research units. She has published widely in the areas of gender, migration, and health.

Brian Hyndman is a Senior Planner with the Health Promotion, Chronic Disease, and Injury Prevention section at the Ontario Agency for Health Protection and Promotion. He has over 20 years of experience in planning and evaluating health promotion initiatives. This was gained through a variety of roles, including 12 years as a consultant with the Health Communication Unit at the Centre for Health Promotion, University of Toronto. Brian has also held key leadership positions in the Canadian public health sector, including that of President of the Ontario Public Health Association and citizen representative on the Toronto Board of Health.

Axelle Janczur has been working in the not-for-profit sector in Toronto for over 25 years. Her interests have been related to addressing systemic barriers to service, grounded in principles of access and equity, working with high-need disadvantaged communities. She is an experienced trainer and public speaker, and a committed volunteer. With an MA in political science and an MBA from the Schulich School of Business, she is currently the Executive Director of Access Alliance Multicultural Health and Community Services.

Margot Kaszap is a Professor in the Faculty of Education at Université Laval. She has worked as a researcher and principal investigator in the field of literacy and health for 15 years. She has published widely in health education, including as a co-author of a chapter in the second edition of *Health Promotion in Canada*.

Ilona Kickbusch is the Director of the Global Health Programme at the Graduate Institute of International and Development Studies, Geneva. She is the chair of Global Health Europe, a platform for European commitment to global health and of the Consortium on Global Health Diplomacy. In Switzerland she serves on the executive board of the Careum Foundation and is the chairperson of the World Demography and Ageing Congress St. Gallen. She advises organizations, government agencies, and the private sector on policies and strategies to promote health at the national, European, and international level. She has published widely and is a member of a number of advisory boards in both the academic and the health policy arena. She has received many awards. She has had a distinguished career with the World Health Organization at both the regional and global level, and has contributed significantly to the development of health promotion. Details can be found on her website: www.ilonakickbusch.com

Michael Krausz is Professor of Psychiatry in the School of Population and Public Health and Providence leadership chair for addiction research at the University of British Columbia. He is also Medical Director of the Burnaby Treatment Centre for Mental Health and Addiction and the regional program of complex concurrent disorders. His research interests include severe addiction and concurrent disorders, especially trauma, psychosis, and their treatment.

Ronald Labonté is Canada Research Chair in globalization and health equity at the Institute of Population Health; Professor in the Faculty of Medicine, University of Ottawa; and

Adjunct Professor in the Department of Community Health and Epidemiology, University of Saskatchewan. He worked in public health and health promotion for over 25 years with municipal and provincial governments and internationally before becoming a full-time, university based researcher in 1999. Recent co edited or co-authored books include *Globalization and Health: Pathways, Evidence, and Policy* (2009), *Health Promotion in Action: From Local to Global Empowerment* (2008), and *Critical Perspectives in Public Health* (2007). Many of his writings are available on his website: globalhealthequity.ca/about/labonte.shtml#

François Lagarde is one of Canada's leading social marketers. After working for a number of community-based organizations, he worked from 1984 to 1991 for ParticipACTION, where he served as vice-president and manager of national media campaigns. Since 1991, he has been a consultant for over 160 organizations, primarily in the health and philanthropy fields. In his capacity as a trainer, he has delivered workshops and conferences in all Canadian provinces and 12 other countries. He is an Adjunct Professor in the Faculty of Medicine at the Université de Montréal and Associate Editor of *Social Marketing Quarterly*.

Daniel Laitsch is an Assistant Professor in the Faculty of Education at Simon Fraser University. His research interests relate to the use and misuse of research to effect change in education policy and practice. He is particularly interested in assessment and accountability policy in K–12 education, and the relationship to education funding and outcomes.

Barbara Losier has been involved in community development for more than 30 years, working in municipal recreation, community radio broadcasting, and community health, on women issues, and in the francophonie movement. She is currently acting as Executive Director of the New Brunswick Acadian Movement for Healthy Communities (MACS-NB) and sits on the board of the New Brunswick Health Council.

Robin Mason is a Research Scientist at Women's College Hospital and an Assistant Professor at the Dalla Lana School of Public Health, with a cross appointment to the Women's Mental Health Program, Department of Psychiatry, at the University of Toronto. She works in health education and research, with a focus on issues of violence, abuse, and trauma.

Raymond Massé is a Professor in the Faculty of Social Sciences, Department of Anthropology, at Université Laval. He worked as a researcher at the Direction de la santé publique of Montreal for 12 years, and has taught medical anthropology and anthropology of ethics since 1994. Since 2008, he has been coordinator of the Ethics and Public Health Researchers Network in Quebec. He has published widely in anthropology and public health, including the books *Culture et Santé publique* (1995) and *Éthique et santé publique* (2003).

Douglas McCall is a scholar affiliated with the Centre for the Study of Educational Leadership and Policy at Simon Fraser University. He has worked in school health promotion since 1985, serving as Executive Director of the Canadian Association for School Health and, more recently, as the coordinator for the International School Health Network. He has written numerous manuals, manuscripts, and peer-reviewed journal articles, as well as pioneered work in web-based knowledge exchange.

Lorna McCue is Executive Director of the Ontario Healthy Communities Coalition. She has over 25 years of experience in developing and managing not-for-profit, community-based organizations and services. She provides training and consultation services to multi-sectoral collaborations working on healthy community initiatives, and has written and contributed to several publications relating to community development and health promotion.

Anika Mendell is a Research Officer at the National Collaborating Centre for Healthy Public Policy (NCCHPP) in Montreal. She has a Master's in community health from the Université de Montréal and, since 2006, has worked on various projects at the NCCHPP, including developing tools for knowledge transfer. She currently works on health impact assessment and policies addressing poverty.

Diane Morin is a Professor at the Faculty of Nursing Sciences, Université Laval, where she acted as dean (2006–2010). She is also Professor in the Faculty of Biology and Medicine at Lausanne University in Switzerland, where she acts as Director of the Institut universitaire de formation et de recherche en soins (IUFRS). Her contribution in research and teaching includes health promotion in aging, continuity of nursing care from hospital to home, as well as determinants and effects of interprofessional practice.

Jodi Mucha is the Director of BC Healthy Communities. She brings a broad range of expertise to the position, including a Master's in environment and management, years of experience working overseas on sustainable development projects in West Africa, New Zealand, and Egypt, and a passion for healthy active lifestyles. Her Master's thesis focused on the connections between spirituality and sustainable development and ways to mobilize them. She has a strong background in public policy research, and worked for several years developing the e-dialogues for sustainable development with Dr. Ann Dale of Royal Roads University. Jodi is also an accomplished triathlete, personal trainer, and leadership coach.

Manon Niquette is a Professor in the Department of Information and Communication, and in the graduate programs in community health at Université Laval. She has served as a consultant in health promotion for a number of governmental organizations and peer-support groups. Specifically, she has been involved with the promotion of breastfeeding and the development of community health services awareness campaigns. She is currently doing critical research on pharmaceutical advertising.

Michel O'Neill has recently retired as Professor in community health and health promotion in the Faculty of Nursing of Université Laval. Michel received his PhD in sociology from Boston University, and has been involved in health promotion at the local, national, and international levels since 1974 as a community health worker, professor, researcher, consultant, and activist. His long-standing teaching and research interests relate to the history as well as to the political and policy dimensions of health promotion, with a special interest in the Healthy Cities movement in Quebec, Canada, and internationally. He is co-editor of four books, including the first two editions of *Health Promotion in Canada*, has published extensively in the scientific and professional literature, and has presented numerous papers in various scientific and professional meetings in Quebec, Canada, and all over the world.

Michelle Patterson is a Research Scientist and Adjunct Professor in the Faculty of Health Sciences at Simon Fraser University. She is a co-investigator on the Vancouver At Home project, and has been involved in numerous other projects that aim to create policy change for marginalized communities, especially people who experience mental health and substance use problems.

Ann Pederson is Director of the BC Centre of Excellence for Women's Health. She was the managing editor of the first edition of *Health Promotion in Canada* and an editor of the second edition, as well as an author in both editions.

Marie-Claude Pelletier is President and CEO of GP²S (Group for Promotion of Prevention Strategies). She also developed and implemented various programs to promote health among individuals and in workplaces when she headed a Quebec company specializing in health promotion. These programs have generated the participation of hundreds of thousands of people, and have resulted in changes in behaviour and significant return on investment.

Kadija Perreault is a PhD candidate in community health at Université Laval. She has a Bachelor's degree in physiotherapy, as well as a Master's in experimental medicine, specializing in adaptation/rehabilitation, and is currently involved in physiotherapy education at Laval. She is particularly interested in the roles of rehabilitation professionals in relation to the fields of health promotion and community health. Her research activities have covered areas such as health promotion and physiotherapy for helping people with pain, agreement between the perceptions of physiotherapists and people with pain, as well as interprofessional education and practice.

Robert Perreault is an Associate Professor of psychiatry at McGill University and a member of McGill's Health Informatics Research Group. He is also Scientific Director of the Clinical Prevention Group at Montreal's Direction de santé publique, the regional public health authority. Dr. Perreault was the co-developer of the web Health Guide, the health information portal of the Quebec government. He is currently in charge of medical and professional affairs for the Health Guide, and active in the development and evaluation of innovative IT solutions.

Louise Plouffe obtained a PhD in psychology from the University of Ottawa, and began teaching gerontology at the Université du Québec en Outaouais. Since joining the Public Service of Canada in 1989, Louise has dedicated her career to translating research on aging into policy and program development. For several years, she managed the policy research program of the National Advisory Council on Aging. She now holds the position of Manager of Knowledge Development in the Public Health Agency of Canada, Division of Aging and Seniors. While on secondment to the World Health Organization from 2005 to 2008, she led the development of the World Health Organization's *Global Age-Friendly Cities Guide*, in collaboration with partners in over 30 cities worldwide. She was a founding member of the advisory board of the Canadian Institutes of Health Research–Institute of Aging.

Blake Poland is an Associate Professor in the Dalla Lana School of Public Health at the University of Toronto, where he is also Co-Director of the Urban Environmental Health Justice Research Network (CUHI, 2008–2010), past Director of the Collaborative Program in Community Development (2007–2008), and past Director of the MHSc Program in Health Promotion (1999–2007). His teaching and research focuses on community development as an arena of practice for health professionals, the settings approach to health promotion, critical social theory and qualitative methods, and environmental health justice.

Pamela Ponic is a post-doctoral researcher at the BC Centre of Excellence in Women's Health and in the School of Nursing at the University of British Columbia. Her doctoral work was a critical analysis of social inclusion as a community-based health promotion strategy when working with marginalized social groups. Through her developing program of research and publications, she is exploring how community action and policy change can address the social determinants of women's health and health promotion.

Nancy Poole works as a provincial research consultant on women's substance use issues with BC Women's Hospital and as a Director with the British Columbia Centre of Excellence for Women's Health, and on research and knowledge exchange relating to policy and service provision for girls and women who use alcohol, tobacco, and other substances.

Louise Potvin holds the CHSRF-CHIR Chair of Community Approaches and Health Inequalities at Université de Montréal. Her main research interests are the evaluation of health promotion programs and interventions that address social health inequalities. She is a member of the Canadian Academy of Health Sciences and a globally elected member of the board of trustees of the International Union for Health Promotion and Education.

Hélène Provencher is Professor in the Faculty of Nursing at Université Laval and a researcher affiliated with Groupe de recherche sur l'inclusion sociale, l'organisation des services et l'évaluation en santé mentale, Partenariat CSSS de la Vieille Capitale—CH Robert Giffard (GRIOSE-SM). For the last 10 years, her teaching and research activities have been mainly oriented toward mental health recovery, including experiential elements and key characteristics of recovery-oriented services.

Dennis Raphael is a professor at the School of Health Policy and Management at York University. The most recent of his over 150 scientific publications have focused on the health effects of income inequality and poverty, the quality of life of communities and individuals, and the impact of government decisions on Canadians' health and well-being. Dr. Raphael is editor of *Social Determinants of Health: Canadian Perspectives* and *Health Promotion and Quality of Life in Canada: Essential Readings*; co-editor of *Staying Alive: Critical Perspectives on Health, Illness, and Health Care*; and author of *Poverty in Canada: Implications for Health and Quality of Life* and *About Canada: Health and Illness*.

Charlotte Reading is an Associate Professor in the School of Public Health and Social Policy, Faculty of Human and Social Development, University of Victoria. Dr. Reading's teaching and research activities are undertaken in areas such as Indigenous health and wellbeing, the social determinants of health, health inequities, and HIV and sexual health among Aboriginal peoples.

Jeff Reading was the inaugural Scientific Director of the Canadian Institutes of Health Research–Institute of Aboriginal Peoples' Health (2000–2008). Presently, Dr. Reading is the inaugural Director of the Centre for Aboriginal Health Research based at the University of Victoria, where he is a Professor in the Faculty of Human and Social Development based in the School of Public Health and Social Policy, and a Faculty Associate with the Indigenous Governance Program. As an epidemiologist, Dr. Reading's research has brought attention to such critical issues as disease prevention, smoking, healthy living, accessibility to health care, and diabetes among Aboriginal peoples in Canada. In 2005, he was elected as a Fellow into the Canadian Academy of Health Sciences, and in March 2008, Dr. Reading was selected by Aboriginal peers to receive a National Aboriginal Achievement Award in the Health category.

Colleen Reid is on the faculty in Child and Family Community Studies at Douglas College and is Adjunct Professor at Simon Fraser University (SFU). Previously, she was Research Director for the Women's Health Research Network and a post-doctoral fellow in health sciences at SFU. She has written widely in peer-reviewed and lay publications in the areas of women's health, intersectionality, the social determinants of health, and community-based research, including three books: *Our Common Ground: Cultivating Women's Health through Community-Based Research* (2009, with E. Brief and R. LeDrew); *Experience, Research, Social*

Change: Methods beyond the Mainstream (2nd ed.) (2006, with S. Kirby and L. Greaves); and *The Wounds of Exclusion: Poverty, Women's Health, and Social Justice* (2004).

Lise Renaud, who trained as a sociologist, obtained a PhD in educational sciences from the Université de Montreal. She has been working in public health for the past 20 years at the Public Health Directorate of Montreal-Center. She is also a Professor in the Department of Communication of Université du Québec à Montréal. She is the Director of Groupe de recherche Média et santé, which combines intervention and research with different target partners from media and health. She devised and produced several media products (videos, written papers) that have won numerous prizes. She is the author of many scientific articles, educational manuals, and popular scientific works.

Lucie Richard is a Professor in the Faculty of Nursing at the Université de Montréal. A FRSQ national scholar, she is currently affiliated with the Institut de recherché en santé publique de l'Université de Montréal (IRSPUM) and the Centre de recherche de l'Institut universitaire de gériatrie de Montréal. Over the last 10 years, she has conducted many projects pertaining to disease prevention and health promotion. She is currently Deputy Director of the IRSPUM.

Barbara Riley is the Director of Strategy and Capacity Development, and Senior Scientist at the Propel Centre for Population Health Impact, a partnership between the Canadian Cancer Society and the University of Waterloo. Her career focus is linking evidence and action in population and public health.

Irving Rootman is an Adjunct Professor in the Faculty of Human and Social Development at the University of Victoria and a Visiting Professor at Simon Fraser University. He has worked as a researcher, research manager, program manager, and educator in the field of health promotion for more than 30 years in the federal government, the World Health Organization, the University of Toronto, and the University of Victoria. He has published widely in health promotion, including as an author of several chapters and as one of the editors of the first two editions of *Health Promotion in Canada*. He is a Fellow of the Canadian Academy of Health Sciences.

Louise St-Pierre is head of projects at the National Collaborating Centre for Healthy Public Policy, located at the Public Health Institute of Quebec. She has a Master's in community health from Université Laval and has studied in the same program at the PhD level. Her research interests include health impact assessment (HIA), intersectoral policy, and governance for health in all policies.

Nathalie Sasseville is a Research Associate at l'Institut national de Santé publique du Québec. She works in the field of research on health in relation to the Quebec program Villes et Villages en santé. She has a doctorate from l'École de Service Social de l'Université Laval.

Martin Shain is founder and principal of the Neighbour at Work Centre, a consulting agency in the area of workplace mental health and safety (www.neighbouratwork.com). He is trained in both law and social science. He worked for many years as a Senior Scientist at the Centre for Addiction and Mental Health (CAMH). Currently, he holds academic appointments in the Dalla Lana School of Public Health at the University of Toronto and Simon Fraser University, where he is involved in research, development, and teaching.

Martine Shareck is a PhD candidate in public health, specializing in health promotion, at the Université de Montréal. She is a CIHR doctoral research award recipient. She has multidisciplinary training, with an undergraduate degree in environmental sciences from McGill University and a Master's in community health from the Université de Montréal. Her research interests include urban health, social and health equity, and the socio-spatial geography of health.

Paule Simard is a researcher at the Québec National Institute for Public Health. She is also an Associate Professor in the Faculty of Nursing and Social Service Department at Université Laval and coordinator of the Quebec WHO Collaborating Centre for the Development of Healthy Cities and Towns. Her work has mostly been directed toward participatory research and evaluation methodologies, as well as toward community development.

Julian Somers is an Associate Professor at Simon Fraser University. He has led provincial and multi-jurisdictional programs in the areas of telehealth, primary health care reform, homelessness, and the corrections system. His previous positions include director of the UBC Psychology Clinic, president of the BC Psychological Association, and inaugural director of SFU's Centre for Applied Research in Mental Health and Addiction.

Sylvie Stachenko is a public health expert in the field of health promotion and chronic disease prevention with over 20 years of experience in academic, community, and government organizations at international, national, and local levels. She has led chronic disease policies at the national level in Canada, including cancer control, diabetes, cardiovascular disease, breast cancer, and AIDS. She was the first Dean of the School of Public Health at the University of Alberta.

Alison Stirling is a knowledge exchange specialist with Health Nexus Santé, a bilingual non-profit organization. She also works with the Public Health Agency of Canada's Best Practices Portal in Health Promotion. Alison has more than 25 years experience in research, writing, practice, and advocating for building health promotion capacity online and at local, provincial, and national levels. She is the founder of the Click4HP health promotion listserv, the Ontario Health Promotion Email (OHPE) Bulletin, and a contributor to the bilingual Health Nexus Today blog and wiki.

Verena Strehlau is a post-doctoral research fellow in the Department of Psychiatry at the University of British Columbia and a Research Scientist at the Centre of Health Evaluation and Outcome Sciences (CHEOS) in Vancouver. Verena's background is in child and adolescent psychiatry and psychotherapy, and she is currently working as field research office manager of a multi-site, randomized controlled trial on homelessness and mental health (At Home-Chez Soi) of the Mental Health Commission of Canada. She is interested in the mental health of youth and marginalized populations, and in psychotherapeutic interventions.

Yanick Villedieu is a science and medicine journalist and has been the host of *Les Années lumière*, the weekly radio show on science of Radio-Canada, since 1982. Since 1983, he has been a regular contributor to the magazine *L'actualité* (science, medicine, and gastronomy). He previously worked for several media, among them the magazine *Québec Science* and Radio-Canada Télévision. He has published three books on health and medicine: *Demain la santé* (1976), *La médecine en observation* (1991), and *Un jour la santé* (2002). He was awarded an honorary doctorate from University of Ottawa in 2005, and nominated Chevalier de l'Ordre national du Québec in 2008.

Marjorie Villefranche is the Program Manager at Maison d'Haïti, a non-governmental organization attending to a diversity of mandates to improve the quality of life of women, men, and families in the close neighbourhoods. Over the years, she has been involved in the defence of the rights of immigrant women and of all those who are misinformed about their rights for personal or contextual reasons, interfacing with health care services, in addition to her constant commitment to work against all forms of discrimination. She has worked on three documentaries: *Port-au-Prince, My City*, *District 67*, and *Small Mothers*, aimed at understanding the importance of the context of one's lives when deriving integration strategies for newcomers.

Bilkis Vissandjée is a Professor in the Faculty of Nursing at the Université de Montréal and a researcher at the CSSS de la Montagne, as well at the Public Health Research Institute of the Université de Montréal. The common theme of her research program is to bring to the foreground the challenges associated with giving quality of care in a multi-ethnic context with a gender and equity-sensitive perspective. Along with NGOs, she has contributed to the implementation of programs aimed at newcomers to Canada in dealing with conditions such as tuberculosis and diabetes. Her publications also illustrate her contribution with internationally based partners regarding the importance of accounting for sex, gender, migration, and ethnicity when deriving strategies for better health in a diversified context.

Bryn Williams-Jones is Associate Professor and Director of the Bioethics Program in the Department of Social and Preventive Medicine, School of Public Health, at the Université de Montréal. An interdisciplinary scholar, he draws on analytic tools from applied ethics, legal and policy analyses, and the social sciences to explore the socio-ethical implications of new health technologies. His current research focuses on ethics in the evaluation of health innovations, the management of conflicts of interest in the context of university research, and conflicts of value or roles that health professionals working in military contexts or humanitarian crises face.

Index

Copyright Acknowledgements

BOXES

BOX 1.4: World Health Organization, "WHO Global Strategy for Health for All by the Year 2000," fi *Plenary Meeting, Resolution 36/43.* Geneva: WHO, 1981. Reprinted by permission of the World Health Orga

BOX 13.2: M. Ghassemi, "Development of Pan-Canadian discipline-Specific competencies for health prc Summary report. Consultation. Toronto: Health Promotion Ontario, 2009. Reprinted by permission c Promotion Ontario.

FIGURES

FIGURE 1.2: Ottawa Charter for Health Promotion. Ottawa: World Health Organization, 1986. Rep permission of the World Health Organization.

FIGURE 1.3: "Population Health Promotion: An Integrated Model of Population Health and Health Prc Ottawa: Public Health Agency of Canada, 2001. Reproduced with the permission of the Minister of H

FIGURE 2.3: C. Rissel, "Empowerment: The holy grail of health promotion," *Health Promotion Intern* (1), (1994): 43

FIGURE 2.4: "Centre for Health Promotion Quality of Life Model," from Quality of Life Resea Toronto: Quality of Life Research Unit, 2011. Reprinted by permission of Quality of Life Research Un

FIGURE 6.1: World Commission on the Social Dimensions of Globalization, A Fair Globalization International Labour Office, 2004. Reprinted by permission of the International Labour Office.

FIGURE 7.1: Adapted by L. McLaren and P. Hawe, Brofenbrenner's ecological theory of Developmen from Santrock et al), "Ecological perspectives in health research," *Journal of Epidemiology and Community* (2005): 6-14. Reprinted by permission of the BJM Group.

FIGURE 8.1: A. Cooke, L. Friedli, T. Coggins, N. Edmonds, J. Michaelson, K. O'Hara, L. Snowden, J. N. Steuer, and A. Scott-Samuel, Mental Well-being Impact Assessment. *A toolkit for well-being*, 3rd ed National MWIA Collaborative, 2011. Reprinted by permission of the National MWIA Collaborative.

FIGURE 8.2: C.L.M. Keyes, The Next Step in the Promotion and Protection of Mental Health. *Canad Nursing Research*, 42 (3) (2010): 21. Reprinted by permission of the Canadian Journal of Nursing Resea

FIGURE 14.2: R. Wilkins, (2007). Statistics Canada, Health Analysis and Measurement Group HAMG Seminar and Special Compilations. Ottawa: Statistics Canada, 2007. Reprinted by permission c Canada.

FIGURE 14.3: R. Wilkins, (2007). Statistics Canada, Health Analysis and Measurement Group (HAMG Seminar and Special Compilations. Ottawa: Statistics Canada, 2007. Reprinted by permission of Statisti

PHOTOGRAPHS

PART I OPENER: "428122 (Old bottles)," by BMPix. From www.istockphoto.com.

PART II OPENER: "1406395 (Repetitive Neighborhood)," by Buzbuzzer. From www.istockphoto

PART III OPENER: "12986192 (People in waiting room)," by Nicole S. Young. From www.istockphoto.com.

PART IV OPENER: "15694899 (Spiry Roots)," by Cunfek. From www.istockphoto.com.